The M

Science and Cultural Theory

THE MALE PILL

• • • • • •

A Biography of a Technology in the Making

NELLY OUDSHOORN

Duke University Press   Durham and London 2003

© 2003 by Duke University Press   All rights reserved
Printed in the United States of America on acid-free paper
Typeset in Quadraat by Keystone Typesetting, Inc.
Library of Congress Cataloging-in-Publication Data appear
on the last printed page of this book.

For Rob

Contents

• • • •

Acknowledgments

· · · ·

The exciting thing about doing research is that there are always many surprises and challenges. When I became interested in the question of why there is no male equivalent of the contraceptive pill for women, I assumed that one paper would be sufficient to answer the question. I soon discovered that there was much more to tell about male contraceptive discourse. The world I discovered in the documents and practices of those involved in this technological innovation turned out to be so rich that I realized I needed an entire book to tell the story.

Apart from the expansion of my research, there was another challenge as well. Whereas most scholars who investigate technological developments write about subjects whose development has been completed, I was faced with a technology that did and does not (yet?) exist. To write this story of a technology in the making, I relied on the invaluable experiences and reflections of the people who work in the field of male contraceptive technology and family planning. Without their willingness to cooperate with me and their permission to use their documents and archives, this book could not have been written. I express my gratitude to Bruce Armstrong, Willem Bergink, Ann Biddlecom, David T. Baird, William Bremner, Judith Bruce, Herjan Coelingh Bennink, Jane Cottingham, Diana Diazgranados, Elof Johansson, T. M. M. Farley, David Griffin, Anton Grootegoed, Wendy Kersemaekers, Herman Kloosterboer, David Kinniburgh, Stephen Matlin, Alvin Matsumoto, Kelly McKracken, Axel Mundigo, Eberhard Nieschlag, Alvin Paulsen, Diana Rubino, J. Mayone Stycos, Ronald Swerdloff, Rosemary Thau, Geoffrey Waites, Christina Wang, J. Weber, Mary Nell Wegner, and Fred Wu.

I am also indebted to Kathy King for providing me with excellent analyses of the British news media's coverage of the clinical testing of male hormonal contraceptives. Karin Ringheim has been generous in sharing several of her unpublished reports describing the experiences of men who participated in the clinical trials organized by the WHO. I am also grateful for the help and encouragement of my colleagues from the Gender and Technology network, the University of Twente, and the University of Amsterdam. In different phases of my research, they gave inspiring and substantial comments on earlier drafts of the chapters of this book. I have also benefited from the insights of many colleagues and friends in the field of sociology of science and technology, in Europe as well as the United States. The conferences of the Society of Social Studies of Science, in particular, have become a warm, intellectual home throughout the years I worked on this book. I want to mention Adele Clarke, in particular, for her friendship, inspiration, and valuable comments on the first draft of this book. I am also grateful to Raphael Allen, who has been an encouraging and helpful editor, and to my two anonymous referees at Duke University Press. Special thanks for technical assistance are due to Gerdien Linde-de Ruiter, Hilde Meijer-Meijer, and Joep van Delft, and to Gene Moore and Lara Tauritz for their skillful and thorough editing of my English.

Last but far from least I am grateful to my mother for her enthusiasm about my work and her impatience to see my new book in print. And I thank my partner, Rob Vrakking, for his unwavering encouragement of my intellectual endeavors and for sharing the responsibilities of contraception. His love and wonderful sculptures always remind me that there are more riches in this world than producing texts.

Some of these chapters are based on previously published materials. Earlier versions of chapter 3 were published in Social Studies of Science 27 (1997): 41–72; and in J. P. Gaudillière and I. Löwy, eds., The Invisible Industrialist: Manufactures and the Production of Scientific Knowledge (London: MacMillan Press, 1998), 345–69. Several parts of chapter 4 appear in G. M. van Heteren, M. Gijswijt-Horstra, and E. M. Tansey, eds., Biographies of Remedies: Drugs, Medicines, and Contraceptives in Dutch and Anglo-American Healing Cultures (Amsterdam: Rodopi, 2002), 79–92. Parts of chapter 5 were published in Sociology of Health and Illness 24 (4) (2002): 436–61. Several parts of chapters 2 and 8 appear in the following publications: A. Saetnon, N. Oudshoorn, and M. Kirejczyk, eds., Bodies of Technology: Women's Involvement with Reproductive Medicine (Columbus: Ohio University Press, 2000), 123–46; U. Pasero and A. Gottburgsen, eds., Gender *und die Konstruktion von Natur und Technik* (Wiesbaden: Westdeutscher Verlag, 2002), 109–26; N. E. J. Oudshoorn, and T. J. Pinch, eds., *How Users Matter: The Co-Construction of Users and Technologies* (Cambridge, Mass.: MIT Press, 2003); and in the journal *Men and Masculinity* (forthcoming). Finally, chapter 9 was published in *Science, Technology, and Human Values* 24, (2) (1999): 265–89.

PART I

. . . .

Overcoming

Resistance:

Constructing

Alternative

Sociotechnical

Networks

1

Designing Technology and Masculinity:
Challenging the Invisibility of Male Reproductive Bodies
in Scientific Medicine

• • • •

We are living in challenging times. For the first time in history, male reproductive bodies are in the headlines, breaking the silence that made them largely invisible in the past. The most compelling sign of this change is the hype in the news media following the introduction of Viagra, a pill for the treatment of male impotence, in the late 1990s. Never before has a drug received such rapid worldwide approval and distribution. Viagra was originally developed to treat high blood pressure, but it has been marketed as a drug for impotence, as a response to its subversive use by test subjects who were reluctant to return their leftover pills after they discovered the "unintended consequences" of the drug. As a pharmaceutical product, it has enjoyed the fastest takeoff ever recorded for a new drug (Handy 1998: 39).[1] On the very day Viagra became available in the United States, urologists and sexologists were overwhelmed by requests from men asking for prescriptions. Month-long waits to see a doctor for a consultation were not unusual (Ibid.). Within a year, Viagra had become one of the best-selling drugs in the United States, doubling the value of shareholders' investments at Pfizer, Inc., the manufacturer of the new drug (Berends 1998: 2).

The story of Viagra illustrates how technology can be instrumental in giving visibility to male reproductive bodies: the drug transformed male impotence from a private matter, confined to the bedroom or the sexologist's clinic and considered the last sexual taboo of the twentieth century, into a health condition firmly entrenched in the public domain (Garschagen 1998).[2] This is not to say that male impotence came to be represented in a manner similar to other dysfunctions of the male body. The manufacturer's promotional materials for

Viagra were carefully designed to avoid any suggestion of failing male bodies. Advertisements in the United States emphasized impotence as "a couple's condition" rather than as a dysfunction of the male body (Handy 1998: 45; Mamo and Fishman 1999: 4). Less spectacular, but equally illustrative, is the attention given by the news media to scientific research that reported a decline in male fertility due to environmental pollution. In the mid-1990s, the book *Our Stolen Future*, dubbed *The Silent Sperm* by journalists, and similar reports were discussed extensively in Western media (Colborn, Dumnoski, and Meyers 1996; Naald 1996).

This increased attention to the male reproductive body is also exemplified by significant developments in the medical world, which did not receive such extensive news coverage. In the mid-1990s, in London, two clinics that specialized in men's health issues emerged: the WellMan clinic and the Andropause Clinic (Nowak 2000). In 1998 the newly formed International Society for the Study of the Aging Male organized the First World Congress on the Aging Male in Geneva. Co-sponsored by the World Health Organization, the congress attracted more than 350 delegates from over forty countries and issued the Geneva Manifesto: "a call for a new initiative to achieve healthy aging for men and calling on support from governments, industry and philanthropic agencies" (Geurts 1998).[3] In the late 1990s Swedish and American manufacturers introduced the first hormonal patch and a gel as testosterone replacement therapies for aging men, both of which received an unexpectedly positive response (Johnson 1997; Kaufman 2000). And, last but not least, reproductive scientists have been involved for more than three decades in the development of a hormonal contraceptive for men, which is the topic of this book.

Female Reproductive Bodies as Natural Objects of Intervention

All in all, developments in contraceptive technology for men must be considered revolutionary. In the twentieth century most of the attention in reproductive medicine has been focused on women rather than men. The century witnessed the introduction of numerous technologies designed to intervene in female reproductive functions, transgressing boundaries which for ages were perceived as natural. Diagnostic procedures and therapies such as in vitro fertilization (IVF), hormone replacement therapy (HRT), screening programs for breast and cervical cancer, the contraceptive pill, and a wide variety of other contraceptives for women have accentuated the distinct reproductive role of women and thus designated the female body as a natural object for intervention (Dyck 1995: 15; Ploeg 1998: 28).

The identification of the female body as the quintessential medical object has a long history.[4] In the late nineteenth and early twentieth centuries, the view that sex and reproduction were "more fundamental to Woman than Man's Nature" (Moscucci 1990) resulted in the creation of a new specialty in the biomedical sciences: gynecology. In her fascinating account of the rise of the "Science of Women," Ornella Moscucci has described how "the belief that the female body is finalized for reproduction defined the study of 'natural woman' as a separate branch of medicine." With the emergence of gynecology women became identified as "a special group of patients" (2). The turn of the last century witnessed the founding of societies, journals, and hospitals specifically devoted to the diagnosis and treatment of the female body. "Woman" thus came to be set apart in the discursive and institutional practices of the biomedical sciences.

Consequently, "woman" became conceptualized as an ontologically distinct category which firmly established the view of Woman as the Other. This meant a definitive rejection of what Thomas Laqueur has characterized as the one-sex-model of medical practice, in which the female body was understood as a lesser version of the male body rather than as a different sex (Laqueur 1990: viii, 4). The growth of gynecology was not paralleled by the establishment of a complementary science of masculinity (Oudshoorn 1994a). "As the male was the standard of the species, he could not be set apart on the basis of his sex" (Moscucci 1990: 32).[5]

This institutional process of othering was continued and reinforced by the rise of sex endocrinology, a discipline that emerged in the 1920s and 1930s and was devoted to the study of sex hormones. In *Beyond the Natural Body* I described how the very existence of gynecology as a speciality facilitated a situation in which the new science of sex endocrinology focused almost exclusively on the female body. The then current gynecological practices transformed the female body into an easily accessible supplier of research materials and a convenient guinea pig for tests, creating an organized audience for the products of sex endocrinology in the process. Both laboratory scientists and pharmaceutical firms depended on these institutional practices to provide them with the necessary tools and materials to transform the hormonal model of the body into a new set of disease categories, diagnostic tools, and drugs. Sex endocrinologists integrated the notion of the female body as a reproductive body into the hormonal model, but not without thoroughly changing it. They provided the medical profession with tools to intervene in processes that had been considered inaccessible prior to the hormonal era. The introduction of diagnostic tests and drugs enabled the medical profession to intervene in the menstrual cycle and menopause, thus bringing these "natural" processes of reproduction and aging into the domain of medical intervention.

With the introduction of the concept of sex hormones, scientists explicitly linked women's reproductive functions with laboratory practice. The study of woman as the Other was thus extended from the clinic to the laboratory and thereby firmly rooted in the heart of the life sciences. The existence of established networks of researchers who were focused on hormones and the female body facilitated the development of hormonal contraceptives for women in the late 1950s. This asymmetry in the institutionalization of female and male reproductive bodies in medicine prevailed until well into the second half of the twentieth century. It was only in the late 1970s that scientists and clinicians established andrology as a medical specialty devoted to the study and medical treatment of male reproductive bodies (Niemi 1987; Moscucci 1990: 32, 33). Today, andrology is still a small and marginal profession compared to gynecology.

Gender Asymmetry in Contraceptives

Bearing in mind this short history of the institutionalization of the female reproductive body in medicine, it will come as no surprise that development of the first physiological contraceptives focused exclusively on women. Since World War II thirteen new contraceptives for women have been developed, including the contraceptive pill. This is in sharp contrast to contraceptives for men (Davidson et al. 1985). In the past century, no new male methods have been developed, except for the improvement of existing methods, namely condoms and sterilization, both of which date from the nineteenth century. Rubber condoms were first introduced around 1860, whereas vasectomy (male sterilization) dates from the late 1890s.[6] In the 1950s improved condoms were developed, and in the 1990s condoms made from polyurethane and other polymers were introduced (Clarke 1998: 166, 167).[7] The "contraceptive revolution" thus remained largely restricted to female methods. In the mid-1990s, only approximately 8 percent of the contraceptive research budget was spent on the development of contraceptives for men (Sachs 1994: 17V).

The gender asymmetry in contraceptives was first challenged in the late 1960s and early 1970s. As in the case of the Pill for women, the request to develop new male contraceptives originated outside the scientific community.[8] In this instance, social pressures came from two different sides: feminists in the Western industrialized world and Southern governments, most

that the reproductive analogies betweer ıle and female end with sperm
transport and egg transport, and that subsequent events potentially
subject to controlled interference occuı nly in the female. (Segal 1972)

It's not easy to design a male contra ɔptive. All you have to do with
women is to knock out the productior of one egg per month, but men
produce something like 250 million ɛ ɔerm cells per ejaculation. Suppressing this gigantic factory of sperm production in men is a lot more
difficult.[10]

Conversely, however, other biologists ırgue that it is easier to suppress
sperm production than the production oı ʒgs:

There is no evidence that it is more ˈficult to prevent "billions" of
sperm from being produced, or actinɡ han one egg. The difference is
not the numbers produced, but the dis tinuity of egg production in the
female and the continuity in the male. nany ways, it is easier to target
a continuous process (where time o ıtment may be unimportant)
than a discontinuous process. (Schwa 76: 248)

These reproductive biologists emphasiz similarities of the reproductive
mechanism in women and men, arguinɡ he same potential sites exist in
women and men for interruption of th ıction of eggs and sperm and
pointing to the similarities in the horr ɛgulation of the reproductive
system (Schwartz 1976; Bremner and d 1975: 390).[11] These contradictory views on the biological constrai development of contraceptives for men illustrate the interpretat bɛ of biological facts. The
same biological phenomena can be inte 199 litating or constraining
the possibilities for intervention in the ı male ˈem.

This book aims to go beyond such es this pɔ ations. By analyzing
male contraceptive discourse, I seek to ɪ 1997). ʒ to perspectives that
create the impression that gender asyn announc ̃tive technologies is
an inevitable result of technical logic. ʼ years. Scɪɛ in social studies
of science and technology has provide when new ɪ ıceptualizations
of the relationships between science, and 1990s th ınd gender. Sociologists of science and technology h time, scientis ̃rnist philosophy in which the interfaces among sciɛ Pill, to avoid cɔ ıre were conceptualized in terms of scientists and They seem to reɛ truth about
nature. Since the work of Thomas Kt they are not sure ɔlogists of
science and technology have gradually media and potentiaɪ exists an
unmediated truth of nature that can b unfulfilled expectatiɔ ıd, they

have introduced the idea that the naturalistic reality of phenomena as such does not exist, but is created by scientists as the object of scientific investigation (Duden 1991: 22). In the last three decades sociologists of science and technology have turned to practice and work to understand the processes of creating facts and artifacts. Instead of focusing on brilliant ideas of scientists discovering the secrets of nature, the analysis has shifted to exposing the concrete and often very mundane human activities that go into the creation of facts and artifacts (Timmermans and Leiter 2000: 214).[13] In this view, technologies do not reflect the essentialistic properties of bodies; they are the materialized result of negotiations, selection processes, contingencies, and technological choices, embodying socially and culturally constituted values and practices.

Adopting this constructivist approach, I view the gender asymmetry in contraceptive technologies as "a reality created in practice" rather than as "a reality rooted in nature" (Kole 1999: 27). The practices of all the actors involved in the development, diffusion, and use of these technologies have been focused almost exclusively on women. As we have seen above, since the late nineteenth century the female reproductive body has become firmly entrenched in the infrastructures of the medical world and beyond. Knowledge, diagnostics, and therapies concerning the female reproductive body have been made robust by alignments among laboratories, gynecological clinics, pharmaceutical companies, family planning policies, family planning clinics, and social movements, particularly the women's reproductive health movement. Since the introduction of the contraceptive pill in the early 1960s, collective actors have focused almost exclusively on women, neglecting men as potential subjects of research, users, and clients. As Adele Clarke has suggested, "It is difficult to conceive of a more sex and gender constructing and maintaining discipline and set of practices and discourses than those of the reproductive sciences" (Clarke 1998: 22). The currently available contraceptive technologies exemplify the argument that "technology is hardened history" (Noble 1984)—hardened in a literal sense: the asymmetry in contraceptive practice is materialized in institutions, medical professions, laboratory techniques, chemicals, and pharmaceuticals. Overcoming the gender asymmetry in contraceptive technologies therefore requires hard work. This book aims to explore all the work that has gone into changing the contraceptive discourse to include men.

The Social and Cultural Construction of Technology

To understand the dynamics of technological change, I will employ the concept of sociotechnical networks.[14] As has been suggested by sociologists of science and technology, a new technology will succeed only when it is able to attract a network of sociotechnical relationships. Social scientists have introduced the concept of networks to capture the heterogeneous social, technical, economic, and political processes involved in the development of a new technology. In order to become successful, new technologies require the stabilization of complex sociotechnical ensembles into networks (Latour 1987; Bijker and Law 1992; MacKenzy and Wajcman 1999). The development of new technologies therefore may involve the creation of new social practices and relations; new clinics and laboratories; new alliances among laboratories, clinics, and industry; new relationships between doctors and patients; and new forms of state regulation. Sociotechnical networks, at least those of successful technologies, once formed, are often highly stable. Networks are not easily disassembled because a large number of elements, including institutions, social groups, techniques, and knowledge, secure their links (Latour 1987). Of course, there are major differences between technologies in the extent to which they require the creation of totally new sociotechnical networks. Many technologies can simply follow the routines and practices developed in previous technologies. Others, however, require drastic transformations of previously established sociotechnical networks. Male contraceptive technology is an example of the latter. As I will show in this book, including men in the contraceptive agenda has meant changing established sociotechnical networks and the vested interests of experts, clinics, the industry, and social movements that were long focused on women rather than men.

Although the concept of sociotechnical networks is an important tool for studying the development of new technologies, it conceptualizes scientific and technological change as a social process and not as a cultural process. Network approaches neglect the fact that cultural conventions are important in securing links of networks. The articulation and accomplishment of the cultural feasibility of technical innovations is as yet a largely overlooked aspect of technological change.[15] The focus on the social rather than the cultural construction of technology is particularly problematic if we want to understand gender aspects of technological innovation. Studying technological innovation from a gender perspective requires a conceptualization of the dynamics of technological development which acknowledges the cultural embeddedness of technology.[16] As feminists and others have argued, technology, as with any other human endeavor, cannot only be understood in terms of social institutions and practices, but should include an analysis of symbolic meanings, the formation of identities, and culturally rooted belief systems (Franklin, Lurey, and Stacey 1991: 181). One way to appreciate the cultural dimensions of technological innovation is to conceptualize technology not only in terms of networks of techniques, knowledge, institutions, experts, and social groups, but also in terms of the relationships between technologies and the identities of users.

The concept of user representations is a useful tool for capturing the work that goes into the cultural construction of technology. As Madeleine Akrich, Bruno Latour, and Steve Woolgar have suggested, scientists and engineers configure users and contexts of use as integrated parts of the processes of technological development (Akrich 1992; Akrich and Latour 1992; Woolgar 1991). If they fail to do this, the technology will fail altogether: without a technology there are no users, and there are no users without a technology. In the development phase of a new technology, designers anticipate and define the preferences, motives, tastes, and competencies of potential users and inscribe these views into the technical design of the new product (Akrich 1992: 208). I suggest that the articulation of the gender identities of users is an equally important but as yet largely unexplored aspect of the processes involved in configuring the user.[17] Although Steve Woolgar has described the process of configuring the user as "defining the identity of putative users and setting constraints on their likely future actions," he describes identity only in terms of "who the user might be." His main concern is to reconceptualize human agency in relation to technology. The analysis is restricted to showing how computers are designed in such a way that they define and delimit the user's actions and behavior (Woolgar 1991: 59, 61). Like Woolgar, Madeleine Akrich restricts her analysis to competencies and actions of users rather than user identities. This scholarship thus reflects a rather narrow view of technological development, which restricts user–technology relations to technical interactions with the artifacts, and thereby neglects the broader cultural dimensions of human agency.[18] My conceptualization of the relationships between technologies and users is broader. I am interested in the identities of users constituted in the discursive practices of male contraceptive technology in laboratories, clinics, family planning policies, social movements, and the media. These identities play an important role in shaping the cultural feasibility of the technology.

The Mutual Adjustment of Technologies and Identities

My point of departure is that technological change requires the mutual adjustment of technologies and gender identities.[19] To study the adjustment of technologies and gender identities, Judith Butler's conceptualization of gender as performance provides a useful approach (Butler 1995). Like technology, gender has no intrinsic qualities. As Butler and many other feminist scholars have argued, gender is not something we are, but something we do.[20] Inspired by J. L. Austin's theory of the speech act,[21] Butler has developed a radical critique of the notion of fixed gender identities rooted in nature or bodies. In her poststructuralist theory of gender, gender is considered as the result of discursive practices that have the potential to produce what they name.[22] Butler emphasizes the role of reiteration in producing and sustaining the norms that constitute gender, which she refers to as a performative process. In this view, gender is not pre-given or fixed but produced as a "ritualized repetition of conventions" (31). Each performance of gender may reproduce existing meanings of gender or represent new, subversive readings of gender which produce the possibility of change. In this performative theory of gender, the seemingly universal dichotomy of gender is the result of a constant maintenance of particular conventions of gender, most notably those of compulsory heterosexuality (25).

Although Butler's work underscores the constraints on the performativity of gender, she does not reflect on the question of how technologies may contribute to the maintenance or transformation of particular gender performances. Rooted in a semiotic and psychoanalytical tradition, her work primarily addresses the forces of prohibition and taboo in sanctioning and unsanctioning particular sexual practices and gender performances (Butler 1993, 1995). I suggest that it is important to address the role of technologies as non-human actors in order to understand the processes involved in producing and sustaining particular forms of gender. Technologies may play an important role in stabilizing or destabilizing particular conventions of gender, creating new ones, or reinforcing or transforming the existing performances of gender.

Contraceptive technologies serve as a specific case in point to illustrate my argument. Prior to the introduction of new contraceptives for women in the 1960s, no stabilized conventions existed concerning the relationships between gender identities and contraceptive use. Since only a limited number of contraceptives were available (condoms, diaphragms, natural methods, spermicides, sponges, and sterilization), neither men nor women had many options for contraception.[23] This situation changed drastically when new contraceptives for women became available—that is, high-tech contraceptives that effectively intervene in the physiological processes that regulate ovulation and conception in female bodies. The introduction of a much wider variety of modern contraceptives for women has disciplined women and men to consider the use of contraceptives a woman's responsibility. Because of the innovation in female contraceptive methods—including the hormonal contraceptive pill, the IUD, and hormonal methods such as Norplant—women's methods have come to predominate in the practice of family planning. Only about 17 percent of contraceptive users rely on so-called male methods, that is, on condoms and male sterilization (United Nations 1994a: 4). Female sterilization, oral contraceptives, and IUDs account for the majority of methods currently in use (Robey et al. 1992: 11). Contraceptives thus function as important tools in delegating and distributing responsibility and control over procreation. In Foucaultian terms, contraceptives are "disciplinary technologies": "they are part of the 'socialization of reproductive behavior', that can discipline such behavior in multiple ways" (Clarke 1998: 165). The predominance of modern contraceptive drugs for women has disciplined men and women to delegate responsibilities for contraception largely to women. Contraceptive technologies thus constituted strong alignments between femininity and taking responsibility for reproduction.

Another illustration of the performative and integrative capacity of technologies to create and sustain gender identities is the emergence of the women's health reproductive movement in the late 1960s and early 1970s. One major reason for the establishment of this social movement was concern about the health risks of the first generation of the contraceptive pill and IUDs (Oudshoorn 1994a). Since then, women's health groups have been important actors in lobbying against the introduction of contraceptives considered unsafe or as having the potential for abuse and in simultaneously advocating for the development of better contraceptives for women (Kammen 2000). In contrast, no men's reproductive health movement exists. This difference in the emergence of social movements concerning the reproductive health of women and men can be understood in terms of a "technosociality": people construct collective identities based on a shared experience with specific technologies, in this case, contraceptive technologies.[24] In the second half of the twentieth century, the idea that women were responsible for contraception thus became the dominant cultural narrative as it was materialized in contraceptive technologies, social movements, and in the gender identities of women and men.

Consequently, contraceptive use became excluded from hegemonic masculinity.[25] Inspired by the Gramscian notion of hegemony, Robert Connell has introduced this concept to refer to the cultural dominance of particular forms of masculinity (Connell 1987). Like Butler, Connell conceptualized gender as a cultural construct, emphasizing the diversity in masculinities and femininities. He explicitly included power as an important aspect of the relationships between genders and within genders.[26] Anticipating, in a way, Butler's performative theory of gender, Connell described gender as "something that does not precede but is constituted in human actions" (Demetriou 2001: 340), emphasizing that the word *gender* should be used as a verb (Connell 1987: 140). According to Connell, hegemonic masculinity implies the subordination of women and subordinated masculinities (185). Hegemony emerges from "preventing alternatives from gaining cultural definition and recognition as alternatives, confining them to ghettos, to privacy, and to unconsciousness" (186). Connell thus identified heterosexuality as the most important aspect of contemporary hegemonic masculinity (186).

Connell's theory of gender is important because it enables me to differentiate between different performances of gender, including hegemonic masculinity and non-hegemonic masculinities.[27] However, like Butler, Connell does not theorize the role of technologies in creating and sustaining particular forms of masculinities. Although Connell occasionally refers to the role of technologies in constituting masculinity,[28] he does not classify technologies as a "gender regime," a concept he confines to the labor market, the state, the family, and, more recently, the "structure of symbolism" (Connell 1995: 357).[29] My point of departure is that in contemporary societies, contraceptive technologies, as with other technologies, constitute a crucial arena for understanding how particular forms of gender gain cultural dominance and others remain marginalized. In the last two decades, feminist studies of technology have suggested that the development and use of technologies are very significant for understanding the social and cultural aligning of technologies and masculinities. Feminist historians and sociologists of technology have shown the strong alignments of technology and hegemonic masculinity in technological practices, particularly in the field of engineering. As Cynthia Cockburn and others have argued, we can never fully understand technology without masculinity and vice versa (Cockburn 1992). In this view, gender and technology are seen as mutually constitutive, or co-produced (Berg 1996; Cockburn 1983; Faulkner 2000; Lie 1995; Oost 2000; Oldenziel 1999; Oudshoorn, Saetnan, and Lie 2002; Wajcman 1991). These studies, however, do not focus on technologies that have weak social and cultural alignments with masculinity, such as contraceptive technologies and reproductive technologies in general.[30] As illustrated by the history of contraceptives presented above, the predominance of contraceptives for women contributed to a stabilization of performances of gender, which constituted a strong alignment between femininity and contraceptive use. Masculinities that might have asked men to take responsibility for their reproductive bodies became excluded from hegemonic masculinity and were constituted as a subordinate form of masculinity. Equally important, the physiological aspect of contraceptives, which separates sexual from reproductive functions, challenges hegemonic views of masculinity that emphasize the intertwining of the male sexual and reproductive body. The development of new contraceptives which would enable men to perform sexually without being fertile would thus conflict with two aspects of hegemonic masculinity: delegating the responsibility for contraception to women and safeguarding the unity of the male sexual and reproductive body (Scale 2002: 1). The "feminization" of contraceptive technologies created a strong cultural and social alignment of contraceptive technologies with women and femininity and not with men and masculinity, which brings the development of new contraceptives for men into conflict with hegemonic masculinity.

The development of new contraceptives for men thus requires the destabilization of conventionalized performances of masculinity. To understand how collective and individual actors contribute to sustaining or transforming conventionalized performances of gender, I differentiate between the performance of gender identities by "end-users" (Saetnan, Oudshoorn, and Kiricjzyk 2000: 16), in this case, the men who participate in the clinical trials of new male contraceptives and the potential male users of the new technology, and the articulation of gender identities by the other actors involved in the sociotechnical networks.[31] Articulating and performing identities that contest the convention of contraception as a woman's responsibility is a major part of the cultural work involved in developing new contraceptives for men. I view the developmental phase of a new technology, therefore, as a cultural niche in which experts and other people participating in the testing of the technology articulate and perform non-hegemonic identities to create and produce the cultural feasibility of the technology.[32] In the development of new contraceptive technologies for men, the construction of masculinities is at the forefront of the design. Technological innovation thus becomes a process of designing technology and masculinity.

This book aims to trace the actions of those who acted as agents of social and cultural change. Or, to put it more precisely: those who acted as gender-benders. I use the term *gender-benders* here to describe the activities of those who consciously try to go beyond dominant narratives of gender. I will explore the social and cultural work required to develop a technology that challenges dominant cultural narratives, particularly those of hegemonic masculinity.[33] It is equally important to make visible traces of resistance. Who acted as opponents of the envisioned technology? What were the major constraints faced by the proponents of new male contraceptive technologies? And, last but not least, how and to what extent have the advocates of the new technology succeeded in overcoming these constraints?

Part I of the book, "Overcoming Resistance: Constructing Alternative Sociotechnical Networks," focuses on the social work involved in technological innovation: the work required to create sociotechnical networks. The chapters in this section describe who the advocates of the new contraceptive drugs for men were, and how they tried to overcome resistance to the new technology.[34] Chapter 2 explores how men came to be included in the contraceptive agenda. Adopting the concepts of path dependence and path creation, I describe how the advocates of new male contraceptives created an alternative research and development (R&D) network to compensate for the pharmaceutical industry's reluctance to participate in the development of this new technology. Due to the resistance of industry, international public-sector agencies became the major actors in promoting and coordinating R&D for male contraceptive technologies. Chapter 3 analyzes how this R&D network created a worldwide laboratory to synthesize hormonal contraceptive compounds, the approach that was selected as the most promising in male contraceptive development. Chapter 4 extends the analysis of the creation of alternative networks from the laboratory to the clinic. In laboratory research, the advocates of new contraceptives for men could not rely on the existing routines and practices for the clinical testing of contraceptives. The chapter describes the work involved in creating the required infrastructure for clinical testing, and analyzes the strategies used by clinicians to overcome problems with enrolling men to participate in clinical trials. Chapter 5 addresses how the reproductive scientists and clinicians involved in the clinical testing of hormonal contraceptives for men tried to overcome yet another constraint: how to make a contraceptive that would meet the standards and norms of safety established in settings both inside and outside the clinic. The chapter analyzes the practices of risk assessment in the male contraceptive community and shows how the use of a specific risk model and the low acceptance of risks, particularly in connection with contraceptive drugs for men, resulted in a rather lengthy period of testing.

In part II of the book, "Configuring the User: Articulating and Performing Masculinities," I focus on the cultural work involved in developing the new technology: the work required to create the cultural feasibility of a technology. To be able to understand the cultural work involved in developing technology, I extend the focus of analysis to locations other than the laboratory and the medical clinic. Chapters 6 and 7 focus on the world of family planning policies and clinics as major locations in constructing the cultural feasibility of the new technology. Chapter 6 addresses how men became included in family planning discourse. The chapter describes how a large part of this work consisted of articulating new identities for men as users of contraceptives to counterbalance the dominant cultural narratives on masculinity, male sexuality, and birth control embedded in family-planning research traditions, policies of national and international family planning agencies, and women's health organizations. Chapter 7 continues to analyze the world of family planning, focusing particularly on the material interventions necessary to change family planning discourse to include men. The chapter shows how configuring men as clients required a drastic reorganization of the infrastructure of family planning clinics, including the founding of special clinics for men, creating separate spaces for men in existing clinics, enrolling new professionals, and defining a new category of patients. Chapter 8 shifts the attention back to the medical clinic. Creating infrastructures for clinical trials, and establishing procedures to enroll trial participants (discussed in chapter 4) are crucial but only preparatory steps for the clinical testing of drugs. Chapter 8 describes the complex work involved in ensuring the cooperation of test subjects. Since men are not accustomed to being subjected to contraceptive testing, and since clinicians are not used to having men as test subjects in contraceptive trials, the clinical testing required specific procedures to discipline men as reliable test subjects. The chapter describes the clinical trials as important cultural niches to develop non-hegemonic masculinities. Chapter 9 extends the analysis of the processes of configuring men as users of new male contraceptives to yet another domain: the world of journalism. The chapter analyzes how journalistic and scientific texts constructed quite different accounts of the technical and cultural feasibility of the technology-in-the-making, including different images of users representing hegemonic and non-hegemonic masculinities. Chapter 10 describes how the pharmaceutical industry eventually became involved in the development of contraceptive drugs for men.[35] Finally, in chapter 11 I evaluate the major conclusions that one can draw from this account of the development of new male contraceptive technologies for the ongoing debate on gender, autonomy, and contraceptive technologies.

2

How Man Came to be Included in the
Contraceptive Research Agenda

· · · ·

Because of the immensity and seriousness of human population growth every avenue
should continue to be explored and we should be unwise to neglect the male approach.
—Harold Jackson, "Chemical Methods of Male Contraception"

If you doubt that there has been sex discrimination in the development of the pill, try to
answer this question: Why isn't there a pill for men? . . . It is because women have
always had to bear most of the risks associated with sex and reproduction.—Barbara
Seaman, *The Doctor's Case against the Pill*

Birth control publications prior to the 1970s are intriguing texts. If we could
read them without further knowledge of reproduction, we would be tempted
to conclude that there is only one sex involved in making babies: the female
sex. Women have been the main focus in the development of new reversible,
physiological birth control technologies in the twentieth century. The major methods of contraception available to men (condom, withdrawal, and
periodic abstinence) are pretty much the same as those available over four
hundred years ago, with only one exception: sterilization—an irreversible contraceptive method (Davidson et al. 1985).[1] Until the 1970s research and development in male reversible contraceptive methods was limited to improvements in the condom in terms of safety, efficacy, fit, and comfort. The almost
exclusive focus on women is reflected in the institutional embedding of contraceptive technological development. As we have seen in the previous chapter, institutional infrastructures, expertise, techniques, and personnel have
been oriented almost exclusively toward the female reproductive body. Since
the late 1950s alliances between reproductive scientists, medical profession-

als, family planning organizations, pharmaceutical firms, and social movements have developed into extensive and stable sociotechnical networks for the development of female rather than male contraceptives. These networks create major barriers to any radical change, which explains the status quo in contraceptive research.

The concept of path dependence, introduced in evolutionary theories of technical change, provides a useful tool to capture the constraints of stabilized sociotechnical networks for technological innovation. Path dependence emphasizes the important implications of history for future developments: due to previous material, social, and symbolic investments, future technologies develop very much in line with existing technologies. Over time, stable paths of development, or "technological trajectories," emerge which set constraints on the development of radically new technologies. This does not imply that "history delivers the inevitable" (Arthur 1989).[2] To avoid a deterministic interpretation of path dependence, sociologists have introduced the parallel concept of "path creation" (Karnoe and Garud 2001; Pinch 2001). Path creation refers to "the enactment of new technological approaches that represent a break from the past" (Karnoe and Garud 2001: 2; Mouritsen and Deehow 2001).[3] Path creation is a useful concept because it draws attention to human agency (Pinch 2001). Human action is not necessarily restricted to reproducing the past; humans have the ability to abandon the past and create something new. Recent studies in technological innovation therefore portray path creation and path dependence as two sides of the same coin of structure and agency (Hirsch and Gillespie 2001; Mouritsen and Deehow 2001; Pinch 2001). Together, path dependence and path creation represent technological change as a "transformative process that entails both reproduction and creation" (Karnoe and Garud 2001: 25).

The conceptual tools of path dependence and path creation enable us to make visible all the work involved in the development of radical new technologies. Technological innovation implies hard work, particularly if it concerns so-called "architectural innovations." Architectural innovations—for example, the development of a new technology for a new market—are the most radical types of innovation (Clark 1985). The development of contraceptive drugs for men could be considered as an architectural innovation since it concerns a new type of drug that requires knowledge in the largely unexplored and poorly understood area of male reproductive biology and since it addresses a largely unknown and culturally contested market.

This chapter analyses the transformative processes involved in including men in the contraceptive research agenda. I will focus particularly on the creative agency of those who would break from a past in which contraceptives were primarily considered drugs for women. First, I will describe those who advocated the idea of contraceptive drugs for men. Then, I will analyze the major barriers to developing new contraceptives for men and the strategies adopted by advocates of the new technology to overcome these constraints.

Articulating the Need for Male Contraceptives

Over the last decade, social studies of science and technology have specified the various ways in which different kinds of worlds are involved in constructing scientific knowledge. These studies have described changes in scientific discourse as a result of "the collective work across worlds with different viewpoints and agendas," rather than merely as a result of the actions of scientists (Fujimura 1992: 169). The history of contraceptive technologies exemplifies these dynamics. Men first came to be included in the contraceptive agenda as a result of social pressures from two divergent groups outside the scientific community: political leaders in Southern countries and feminists in Northern countries. In the 1960s Chou En-lai in China and Indira Gandhi in India first articulated the need to include men as a target for birth control technologies. In China, Chou En-lai announced at a meeting of the Chinese Academy of Science that research should be directed to the development of new male contraceptives. Alvin Paulsen, a professor in reproductive physiology at the University of Washington's Medical School Population Centre for Research in Reproduction and one of the pioneers in male contraceptive research, remembered this event: "If you have an authoritarian society like China and the second man in charge says: 'Let there be more work in the Male,' all of a sudden everyone started working on Gossypol [a male contraceptive agent introduced by Chinese scientists]" (Paulson interview 1994).

Population politics in India went one step further. In 1961 Prime Minister Indira Gandhi attempted to pass a law which would have implemented a large-scale forced sterilization program for men (Stokes 1980: 31; Berelson 1969: 534, 535). The proposed measure proved to be one step too far: it generated such enormous protest that it resulted in the fall of Gandhi's cabinet. Despite this failure, Gandhi continued to promote a role for men in family planning, now placing her faith in the development of new, reversible contraceptives for both women and men: "Family planning programs are awaiting a big breakthrough; without a safe, preferably oral drug which women and men can take, no amount of governmental commitment and political determination will avail" (Diczfalusy 1985: 5).

The fact that India and China entered the history of birth control technologies as advocates for male contraceptives is not just a coincidence. Both countries were facing rapid population growth, and even more crucial, both had strong state traditions. Governmental control over family planning thus fit seamlessly into the dominant politics of state control over the lives of citizens. By the 1960s, India and China had well-established governmental birth control programs.[4] The first articulation of the need to include men as a target for birth control technologies thus came from Southern countries: men should no longer be neglected because they are a necessary tool for reducing the population growth.

In the early 1970s the Western industrialized world witnessed the emergence of a similar articulation of the need to develop new male contraceptives. In this case, it was the feminist movement which first put men on the contraceptive agenda. Feminists became advocates of birth control technologies for men when the health risks of the female contraceptive pill, increased risks of cancer and diseases of the circulatory system, became apparent (Seaman and Seaman 1978). Feminist essays with titles such as "His safety or hers?" illustrate their major concern: that the use of contraceptives is a risky business that should not be placed exclusively on the shoulders of women. Consequently, they pleaded for the development of male contraceptives that would make it possible to share the health risks of technological birth control. Feminists not only demanded a sharing of risks, they also emphasized the need to share the responsibility for family planning. They were opposed to the idea that family planning was a woman's responsibility, and they argued that men had a "personal and social responsibility for their own sexual behavior and fertility" (International Women's Health Coalition 1994: 2).

The impetus to change the status quo in contraceptive research so as to include male methods thus grew out of two contrasting sets of motives, which entailed two different types of discourse: population control discourse, which framed the need for male contraceptives in terms of the technology's contribution to limiting population growth, and emancipation discourse, which articulated the need for male contraceptives in terms of sharing the responsibilities and the risks of contraception between the sexes. The history of contraceptive technologies thus illustrates the importance of social movements for technological innovation. These movements are, however, largely overlooked in the literature of innovation, which emphasizes the role of economic change and government policies in technological development.[5] Feminists have not only been important in articulating the need for new male contraceptives; they have been critical agents of change for female contraceptives as well. Contraceptive research and development was traditionally a major concern for the women's movement in the twentieth century. As we saw in chapter 1, the need to develop a contraceptive pill for women was first articulated by Margaret Sanger, a women's rights activist and pioneer of birth control in the United States throughout the first half of the twentieth century. During the second wave of feminism in the 1970s, the women's health movement campaigned for a woman's right to make informed choices about her fertility, for improved services, and for appropriate technologies. The articulation of the need to develop new contraceptives for men thus shows a peculiar pattern in which political leaders and feminists acted as spokespersons for men, even as the latter remained remarkably silent. The need to develop male contraceptives was never articulated by the potential users of any new technology: men. Rather, the advocates of male methods were political leaders and feminists, who spoke for, but did not necessarily represent, the demands of men.

Barriers Against Male Contraceptive Innovation

Lack of Expertise and Material Resources

Advocacy for new male contraceptives challenged the status quo in contraceptive development in the 1970s. The request for technological innovation, however, fell on almost completely deaf ears. Path dependence in the field of contraceptive technology and reproductive biology had created a situation in which the basic knowledge of male reproductive biology, the expertise and techniques needed to synthesize male contraceptive drugs, and the infrastructure for clinical testing of any new male contraceptive technologies had remained largely unexplored, underdeveloped, and marginal.

Let us first take a look at the available expertise in male reproductive biology. When the need for the development of new male contraceptives was first articulated, there existed, worldwide, only a handful of researchers who specialized in male reproductive biology and contraceptive development. In Europe, the field consisted of two major research groups: the Max Planck Research Institute for Reproductive Medicine in Germany and the Medical Research Council's Center for Reproductive Biology in Edinburgh. In the United States, there were three research centers which devoted a part of their research program to male contraceptive research: the Department of Endocrinology at the Harbor–UCLA Medical Center in Torrance; the Population Council's Center for Biomedical Research in New York; and the Department of Medicine at the University of Washington School of Medicine in Seattle. Outside Europe and the United States, the only other country in the Western world that was known to be involved in male contraceptive research was India, where research was taking place at the Department of Reproductive Biology of the All India Institute of Medical Sciences in New Delhi.[6]

In the 1950s and 1960s these research groups pursued two lines of research: the impact of chemicals on male fertility and the role of hormones in male reproductive functions. The interest in chemicals can be traced back to two earlier research programs in the reproductive sciences: research on spermicides (chemical contraceptives used by women that worked topically on sperm) in the 1920s and 1930s, and research on the adverse effects of chemical drugs on fertility in the 1950s (Borell 1987: 53; Knight and Callahan 1994: 289).[7] Although they had not been involved in generating knowledge for the development of male contraceptives, both research programs had provided the first leads and expertise for the emerging field of male contraceptive research.

As with chemical agents, research on the contraceptive activity of hormones emerged in the context of infertility studies. In the early 1950s American reproductive scientists were focused primarily on the possible use of hormones as drugs in the treatment of infertility (Knuth and Nieschlag 1987: 42; Heckel 1939). These studies had the unintended side-effect of generating knowledge on the role of hormones as possible contraceptive agents. Interest in hormones as male contraceptives emerged in the mid-1950s when steroids (progesterones) were being tested as possible contraceptives for women. These hormonal preparations were also examined for their effects in the male by Gregory Pincus, one of the "fathers" of the Pill for women, and by other American reproductive scientists who had previously focused on infertility research.[8] The emergence of hormonal approaches to male contraceptives clearly shows a path dependence: previous practices in the field of female contraceptive development directed male contraceptive innovation to hormonal approaches.

In the 1950s and 1960s initiatives to increase expertise for intervention in male reproductive functions remained marginal. Except for Pincus's work in the 1950s, most research in male reproductive biology was directed primarily at understanding the fundamental control mechanisms of male reproduction rather than at trying to develop methods for intervening in those mechanisms (Paulsen 1977: 458). This preference for basic knowledge of the male reproductive system did not necessarily provide the best chances of success. The history of drug development shows that most drugs are selected not by fundamental research but by blind screening (Ericsson 1973: 301). As had happened in the field of female contraceptive development, basic research in reproductive functions was considered more respectable than applied research aimed at the development of contraceptives. This difference in respectability between basic and applied research has been one of the major constraints in contraceptive research since the 1920s.[9] For male contraceptive research, the situation has been even worse than for female contraceptive research. Scientists who decided to work on new male contraceptives entered the politically and culturally contested zone of sexuality, contraception, and emancipation. In the 1970s male contraceptive research was largely considered something of an illegitimate specialty, as is exemplified by the experience of Ronald Ericsson, one of the researchers active in the field in the 1960s:

> Male contraceptive research has a dismal past. It is almost an illegitimate specialty within reproductive biology. For the most part, the brightest workers avoid it and those who do work in the area are looked on as rather strange fellows. Scientific meetings . . . held on human fertility control invariably have the one paper devoted to male contraception. Not that much was happening but this one paper gave credence to the mere existence of the field. (Ericsson 1973)

Even in the 1990s male contraceptive research had a negative image. Researchers who became involved in mission-oriented research in reproduction risked being classified as "second-class scientists." Or, as one young researcher noted: "There is also a tremendous push to do more basic research, and pooling laboratory-based molecular biology type of research is the most useful credential for making it in academic medicine" (Matsumoto interview 1994).

For the first and second generation of reproductive scientists, who took these risks, the benefits seemed to have outweighed the risks. Pioneers such as R. John Aitken, Alvin Paulsen, and Eberhard Nieschlag, who initiated research on male contraceptives in the 1950s and 1960s, and William Bremner, Alvin Matsumoto, and Fred Wu, who joined the field in the 1970s and early 1980s, have succeeded in building their reputations by specializing in male fertility research. For these researchers, the availability of funds and the awareness that they were joining a young but growing field obviously outweighed the possible negative consequences for a career in science. In the 1990s prospects seemed to become much worse: "I don't see the next generation of researchers. I'm relatively young yet, but I'm on the fringes of being a senior investigator and have gotten lots of grants and things, but I don't see the next generation below me. My fellows and the fellows that are just coming into the program don't see this as a way to make a career in academic medicine" (Matsumoto interview 1994).

In the early 1970s the lack of clinicians with male reproductive expertise demonstrates a path dependence similar to that in reproductive biology. The orientation of the medical profession to female reproductive bodies had resulted in a lack of clinical investigators and clinicians trained in all aspects of male reproduction. The existing structure of medical education and the organization of clinical research were major barriers to the development of clinical expertise in male reproduction. The institutionalization of clinical expertise concerning the male reproductive body exhibits a fragmented picture, in which practitioners with specific knowledge of the male reproductive system were distributed over a variety of medical specialties, particularly urology, endocrinology, gynecology, and andrology, rather than being concentrated in one specialty, as was the case for the female reproductive body. Traditionally, urologists specialize in the urinary system and the prostate gland. Endocrinologists deal with the testes and testosterone replacement therapy. The treatment of infertility is largely delegated to gynecologists, a situation which has been strengthened by the introduction of in vitro fertilization techniques for the treatment of male infertility (Wu interview 1994). In practice, it is usually the urologist who is expected to treat all diseases of the male reproductive system. Departments of urology, however, have only a few clinicians specialized in the medical aspects of male reproduction. Prior to the 1970s, medical education largely neglected male reproductive physiology (Diller and Hembree 1977: 1272, 1273).

This situation has improved a little since the late 1960s, when clinicians in Europe and the United States took the initiative to establish andrology as a medical subspecialty devoted to research and medical treatment of the male reproductive system. The first andrological journal (*Andrologie*) was founded in 1969, and the first andrological societies were established in 1973—the Nordic Association for Andrology and the American Association of Andrology (Niemi 1987). Since the 1970s programs in andrology have been based in departments of medicine, gynecology, or in independent divisions of research hospitals (Diller and Hembree 1977: 1272). Currently, andrology as a clinical and scientific discipline is still rather marginal compared to its bigger sister, gynecology. Although the male reproductive body thus became embedded in the medical infrastructure, clinical expertise in male contraceptive research remained underdeveloped. As was the case for research in human reproductive biology, andrologists oriented their activities mainly in the study of infertility, which became fashionable in the 1980s (Djerassi 1989: 358). In sum, the lack of a critical mass of trained basic scientists and clinical investigators was a major barrier to male contraceptive innovation in the early 1970s.

A second barrier to male contraceptive innovation was a lack of suitable compounds. The development of hormonal contraceptives for men, one of the approaches that became dominant in the field in the early 1970s, depended largely on the availability of androgens. The paucity of available androgens is yet another example of path dependence in contraceptive research. Because of previous material investments in the development of hormonal therapy and contraceptives for women, the synthesis of new hormonal compounds had been largely restricted to progesterones and estrogens. When Gregory Pincus began the testing of hormones as female contraceptives, he could rely on a wide variety of available estrogens and progesterones produced by a number of American and European pharmaceutical firms (Oudshoorn 1994a). In contrast to Pincus, researchers and clinicians who took up the development of male hormonal contraceptives had to start from scratch. Although the first synthesis of testosterone dates from the 1930s, innovation in androgenic synthesis lacked any serious attention, both in the academic and industrial world (Wang interview 1993; Oudshoorn 1994a). Even in the late 1990s, investigators involved in male contraceptive research considered the lack of a suitable androgen as a major bottleneck and described the synthesis of androgens as "a 1960s technology" (Baird interview 1998).

Lack of Industrial Involvement, Cultural Resistance, and Limited Funding

The pharmaceutical industry has traditionally been a major resource in drug innovation. It is thus not surprising to note that pharmaceutical companies became involved in developing drugs for contraceptive purposes in the early 1960s. Although pharmaceutical firms were initially reluctant to enter the field of contraceptive R&D, they gradually became aware of the promise of this new market. When Gregory Pincus approached two pharmaceutical firms—Syntex, a Mexican company, and Searle, an American company—to collaborate in the development of what came to be known as "the Pill," both companies provided him with the requested compounds for animal testing. Although it took Pincus more effort to eventually persuade Searle to manufacture this first oral contraceptive, the Pill was brought to market within two years of its initial clinical testing (Oudshoorn 1994a). Due to its success, industrial R&D of new contraceptive agents became a booming business, attracting major American and European pharmaceutical firms to this new area of drug development.[10]

The first clouds in this apparently blue sky appeared when reports began to circulate about the health risks of oral contraceptives, most notably increased risks of cancer and diseases of the circulatory system (Seaman and Seaman 1978). Both consumer advocates and the women's movement criticized the rapid introduction of the Pill and suggested that reproductive science and industry had shown inadequate concern for the health of women (Gelijns and Pannenborg 1993: 227; Seaman and Seaman 1978). The strong public demand to reduce health risks had two major consequences which eventually led to a decline in industrial activity in contraceptive R&D. First, concerns about the health risks of contraceptive technology generated an enormous increase in the number of liability suits, initially against the U.S. manufacturers of the Dalkon Shield intrauterine device, and later against manufacturers of oral contraceptives. In the 1980s, "there were more liability suits for oral contraceptives annually than for any other drug category" (Gelijns and Pannenborg 1993: 227; Djerassi 1989, 1992). In the United States this dramatic increase in lawsuits led to a situation in which liability insurance for manufacturers became temporarily unavailable. Even today, the cost of liability insurance in the field of contraceptive research is higher than for any other drug category (Djerassi 1989: 357).[11]

Second, the public demand to reduce the health risks of new drugs led to more stringent rules and procedural regulations for the production and approval of new drugs. This happened generally for all drugs, one result of the thalidomide tragedy of the early 1960s, and drug regulatory requirements became more stringent both in Europe and the United States (Greep 1976: 352). Presently, "extensive requirements . . . must be met before a company is permitted to test or market a new drug" (Greep 1976: 352). In the United States, the role of the FDA shifted from one of protecting the consumer to one of guaranteeing the safety of a drug (Diller and Hembree 1977: 1275). Since 1962, the FDA's mandate has been extended; it now includes evaluating the "efficacy and appropriateness of proposed research designs to investigate new drugs and to monitoring of marketed drugs" (Greep 1976: 352).

The requirements for contraceptives are even more stringent than for other types of drugs (Greep 1976: 352) because contraceptives are normally used by healthy people over the course of many years. In response to concerns about the long-term effects of oral contraceptives, the FDA placed pre-marketing requirements on long-term animal research, even to the point of specifying animal models.[12] Moreover, the FDA introduced requirements for the clinical testing of all drugs in which the length of time from phase I to phase III trials is specified (Djerassi 1970). These more extensive testing requirements significantly increased the R&D costs for drugs and contraceptives: within two decades the average R&D cost of developing a new chemical compound increased from $65 million to $344 million.[13] As a result, most contraceptive R&D has become increasingly dependent on government funding.[14] The more stringent drug regulatory requirements also led to an increase in the development time for new contraceptives, which decreases the effective life of patents (Gelijns and Pannenborg 1993: 227).

These changes in the drug regulatory system have transformed contraceptive R&D into an area of innovation with a high risk of failure.[15] Industry representatives often cite these changes to explain the decline in industrial activity in contraceptive development. The past three decades have witnessed the virtual withdrawal of the U.S. pharmaceutical industry from contraceptive R&D (Mastroianni, Donaldson, and Kane 1990). In the 1970s at least thirteen major U.S. pharmaceutical firms were actively involved in contraceptive research. Currently, only Ortho maintains a significant R&D program (Fraser 1988). As a result, contraceptive R&D has largely shifted to Europe, where three major drug companies, Organon, Schering A.G., and Roussel-Uclaf, maintain sizable R&D programs (Gelijns 1993: 216). The European industry is able to continue research in contraceptives since liability issues have not played such an important role in Europe as in the United States (WHO/HRP 1990a: 14).

However, the overall impact on innovation in contraceptives is drastic: no contraceptives are ranked among the top-35 leading R&D therapeutic agents (Djerassi 1989: 360). In 1993 investments by the pharmaceutical industry accounted for only 39 percent of the global funding for contraceptive R&D (Service 1994: 1489). Obviously, the industry has largely turned to less risky and more lucrative non-contraceptive products.[16] Most current R&D activity in Europe is focused on the improvement of existing methods, such as the development of third-generation steroidal contraceptives for women, in order to retain the companies' share of the market (WHO/HRP 1990a: 14, 17). The stringent drug regulation requirements thus strengthened patterns of path dependence, in which most R&D remains focused on the development of so-called "me-too" products rather than on radical new technological innovation (Diczfalusy 1985: 47). The only new technology developed by the pharmaceutical industry during the 1980s was the abortion pill RU-486, a Roussel-Uclaf product. Another area of innovation in which the industry has gradually become involved is the development of contraceptive vaccines (Kammen 2000).

Other major areas for innovation, such as the development of new contraceptive delivery systems for use in developing countries or research into male contraceptives, have not received any substantial industrial R&D activity (Thau interview 1993).[17] Until the late 1990s, pharmaceutical firms showed hardly any interest in the emerging field of male contraceptive research, which was restricted to the delivery of hormonal compounds for clinical trials to academic centers and public sector agencies, and, only incidentally, to the organization of a workshop devoted to male contraceptive research. In 1972 the German pharmaceutical company, Schering A.G., organized the "Schering Workshop on Contraception: The Masculine Gender" (Raspe and Bernhard 1973). The pharmaceutical industry can thus be characterized as a reluctant actor in male contraceptive research.[18]

In addition to regulatory constraints, innovative work on male contraceptives also faced serious cultural resistance. Ever since the idea of male contraceptive drugs was first introduced, various groups, including feminists, scientists, journalists, and pharmaceutical entrepreneurs, have questioned whether men and women would accept a new male contraceptive if one were available. The complex cultural implications of new male contraceptives is particularly visible in the reactions of feminists to the new technology. On the one hand, the development of new contraceptives for men would enable feminists to realize two central aims of the women's health movement: a reduction of the health risks of contraception for women and an increase in male responsibility in the use of contraceptives. On the other hand, the new technology would delegate less autonomy to women, which conflicts with another major aim of the women's movement, that is, to give women control over their own fertility. In the 1970s women's rights to easy access to female contraceptives became a cornerstone of the movement. The shift toward contraceptives for men implies that women would "once again place their fate in a man's hands" (Stokes 1980: 41). To this day, the choice between autonomy and trust is still a feminist dilemma (I will analyze these debates in greater detail in chapter 6.) As well as feminists, journalists have also played a major role in contesting the cultural feasibility of new contraceptives for men, primarily as opponents of new contraceptives for men (see chapter 8). Because of this cultural resistance, the potential market for new male contraceptives was increasingly represented as "recalcitrant," or even non-existent.[19] As I will show in chapter 10, this negative view of the cultural acceptability of male contraceptive drugs dominated the R&D policies of pharmaceutical firms until the late 1990s.[20]

Finally, a lack of financial support provided yet another barrier to male contraceptive innovation. Over the years, the amount of money delegated to male contraceptive research has been small compared to that for female contraceptive research and drug development, in general (Diller and Hembree 1977: 1275, 1277).

Building an Alternative Sociotechnical Network

Advocacy of the development of new contraceptives for men thus began at a time when the conditions for radical technological change were very poor. Expertise, funding, laboratory and clinical infrastructures, drug regulatory procedures, the disinterest of the pharmaceutical industry, and cultural resistance constituted major barriers to initiating male contraceptive R&D. In the early 1970s male contraceptive research was an illegitimate line of research, conducted by a handful of researchers facing a recalcitrant market. In this context, path creation would seem to be an almost undoable job. The question thus becomes: How do radical new technologies, such as male contraceptives, ever manage to emerge, since they will always face a broad range of social, economic, cultural, and material barriers? The concept of the "niche," introduced in the evolutionary theory of technological change, provides a useful tool to capture the dynamics of radical technological innovation (Dosi et al. 1988). A "niche" refers to a protected space in which technological innovation can take place. Protection is needed because knowledge, expertise, techniques, market, societal infrastructures, and cultural acceptability have yet to be developed (Schot, Hoogma, and Elzen 1994). Laboratories, for example, provide one such space. As I will show in this section, R&D networks initiated and coordinated by agencies in the public sector are another type of niche in which technological innovation can emerge. In the case of male contraceptive innovation, path creation depended largely on the creation of alternative sociotechnical networks, a task in which public-sector agencies played an important role.[21]

Creating a Protected Space

Since the late 1960s international public-sector agencies, most notably the World Health Organization (WHO),[22] have become major actors in the promotion and coordination of contraceptive research worldwide. WHO first adopted this role in 1951, when it responded to a request from India to help with organizing pilot studies on the introduction of the rhythm method of fertility regulation. In 1952 WHO extended its role in the area of human reproduction research when the agency promoted its own participation in the World Population Conference being planned by the United Nations for 1953. Family planning was both politically and culturally controversial in this pe riod. Due to its activities, WHO came under heavy attack: some member states of the World Health Assembly "threatened to leave the Organization if it pursued any activities in the area of family planning and population. For the next decade the subject of family planning was to remain a taboo in WHO" (Kessler 1991: 43). By 1962, WHO considered that the situation was ripe for a second attempt to include family planning as one of the targets of its organization. This time the agency adopted a remarkable strategy to circumvent its critics. Dr. Kessler, who was involved in the effort to make family planning part of the agency's mission, and who eventually became the first director of WHO's special branch for human reproduction research, explained: "It was felt that a soft entry point for international collaboration in this area might be found through research in human reproduction. In a speech to the Fourth World Congress on Fertility and Sterility held in Rio de Janeiro, Brazil (1962), without ever mentioning the words family planning or fertility regulation, the Director-General stressed the great deficiencies in knowledge about reproduction and the fact that only a small number of scientists were engaged in its study." Moreover, the director-general emphasized that human reproduction ought to be considered "a major public health problem" (Kessler 1991:43). WHO thus circumvented the controversial subject of family planning, using the lack of information in the field of reproductive science as the rationale to expand into this new area. In the next few years, WHO gradually integrated its new mission into its organization, first by preparing an extensive review of human reproduction research, and later by appointing a staff member to work exclusively on this subject. In 1963 the agency began to support research in human reproduction by giving small grants to a broad spectrum of research projects in several countries in Europe, India, Latin America, and the United States.

In the meantime, a host of other organizations, including several national research councils, the International Planned Parenthood Federation, the World Bank, several agencies of the United Nations, the Ford Foundation, the Rockefeller Foundation, and the Population Council had also become very active in the area of family planning (Kessler 1991: 47). In June 1970 WHO took the initiative and convened a meeting with representatives of these organizations in order to coordinate all their activities. The agencies agreed that there was a need to develop new fertility-control methods, particularly for developing countries, and that further coordination of work was needed to make optimum use of the limited resources available for research in reproduction (Kessler 1991: 56). In the late 1960s the field of reproductive sciences was still a marginal, poorly financed field within the biomedical sciences. As a result of the 1970 meeting, WHO established a new branch specifically devoted to reproductive R&D: the Special Program for Research and Development and Research Training in Human Reproduction (shortened to the Human Reproduction Program, or HRP).[23]

By launching the HRP, WHO explicitly aimed to create alliances between governments and scientists:

> The Program is unique in the area of family planning research in that it brings together governments and scientists in a collaborative effort in both research and institution-strengthening. The HRP is the main instrument within the WHO for promoting and coordinating international research on the provision of family planning care and development of better methods of fertility regulation, and dissemination of information on research in family planning to policy makers, program administrators, service providers, scientists and the public. (WHO/HRP 1981: 10)

National governments are represented in WHO as member states of the World Health Assembly, and some of these states make special financial contributions to the HRP. Since 1988, the HRP has also been sponsored by the U.N. Development Program, the U.N. Population Fund, the World Bank, and WHO. The HRP has thus achieved status of "the research arm of the United Nations System in the field of human reproduction" (WHO/HRP 1991: ix). Thus, the WHO initiative to bridge the worlds of family planning and science resulted in the creation of a new research organization:

> In the first year of operation (1972) 150 scientists from 46 countries participated in planning meetings and began to initiate research . . . and by 1976 about 650 scientists from 62 countries, of which 34 were developing, were working with the Program in goal-oriented research. Funding to the Program rose from about US$4 million contributed by four donors in 1972 to over US$12 million in 1976 from nine donors. (Kessler 1991: 50)

The HRP's main emphasis in the 1970s was on the development of new birth control technologies. Since its foundation, it has established several task forces, each devoted to a specific contraceptive technology, including a task force for male contraceptive methods (Atkinson and Schearer 1980). This task force was initiated in response to a request from several WHO member states, most notably China and India, and strongly supported by Canada and

Sweden (Nieschlag interview 1995). In 1968 the WHO Scientific Group on Fertility Control, in Geneva, which was convened to review developments in contraceptive technologies, listed male fertility control methods as the first subject in its report (WHO 1987b: 5). During its first year in existence, six-teen scientists from ten countries were involved in the activities of the Task Force on Methods for the Regulation of Male Fertility (shortened to Male Task Force), whose budget was US$300,000 (WHO/HRP 1988: 1). Within two years, the number of participating scientists had doubled and the budget had increased to US$408,000 (WHO/HRP 1973: 9).

Beginning in the late 1960s research and funding for male contraceptive research have been included in the programs of other agencies as well, par-ticularly in the United States. The Population Council, a family planning organization funded by the Rockefeller Foundation, with a laboratory for research in reproductive physiology and contraceptive methods, began devot-ing a part of its budget to the study of male contraception (Seaman and Seaman 1977). The Contraceptive Development Branch of the National In-stitutes of Health, another American, goal-oriented program to develop con-traceptive methods, also includes male contraceptive R&D in its budget (WHO 1987b: 11). Other funding agencies, particularly the Center for Population Research, which was established as part of the U.S. National Institute of Child Health and Human Development in 1968, and the Agency for International Development, gradually began to support research in male contraceptives, although budgets remained modest compared to support for research in con-traceptives for women.[24] Despite limited funding, such initiatives, particularly the establishment of WHO's Male Task Force, have had a definite impact, as can be seen in the gradual increase in the number of publications on male contraceptives. In 1974 the first review of literature devoted exclusively to male reproduction appeared in the *Annual Review of Physiology*, and in 1975 three workshops on male reproduction took place, events that signaled the growing interest of the scientific community in the subject (Gomes and Van Demark 1974: 32, 91). Since 1974 there has been a small but steady flow of about ten papers per year on this subject in family planning journals, basic science journals, and clinical journals.[25]

The creation of WHO's Male Task Force thus succeeded in creating a pro-tected space for technological innovation in male contraceptive methods. WHO provided contraceptive researchers, particularly those who participated in the Steering Committee of the Male Task Force, with an infrastructure through which they could exchange ideas and experiences on male fertility research, and which enabled them to transcend the competitive environment of the academic world. Eberhard Nieschlag, chairman of the Steering Committee during the period 1985–1990, observed:

> The major achievement of the program is not so much spending money in research, but getting the people together. I think the idea of the Task Force and the idea of the Steering Committee is tremendous, for you get world experts in the field to sit around the table for several years and think about the project. What the scientists normally do is competing with each other, and not telling what you think because you want to do it before anyone else. In the Steering Committee you really put your brains together in a constructive way. I think therefore that this program has borne a lot of ideas. (Nieschlag interview 1995)

Like the scientists, WHO also benefited from these alliances. The participation of the scientists legitimated the organization's involvement with family planning. WHO's decision to invest in (male) reproductive research was, as described earlier, part of its policy to circumvent opposition to the decision to include family planning in its activities. The close collaboration with scientists enabled WHO to define itself as an organization that was contributing to solving "the world population problem," which was, and still is, perceived as an urgent health-threatening and socioeconomic problem. WHO's commitment to the field of family planning, and particularly its involvement with contraceptive R&D, however, was by no means unproblematic. From its inception, the HRP had to defend its decision to include the development of new contraceptives in its program against critics who rejected such a "technological fix" and advocated socioeconomic solutions to population problems. Equally problematic, WHO's decision to invest in male contraceptive research was an act of faith, because nobody knew when such an R&D program might eventually bear results.

Although WHO embarked upon a project with a highly uncertain future, the establishment of the Male Task Force can be considered an important attempt to overcome the barriers to male contraceptive research. First, the task force played a major role in coordinating the limited and widely dispersed expertise in male reproductive biology and contraceptive research, while at the same time stimulating new research in the emerging field of male contraceptive research. Compared to other organizations, such as the Population Council and the U.N. Family Planning Association (UNFPA), WHO's role consisted not so much in financing research but in bringing the required experts together (Nieschlag interview 1995). In its early years, the Male Task Force successfully recruited reproductive scientists whose expertise and skills lay in research on chemical and hormonal contraceptives. WHO promoted close cooperation among scientists by inviting leading experts in the field to become members of the task force's Steering Committee. Alvin Paulsen, who we have seen was one of the pioneers in male contraceptive research in the United States, agreed to act as coordinator and chairman of the Steering Committee.[26]

One of the first activities of the Male Task Force was to launch a basic research program, which it justified thusly: "In acknowledging that the drugs with an action on sperm maturation were largely made available by serendipity, the Task Force became convinced of the need for a coherent research strategy based on fundamental biomedical science" (WHO/HRP 1988: 27). The first sixteen contracts issued were for research to improve knowledge of two aspects of the male reproductive system: sperm maturation in the epididymis and the ability of mature sperm to penetrate the ovum (Diezfalusy 1985; WHO/HRP 1988: 1). Another major project, the inhibin research program, consisted in the isolation of peptides of testicular origin and the development of bioassay systems (WHO/HRP 1988). In the late 1980s the task force expanded its funding for fundamental biomedical research by initiating an "open program of basic research" (WHO/HRP 1988: 27). The decision to fund basic research can be seen as a strategy to reconcile two different constraints on male contraceptive innovation. On the one hand, the choice of basic research was a concession made to reproductive scientists who were reluctant to engage in applied research. As previously described, reproductive scientists preferred basic research because it facilitated their academic careers. On the other hand, the decision to encourage basic research could also be considered as a form of path creation, by which the Male Task Force tried to stimulate new approaches in the emerging field of male reproduction. Due to the path dependence of female contraceptives, most research on male contraception was focused on hormonal approaches. The decision to focus on the role of inhibin in male reproductive functions, a little studied area, implied a break with this tradition. It also meant a commitment to a line of research that implied a long road to the development of a new contraceptive agent. Indeed, although the Male Task Force has spent much time and money in inhibin research, the program has not yet resulted in a new contraceptive agent.

A second example of the role of WHO and other agencies, such as the Population Council, in stimulating new approaches to male contraceptive R&D is the development of antifertility vaccines, which was added to the agendas of these agencies in the early 1970s. The development trajectories of these new contraceptives illustrate processes of path creation as well as path dependence. On the one hand, public-sector agencies, scientists, and funding agencies have been able to introduce a new potential lead into contraceptive development. Currently, approximately 10 percent of public funding for contraceptive research is spent on antifertility vaccines for both men and women. On the other hand, previous material and symbolic investments have directed the development of antifertility vaccines, again, mostly to women. Although public-sector agencies and the small research community initially focused on the development of a vaccine for both sexes, most research has been devoted to developing a vaccine for women (Kammen 2000).[27]

In addition to its role in stimulating and coordinating basic research in male contraception, the HRP also played an important role in overcoming some constraints that were caused by a lack of available research materials. In the 1970s the HRP initiated a program for the synthesis of hormonal contraceptive agents. The Steroid Synthesis Program drew heavily on the expertise and skills of chemistry and pharmaceutical laboratories in Western and Southern countries. What WHO brought to this field was the creation of an infrastructure to mobilize resources. The synthesis of new steroids was allocated to a network of nineteen laboratories, initiated and coordinated by WHO. For the most part, these were chemistry labs and some pharmacy labs, with locations all over the world. This worldwide effort succeeded in the synthesis of approximately 380 steroids: 310 progestin esters for female contraceptives and 70 androgen esters for male contraceptives (WHO/HRP 1981: 2; Oudshoorn 1997a). This work will be analyzed in more detail in the following chapter.

Finally, WHO played a major role in overcoming barriers to male contraceptive research by creating a network of academic centers with the expertise, skills, and facilities to conduct clinical studies. Because the study of male reproductive functions had not yet been institutionalized as a medical specialty, facilities to conduct clinical trials were very limited in the early 1970s:

> Another important limitation to progress has been the general neglect of andrology as a medical discipline. Virtually every medical school and hospital devotes a substantial part of its resources specifically to female reproductive medicine, but rarely is there any provision at all for andrology, the male equivalent. The consequence of such neglect is the very limited availability of a suitable expertise and facilities to conduct the necessary high-quality clinical studies. (Handelsman 1991: 232)

WHO recognized this weakness and put great effort into creating the required infrastructure for clinical trials. These efforts resulted in the establishment of a worldwide network of eleven clinics, which cooperated in multi-center clinical trials on gestagen–androgen combinations and cyproterone acetate (WHO/ HRP 1988: 30). In the mid-1980s, this network of clinics was extended to facilitate two large-scale clinical trials (described in chapter 4). Many of these contacts with academic institutes, established in these early years, evolved into long-term collaborations. In the 1980s WHO named these institutes "Collaborating Centers for Research of Human Reproduction." The Institute of Reproductive Medicine in Münster provides an example of the mutual benefits derived from this collaboration: "The status of WHO–Collaborating Center allows the Institute to employ two scientific workers or two physicians-in-training using Federal Health Ministry funds, following an annual grant application. In addition, scientific projects are financed directly by the WHO. . . . Within the framework of such collaboration Institute members prepare reports and statements, sit on committees, develop research projects and carry out studies on behalf of the WHO" (Nieschlag, Lerch, and Nieschlag 1994: 7, 8).

By creating networks for collaborative laboratory research and clinical testing WHO achieved a major change in the usual pattern of collaboration in the academic world. It was WHO's explicit policy to include institutes from developed and developing countries, which thereby gave an important stimulus to the improvement of communication and collaboration between labs and clinics that previously had not had any contact. This "institution-strengthening" policy was, and still is, one of the cornerstones of WHO. Most importantly, this policy proved to be beneficial, both for WHO and for the field of male contraceptive research. It helped realize one of WHO's central aims: to distribute expertise in male reproductive research, particularly in developing countries. For the field of male contraceptive research, it meant a substantial increase in the number of scientists involved in R&D and basic research, and the creation of an infrastructure in which large-scale laboratory research projects and clinical trials could be conducted.

Governments as Agents of Path Creation

In 1979 the promising first phase of the Male Task Force's mission came to an abrupt end. The Advisory Group to HRP recommended that the task force's research program be phased out by 1980, after a number of limiting factors for research in male contraceptive methods, which hampered the activities of the task force, were identified in WHO's 1979 Annual Report. These were, specifically:

—the need for long-term, large-scale investment in basic science,
—the relatively few investigators involved in this area,

—the lack of well-funded research establishments capable of working in this area,

—the extent to which a male "pill" or injectable would be used by men. (WHO/HRP 1988: 5)

This last concern exemplified the still fragile belief in the whole mission about whether the development of new male contraceptives would eventually be effective in changing attitudes toward contraceptive use by men. The decision to terminate the activities of the Male Task Force was part of the HRP's effort to concentrate manpower and financial resources on a smaller number of lines and products (WHO/HRP 1979a). The cancellation of the Male Task Force did not imply that the HRP was definitely withdrawing its interest in male contraceptives since it also decided to "continue to monitor the field and be alert for developments which would justify the re-initiation of 'mission-oriented' research by the Task Forc" (WHO/HRP 1988: 6).[28]

The decision to phase out the activities of the Male Task Force did not go unnoticed. Both reproductive scientists and several WHO member states, most notably India and China, objected quite strongly to this decision (Paulsen interview 1994; WHO/HRP 1981b). The HRP's Advisory Group responded to these adverse comments by saying that they "needed to see new features before agreeing to reinstate the Task Force" (WHO/HRP 1988: 8). At that point in its history, WHO's affiliation with governments turned out to be of crucial importance for the survival of the Male Task Force: it was the Chinese government, one of the earliest advocates of male contraceptive research, which eventually came to its rescue. Prior to 1976, China had been a closed society. In 1966 the Chinese political leaders Mao Tse-tung and Chou En-lai had adopted a strong anti-internationalist policy which prohibited all contact with the rest of the world. In this period, known as the Cultural Revolution, many intellectuals lost their positions and jobs because their work did not further the "proletarian revolution." In 1972, when China became a member of the United Nations, the Chinese leaders opted for a more liberal policy and exchanges with the Western world became more frequent. China now wanted to join the world community, which resulted in collaborative projects in business and science, although it was only after the death of the Mao and Chou, in 1976, that the situation of China's more highly educated citizens, for example, scientists, technicians, writers, and artists, gradually improved (Das and Oerlemans 1984: 259, 260).

The opening of China seemed to promise a revolution for the Western male contraceptive research community. China claimed to have developed the artifact the Western world still dreamed of: a male oral contraceptive. "When a group from the United States visited China, I think in 1979, they became aware that about 14,000 Chinese men were participating in clinical trials on Gossypol. Well, it hit the Associated Press. I must have had in two days over a hundred phone calls, saying: 'What's this on Gossypol, I've never heard of it.' I remember in 1980 at an andrology meeting in Chicago, everyone was really excited about Gossypol" (Paulsen interview 1994). Although clinical trials of Gossypol (a component of cottonseed oil, whose contraceptive properties were discovered accidentally by Chinese scientists[29]) had been taking place in China since 1972, the news did not reach the Western scientific press until the early 1980s.[30] In 1980, the *American Journal of Chinese Medicine* published the results of the trials in a paper with the intriguing title "China Invents Male Birth Control Pill":

> China, famed for its historical inventions, is on the verge of adding another "first" to the history of human discovery—an oral contraceptive for men. Tests carried out over a six-year period and involving some 10,000 volunteers using a drug known as Gossypol have proved 99.89% effective, with no appreciably harmful side effects. . . . The National Coordinating Group on Male Anti-fertility plans to call a meeting this summer (1979) to give a complete and overall assessment of Gossypol's results. If agreement is reached on the safety and effectiveness of the pill, it will go into production immediately and could be in general use by the end of 1979. (Wen 1980: 195, 197, emphasis in original)

When the news finally spread, reproductive scientists, public-sector agencies, and pharmaceutical firms jumped on the bandwagon: several research groups in the United States, including the Biomedical Research Unit of the Population Council and the American firm Upjohn, began to conduct animal research to evaluate the contraceptive potential of Gossypol (Benditt 1980: 154). In October 1979, ironically at the last meeting, in Geneva, of the Male Task Force prior to its suspension of operations, Chinese scientists were invited to report on their experiences with Gossypol (WHO/HRP 1979a). High hopes concerning Gossypol were dashed, however, when it was revealed that the drug's toxic adverse effects included diarrhea, circulatory problems, heart failure, and permanent sterility (Diczfalusy 1986). When WHO representatives visited China in 1979, they raised these concerns about the potential dangers associated with taking Gossypol. In 1981 the Director of the WHO Human Reproductive Program decided that "WHO could not be associated with new prospective clinical studies with Gossypol until these concerns were resolved"

(WHO/HRP 1988: 7). Since then, WHO has no longer been involved in studies of this contraceptive (Waites, Wang, and Griffin 1998). Despite this cautious attitude, the HRP acknowledged that the Chinese drug represented a possible new lead for the development of male contraceptives (Diczfalusy 1986).

During the Second International Congress of Andrology, held in Tel Aviv in 1981, HRP representatives convened a meeting of experts to review the state of knowledge in male contraceptive research. The result was a request to the Advisory Group of the HRP to reinitiate the research activities of the Male Task Force and a proposal to initiate studies in new areas of male contraceptive research: studies of Gossypol and of vasectomy (WHO/HRP 1988: 8). As with Gossypol, Western scientists had become interested in new vasectomy techniques after work in this area was reported by Chinese clinicians. In the 1970s China had developed new non-surgical and reversible techniques in vasectomy (WHO/HRP 1988). News of these new techniques came at the same time as the Western world was becoming more concerned about the long-term safety of vasectomy. Nevertheless, the Chinese experience increased Western interest in these new vasectomy techniques.

The opening of China to the West gave the HRP the arguments it needed to convince WHO to continue its involvement in male contraceptive research. The Gossypol adventure had an enormous impact on the field of male contraceptive research: although China could not keep its promise to develop a new, safe, reversible contraceptive, it showed that it had at its disposal a substantial number of scientists and clinicians with a long-established expertise in male reproductive research in two new areas: Gossypol and vasectomy. The "Chinese connection" thus provided the HRP with an even stronger argument to counteract one of the major concerns that had led WHO to phase out its male contraceptive research program, that is, the relatively small number of scientists working in this field. In 1982 WHO decided to reinitiate the activities of the Male Task Force, which heralded a new phase in male contraceptive research in which China became an important actor.

In the meantime, WHO had committed itself quite strongly to collaboration with China. In 1979 the People's Republic of China had approached the HRP to collaborate "in the development of capabilities for basic, clinical and epidemiological research in fertility control" (WHO/HRP 1988: 6). China had received major funding for family planning research from the U.N. Fund for Population Activities, in which WHO was asked to assume the role of Executing Agency. WHO accepted this invitation and charged the HRP with day-to-day responsibilities for this program. The in-depth report which evaluated the activities of the Male Task Force in 1987 described these events: "There were immediate major consequences for male research related to Gossypol and vasectomy. But equally important, these developments heralded the start of a process of institution strengthening which was to go some way toward allaying two of the concerns expressed earlier about male research i.e. the relatively small number of personnel and of well-founded centers working in the field" (WHO/HRP 1988: 6).

For WHO, the collaboration with China provided a substantial broadening of the activities of the HRP. The WHO Ninth Annual Report (1980) evaluated this collaboration:

> The request for collaboration in institution-strengthening from the People's Republic of China, which already a year ago could be clearly seen to entail a major effort, comprising the setting up of a large research institution in Shanghai, the involvement of Chinese scientists in several Task Force Steering Committees and providing journals, standard reagents and small supplies to more than a dozen other institutes in all parts of China, expanded further during the year. The Chinese Government and the United Nations Fund for Population Activities asked the Program to be the Executing Agency for the setting up in Beijing of the National Research Institute for Family Planning and also to explore the possibility of strengthening a number of other research institutes in the provinces. The funds for the Beijing Institute alone amount to some $3.5 million over a four-year period, and are being provided by UNFPA in addition to UNFPA's contribution to the Program as a whole. (WHO/HRP 1979B: 3, 4)

For the Chinese scientific community, the collaboration with WHO thus meant a firm entrance into the Western scientific world. For the field of male contraceptive research, the Chinese connection provided a challenge to the dominance of hormonal approaches to male fertility control. In the 1980s non-pharmaceutical approaches, that is, plant products and new vasectomy techniques, gained acceptance as promising new leads to male contraception. Before the 1970s WHO's activities had been oriented almost exclusively toward Western methods. The dominance of Western medical approaches was first challenged when China was accepted as a member of WHO. China contested WHO's preference for Western medicine and helped it to develop a policy that was more open to traditional medical practices (Lee 1997). The inclusion of non-pharmaceutical approaches to male contraceptives can thus be understood as a first challenge to the dominance of Western medicine in contraceptive development.

The research budgets of the Male Task Force illustrate this shift to non-Western approaches. Major expenditures in the 1980s were on Gossypol research, whereas expenditures on hormonal methods declined from 69 percent of the total budget in the period 1972–1979 to 25 percent in the period 1982–1986 (WHO/HRP 1988: 38). In 1982 the Male Task Force initiated a large-scale program to synthesize active, non-toxic analogues of Gossypol. Thirteen centers cooperated, including two Chinese centers (Waites 1986: 156, 157). Although WHO invested much time and money in this project, the problems with toxicity were not easily solved. WHO therefore decided not to initiate clinical studies of these newly synthesized Gossypol analogues, as it had done with the products of the steroid synthesis program. In 1990 the Gossypol research project was terminated (WHO/HRP 1988). In the context of WHO, the technological trajectory of Gossypol provides a clear example of path destruction. Despite WHO's investment in this line of research, the organization decided to stop this trajectory. However, Gossypol did not completely disappear from view. The Population Council, which had also included Gossypol research on its agenda, continued its involvement with this research and initiated clinical trials in the so-called "South to South" research groups, a collaborative program among Southern countries (Male participation 1995).[31] Another plant product that came to be included in the male contraceptive research agenda was *Tripterygium wilfordii*. Beginning in 1986 the Male Task Force had funded collaborative studies with Chinese scientists aimed at the chemical isolation and identification of pure compounds from this plant, as well as animal testing of these compounds (WHO/HRP 1993: 67). In addition to plant products, the development of new, reversible vasectomy techniques became more central to the research agenda. Due to the Chinese connection, new approaches to vasectomy, such as non-scalpel techniques, percutaneous injections with silicone and polyutherane, and microsurgical techniques to reverse vasectomies and to reach the vasa through puncture rather than incision, came to be adopted as new research lines by the Western scientific community. The Male Task Force developed a research program, including animal studies and clinical trials, to test the efficacy of a silicone plug (Vasoc) which had already been used for female sterilization. Equally important, the Task Force initiated a program to transfer the experiences and skills of Chinese clinicians with vasectomy techniques to the Western world by organizing training workshops in these techniques for non-Chinese surgeons (WHO/HRP 1993: 64, 68). Networks between governments and scientists thus played an important role in introducing new lines of research in the field of male contraceptive research. Although the hormonal approach remained dominant,[32] other approaches, that is, plant products and vasectomy, came to be accepted as relevant new leads in the development of male contraceptives. In the WHO/HRP biennial reports of the late 1990s, hormonal approaches and new non-surgical methods of vasectomy appear in the program's list of most promising, high-priority product leads (WHO 1990–1999).

Feminists as Agents of Cultural Change

As we have seen, governments, and most notably the government of China, have been important actors in changing the status quo in contraceptive development. Due to the advocacy of governments, male contraceptive technological innovation came to be included in the contraceptive research agenda. Most importantly, the support of governments enabled WHO to create an alternative sociotechnical network to stimulate and coordinate male contraceptive R&D. The Chinese government turned out to be of crucial importance once again when WHO decided to withdraw its support for male contraceptive research. Governments and public-sector agencies have thus been important in creating new sociotechnical networks to overcome problems of path dependence. The development of new male contraceptives was, however, constrained, and not only by the lack of expertise and research materials and infrastructure. As I have indicated, there was yet another important barrier to technological innovation in this area: that is, disbelief in the cultural feasibility of the technology. The final part of this chapter therefore focuses on the transformative work of the other agent of change, namely, the feminist movement. In the early 1970s feminists, and particularly women's health advocates, were important in reframing the need for new male contraceptives in such a way as to open a potentially broader market, thus making the endeavor more attractive to pharmaceutical firms. As we have seen, feminist advocacy of male contraception grew out of criticism of the role of scientists and industry in the introduction of new contraceptives for women, most notably the oral hormonal contraceptive and the Dalkon shield, an intrauterine device. In the late 1960s feminist health advocates campaigned against the Pill because of its side-effects and accused the scientific community of not taking seriously the many complaints of users. In *The Doctor's Case Against the Pill* (1969), Barbara and Gideon Seaman, leading American women's health experts, documented the experiences of women using the Pill. One year later, on 23 January 1970, feminist health advocates in the United States interrupted Senator Gaylord Nelson's hearings on the Pill, demanding to know: "Why is there no pill for men?" (Seaman and Seaman 1978: 325).[33] In 1972 Barbara Seaman continued her criticism of the Pill in *Free and Female*, in which she charged scientists with sex discrimination for developing contraceptives for women and not for men.[34] Since the early 1970s, scientists working in the area of male reproduction have increasingly been confronted with critical questions about the reasons for the discrepancy between the available contraceptives for women and men. In "Contraceptive Research: A Male Chauvinist Plot?" Sheldon Segal, vice-president of the Population Council in the 1970s, complained: "I think that I have not attended a single nonscientific meeting in the last two years at which the progress of contraceptive development was discussed that someone—usually a woman—has not asked: What about the men? Why aren't scientists trying to develop a new male contraceptive?" (Sheldon 1972: 21). In his essay Segal simply rejected the criticism of feminists, and particularly the work of Barbara Seaman. In 1975 two other American reproductive scientists, William Bremner and David de Kretser, braved the lion's den to report similar experiences. Writing in the journal *Signs*, they described these confrontations with feminists:

> As a general comment on the history of research in fertility control, it is of interest that contraceptive techniques for men seem to have lagged somewhat behind those available for women, particularly in the area of oral preparations. Questions about the reasons of this discrepancy are often asked of workers in the area of male contraception. The questions are occasionally asked with a certain degree of hostility, with the implication that scientists in the area of reproduction research have been responsive to male opinion, which is held to regard the female as the sex responsible for contraception. (Bremner and de Kretser 1975: 395)

Except for these kinds of confrontations, there was no direct interaction between feminists and scientists. Feminists depended on the media, which played a major intermediary role between the worlds of feminists and scientists. In the 1970s and 1980s newspapers regularly repeated the question first posed by feminists: What about the male Pill?

These criticisms shaped reproductive discourse in the 1970s. Review papers describing the state of the art in contraceptive research usually included a section which explained why there was as yet no male equivalent to the female pill. The initial reaction of most reproductive scientists was to defend their field against accusations of male chauvinism by arguing that their work simply reflected fundamental biological differences between the sexes. Other scientists adopted similarly natural explanations but agreed with feminists that there had been prejudice (Fawcett 1978: 57). However, not all scientists shared these biological explanations. Roy Greep is a leading reproductive scientist at Harvard Medical School and project director and one of the editors of *Reproduction and Human Welfare: A Challenge to Research*, the first extensive review of the reproductive sciences and contraceptive development, initiated and funded by the Ford Foundation in 1976. Greep turned the tables on the scientific community by suggesting that if scientists had simply followed nature, they would have developed male contraceptives rather than female methods:

> The paucity of contraceptives available to the male and the inexcusable delay in developing a research program to correct this deficiency is not a readily understandable circumstance since there are potent biological reasons why the burden of responsibility for conception control should rightfully fall on the male. Firstly, it is the male that plays the initiating role in the procreation process. Procreation involves the union of egg and sperm, but it is only the sperm that must be transferred between the sexes. It is the sperm that comes calling on the egg at home. . . . There is another and much overlooked circumstance that makes the practice of conception control by the male an imperative matter. This is the fact that men have a much longer fertile life than that of their female counterparts. . . . Men, therefore, constitute a target population for the implementation of conception control that could be of unparalleled significance to the future welfare of the human species. (Spilman, Kirton, and Kirton 1976: 2–3)

Greep and other scientists ascribed the gap between female and male methods to a lack of fundamental knowledge of the male reproductive system, caused by institutional reasons. In *Reproduction and Human Welfare*, the authors concluded:

> The number of basic and clinical investigators interested in andrology as opposed to gynecology is very small, and the investment in basic research on the male has been only a very small fraction of that devoted to the female. . . . The state of our knowledge of the male is now nearly comparable to that preceding the development of oral contraceptives for the female. If adequate research support can be sustained, there is every reason to expect that the next fifteen years will see the development of safe effective means of fertility control in the male. (Greep, Koblinsky, and Jaffe 1976: 251)

The ways in which feminist criticism shaped reproductive discourse thus evolved from a debate on male bias to a debate in which scientists used feminist criticism as a resource to argue for more funding of male reproductive research. Since the mid-1970s publications have appeared with titles that explicitly refer to the emancipation of women—for example, *Contraception: Equality for the Sexes?* (Aldhous 1990) and *Bridging the Gender Gap in Contraception: Another Hurdle Cleared* (Handelsman 1991). Reproductive scientists explicitly framed the relevance of male contraceptive research in feminist terms, which culminated in the organization of three workshops on male fertility control in 1975, the year declared by the United Nations as the Year of the Woman. The Foreword to the published proceedings of one of these workshops exemplifies this change in discourse: "As one of our main practical concerns is the control of human fertility, the last part of the book is devoted to the still scarce knowledge gained in male fertility control in the recent years. Actually it was the purpose of the entire meeting which would have culminated during the Year of the Woman into the round table on 'Perspectives in male fertility control'—as a contribution to a shared responsibility in responsible parenthood" (Hermite, Hubinont, Schwers 1976: xi, xii).

Although feminists and scientists disagreed on many things, there was one mutual concern which brought these worlds together: the health risks of contraceptive methods for women, particularly of the Pill. The major impact of feminist advocacy for male contraceptive innovation was that the discourse on the need to develop male methods became increasingly framed in terms of sharing health risks between the sexes. In the late 1970s both the Population Council and WHO evaluated their research efforts in this field in health terms (Kretser 1978). A piece in the WHO *Bulletin* in 1978 clearly exemplified this discourse:

> In the past, emphasis has been placed on the development and use of contraceptive methods for women but, with increasing publicity on the problems associated with the use of oral estrogen-gestagen contraceptives, the role of the male in contraceptive practice is re-examined. . . . Consequently, over the past decade increasing effort has been devoted to a re-examination of the male role in contraception and research into new methods is being stimulated. . . . It is against this background that agencies interested in contraceptive development have been attempting to stimulate research in the development of contraceptives for males. Through its Special Program of Research, Development and Research Training in Human Reproduction, the World Health Organization has been able to increase significantly the research effort in male contraceptive development, by initiating a task force to develop methods of regulating male fertility. (Kretser 1978: 353)

Feminist advocacy for new male contraceptives thus provided scientists and WHO with rhetorical devices to increase the legitimacy of male contraceptive research. Even in the 1990s, the legitimacy of the quest for male contraceptives needed to be articulated explicitly, and, again, scientists and WHO relied on the feminist demand for male contraceptives, as exemplified in the WHO Biennial Report for 1992–1993: "Recently, through increased public awareness, statements supporting research on male methods and the greater involvement of men in reproductive health have been forthcoming from several quarters, including the women's health movement" (WHO 1992–1993: 129).

Feminist activism has not been restricted to science. The feminist quest for male contraceptives was, however, eventually much broader than the development of a new technology. The feminist movement was a social movement that aimed to change the norms and attitudes of men and of society at large toward the family and the child-rearing responsibilities of men. The endeavor to make new male contraceptives included the making of a New Man. Through the years, feminists have been crucial in mobilizing heterogeneous groups such as family planning organizations and the United Nations to include male responsibility for family planning on their agendas. In the 1980s women's health activists lobbied successfully in the United Nations to give more priority to research on male contraceptives and the design of family programs for men. Both issues were included in the policy recommendations of the U.N. Population Conference in Mexico (U.N./ICPD 1984), and they were even more central during that organization's last conference in Cairo (U.N./ICPD 1994a). Feminists thus not only demanded a new technology, they emphasized the need for broader cultural transformations and political reforms in the arena of family planning services. In chapter 6 I will describe this transformative work in more detail.

What feminists brought to the world of contraceptive research was the demand to develop new contraceptives for men in the Western industrialized world. Whereas the major objective of the Male Task Force was initially "to develop practical methods of male contraceptives, preferable applicable to developing countries" (WHO 1987b: 11), feminists added the demand to develop new contraceptives for men in developed countries. The intervention of feminists resulted in a shift toward a wider and financially more substantial market with two categories of users: Southern men who want to limit the size of their families because they were responsible heads of households, and Northern men who were willing to share health risks and family responsibilities with their partners. Feminists thus mobilized stronger and broader support, both in developing and developed countries.

Conclusions

Reflecting on this reconstruction of how men came to be included in the contraceptive research agenda, we can conclude that governments and social movements have played an important role in challenging the status quo in contraceptive research. The advocacy for new male contraceptives articulated by Chinese and Indian political leaders and feminists in the Western in-dustrialized world resulted in the formation of new sociotechnical networks that included reproductive scientists, clinicians, feminists, and public-sector agencies, most notably WHO. By creating this alternative network, male con-traceptive proponents tried to overcome the barriers resulting from path de-pendence and cultural resistance toward the new technology. The network provided a protected space in which scientists could break away from the routines, practices, agendas, and norms that had directed the development of contraceptive drugs exclusively toward female users and contraceptive meth-ods. Most importantly, the creation of new sociotechnical networks set in motion transformative processes within and between heterogeneous groups. Alliances among governments, scientists, feminists, and public-sector agen-cies were potentially powerful because they gave access to the skills and resources to realize changes in the research agenda of academic laboratories and public-sector research centers, in the programs of family planning orga-nizations, and in the cultural attitudes toward male responsibility in con-traception among men and society at large. Those who had not been pre-viously involved in contraceptive development, that is, WHO, governments, and feminists, enabled the network to mobilize different resources to over-come the barriers to male contraceptive research.

WHO played an important role in giving credibility and respectability to the quest for new male contraceptives. WHO's imprimator granted the project the recognition of an international health agency with a well-known reputation, both in developing and developed countries. This was a crucial contribution, because reproductive research in general, and male contraceptive research in particular, were marginal, not highly respectable fields in the academic world. Most importantly, WHO provided the project with the required infrastructure and momentum. Since the early 1970s, the field of male contraceptive re-search has been transformed from a collection of small, scattered research projects into large-scale, multi-center laboratory research projects and clinical studies, a process in which the Male Task Force has played a crucial role. The initiation and coordination of large-scale collaborative projects transformed the usually competitive norms of the academic world. WHO provided a context in which laboratories and clinics with no previous contacts could collaborate to overcome the limited research and clinical testing facilities in the field. Moreover, WHO's policy to include researchers from developing countries meant a substantial increase in the number of scientists involved in male contraceptive research and transformed the Western-dominated research field into a multi-cultural endeavor.

Governments, particularly China and India, were equally successful in mobilizing another important resource to strengthen the endeavor to develop male contraceptives. The Chinese and Indian governments were key figures in granting relevancy to the project. They were the first to emphasize the need to improve male responsibility in family planning and to argue that this goal could be achieved by increasing the number of contraceptive methods available to men. Both China and India played an important role in the establishment of the Male Task Force, and China also contributed in rescuing the Task Force from an untimely death. Equally important, the contacts with China transformed the field of male contraceptive research from a field dominated by research on hormonal methods to one that included plant products and reversible vasectomy techniques as promising leads for new contraceptives.

Finally, feminists, initially considered troublemakers, were able to mobilize resources that were beyond the capacities of the other members of the sociotechnical network to promote the transformation of cultural norms toward men and contraception. The often repeated demand for the male Pill made the whole endeavor of developing new male contraceptives into a publicly debated issue in many societies. Never before had a product seen such an intensive promotion even before it actually existed. Feminists added yet another resource to the project. Whereas governments in Southern regions had provided the resources to legitimate the relevancy of new male contraceptives for developing countries, feminists legitimated the relevance for men in the Western industrialized world. The women's health movements were able to mobilize family planning organizations and even the United Nations to include male responsibility for family planning on their agendas. These were crucial transformations, because the quest for new male contraceptives would ultimately fail if men were not willing to use them or if family planning organizations were not inclined to include them in their programs.

Evaluating the achievements of governments, feminists, and WHO, we can conclude that the emerging sociotechnical network was quite successful: it established new research lines for the development of male contraceptives, it provided the infrastructure required for the synthesis and the clinical testing of contraceptive drugs, it made male responsibility for fertility control one of the priorities in family planning, and it succeeded in putting the New Man on the cultural agenda. These processes of change were by no means easy to achieve. The following chapters will analyze these transformative processes in greater detail.

3

Creating a Worldwide Laboratory for Synthesizing
Hormonal Contraceptive Compounds

· · · ·

The pharmaceutical industry has played a dominant role in the research and development of drugs. Most modern prescription drugs have been developed by pharmaceutical companies in the Western industrialized world (Djerassi 1970: 943).[1] Contraceptives are, however, a major exception. In the last three decades, the pharmaceutical industry has virtually withdrawn from contraceptive R&D, particularly in the United States (Djerassi 1989; Gelijns and Pannenborg 1993). Innovation in contraceptive technologies, particularly where contraceptives for men are concerned, has become increasingly dependent on alternative sociotechnical networks, in which the role of the pharmaceutical industry is replaced by public sector agencies, most notably WHO. As I argued in the previous chapter, these alternative R&D networks can best be described as niches: protected spaces in which technological innovation can take place to overcome the constraints and resistance of traditional R&D organizations. An important question is the extent to which WHO has succeeded in creating such a protected space for male contraceptive R&D. What alternative structures need to be in place when industry does not participate directly in drug development? One of the major activities of the pharmaceutical industry in drug development consists of the synthesis of new compounds that may eventually result in the development of new drugs. As we saw in the previous chapter, the lack of suitable compounds for male contraceptives was a major obstacle to innovation. Due to investments in the development of hormonal therapies and contraceptives for women, the synthesis of new hormonal compounds has been largely restricted to progesterones and estrogens. In contrast to the pioneers in female contraceptive development, who could rely on a

wide variety of available steroids produced by pharmaceutical firms, the pioneers of male contraceptives had to start from scratch.[2] One of the first WHO
initiatives in coordinating and stimulating the development of male contraceptive drugs, therefore, was a program for the synthesis of hormonal
contraceptive agents: the Steroid Synthesis Program. Although this program
also included the synthesis of steroids for female contraceptives, it can be
considered a major first step in male contraceptive innovation.

In this chapter I explore the ways in which WHO tried to establish an R&D
network outside of traditional pharmaceutical channels. A quick glance at
WHO's initiative to coordinate the synthesis of new hormonal compounds
shows that this task was by no means easy: the synthesis of steroids required
the organization of a worldwide research network involving nineteen laboratories. It can easily be imagined that the coordination of such a decentralized
network required a great deal of extra work, especially when compared to
what might be required to coordinate a research organization consisting of
just one or two large research laboratories. In the first part of this chapter,
therefore, I analyze WHO's efforts to standardize and synchronize the activities of local laboratories so as to achieve translocal laboratory practices.
I then proceed to examine the ways in which WHO tried to become influential
in the field of contraceptive development.

Building an Alternative R&D Network

In 1975 the WHO Special Program for Research and Development and Research Training in Human Reproduction (HRP), working outside the traditional channels of the pharmaceutical industry, initiated a task force for the
development of long-acting contraceptives. This decision was a response to
appeals from population control organizations and several governments in
developing countries who stressed the need for alternative contraceptives that
would last for up to six months (Crabbé et al. 1983). Long-acting contraceptives were expected to provide a better tool for population control programs.
This type of contraceptive is a good example of a "technical delegate": an
artifact that is designed to compensate for perceived deficiencies in its users,
in this case, users' tendencies to "forget" to use contraceptives.[3]

Initially, the development of long-acting contraceptives had been taken up
by industry. In the 1960s the American pharmaceutical company Upjohn had
developed a long-acting injectable contraceptive (medroxy-progesterone acetate, or MDPA). The contraceptive had not been approved by the FDA, however, because of feminist lobbying in the United States. Feminist health advo-

cates took the view that the new contraceptive might undermine women's rights, since injections might easily be abused in certain societies. The "ban the jab" political lobby was an important factor in discouraging industry from further research of this kind (Matlin 1994a: 125). According to Stephen Matlin, a professor of biological chemistry at Warwick University in Coventry and one of the central investigators in the HRP's program for the development of long-acting contraceptives,[4] it was the vacuum created by the absence of a long-acting injectable that brought WHO into the field:

> By the mid 1970s it was clear that many developing countries saw [long-acting injectables] as a very desirable approach to contraception. There was a demand for this product. The only other product available was Schering's oily solution of Norethisterone enanthate, which is only a two-month injectable. It was less advantageous to use in a variety of ways, and so there was perceived to be a need for long-acting methods of contraception that would be suitable for a mass-market in developing countries, easy to apply and with infrequent contacts [with health-care workers]. And the pharmaceutical industry was absolutely unwilling to touch it, because they had seen what had happened to Upjohn and the feminist movement. So that was the gap in the market that WHO was trying to fill. (Crabbé, Diszalusy, and Djerassi 1980: 992)

WHO launched its program with the following statement: "The development of new injectable contraceptives requires that a concerted effort be made to synthesize novel steroid compounds and subject them to thorough biological evaluation. Since such an effort was not being made by international pharmaceutical companies, the World Health Organization as part of its Special Program for Research Development and Research Training in Human Reproduction established a task force to determine whether such a development program could be launched outside the pharmaceutical industry" (WHO/HRP 1981a). The HRP thus transformed and specified the demand for long-acting contraceptives according to two explicit criteria: they should be injectable and they should be steroids.[5]

The next step was to build an R&D organization. WHO did not have laboratories, nor did it build them. Rather, in July 1975 the organization consulted a group of leading steroid chemists with past or current experience in industry.[6] These experts—"boundary elites," to use Hoch's felicitous phrase[7]—provided the HRP with precisely what it needed: a list of approximately 150 hypothetical steroid compounds, and a proposal involving a number of laboratories with the ability to synthesize these new compounds. Geoffrey Waites, manager of the Task Force for the Regulation of Male Fertility, described the birth of what would eventually be called the Chemical Synthesis Program of Steroids, as follows: "This Program was initiated because of the realization that, unless we have drugs developed in the public sector, we would always be at a disadvantage by being left to negotiate with the drug companies for drugs that they are developing" (Waites interview 1994). WHO thus explicitly opted to become an independent R&D organization, particularly independent from industry.

The actual design of the program and its consequent realization exemplifies how many things and people need to be organized when industry does not participate directly in drug development. The first problem was to find laboratories with the necessary expertise and willingness to cooperate in a program for the synthesis of novel steroid compounds. The program got off to a promising start. WHO staff in Geneva did not have to begin from scratch. Pierre Crabbé, named coordinator of the steroid synthesis program, could rely on his informal contacts with the chemists who had designed the program.[8] Crabbé approached the laboratories mentioned at the consultancy meeting in July to determine whether they would be willing to participate in the program. Most importantly, he did not approach these laboratories with empty hands. Crabbé proposed an arrangement by which, "in addition to supplying literature, material, and chemicals," WHO would fund "each laboratory to the extent of $10,000 to $15,000, the sole requirement being that 5-gram quantities of pure steroid would have to be delivered to WHO headquarters. Patent rights would remain with WHO" (Crabbé, Diszalusy, and Djerassi 1980: 992). The proposed arrangement was quite effective: eventually, sixteen laboratories agreed to participate in the program. These laboratories, for the most part chemistry labs and some pharmacy labs, were located in Australia, Brazil, Bulgaria, China, East Germany, Iran, Israel, Korea, Mexico, Nigeria, Poland, Singapore, Spain, Sri Lanka, Thailand, and Yugoslavia. The choice of such a decentralized and multinational R&D network was not a necessary step toward building an effective research organization for the synthesis of contraceptive compounds, but it can be understood in terms of WHO's broader institutional goals.

As much as anything, choosing a large array of decentralized laboratories fit with another aspect of WHO's profile. It certainly would have been possible to utilize only one or two laboratories, with each laboratory receiving a contract for a couple of hundred thousand dollars. But, particularly in the 1970s, when the HRP program was in its infancy, one of the fairly perceived aims of the program was the strengthening of institutions and the distribution of expertise. I suspect that the placement of smaller sums of money ($15,000 per year) into a larger number of laboratories was aimed at expanding interest in the synthesis of antifertility compounds. WHO was thus committed to trying to increase interest in antifertility work in developing countries (Matlin interview 1994).[9]

As Pierre Crabbé has written:

> Excluding efforts by the military establishment,[10] this is probably the first instance in which an international public sector agency has launched successfully a program of this nature, and it is reasonable to ask how economical the program is. In terms of time, the chemical synthesis has taken longer than it would have in the steroid synthesis laboratory of a large pharmaceutical firm in the U.S., Western Europe, or Japan. However, part of that extra time was consumed in institution building and in creating technical capability in developing countries—two features that will be of long-lasting benefit. . . . What is important is that societal goals rather than pure economics have become the driving force. (Crabbé, Diszalusy, and Djerassi 1980: 992)

WHO's steroid synthesis program thus functioned as an important mediator in transferring knowledge, skills, and equipment to Southern and Eastern countries. To realize this goal, there was, however, a price to pay. Crabbé noted the development of a decentralized network of laboratories with locations all over the world was time-consuming. The major challenge was how to manage this worldwide network. It can easily be imagined that the coordination of laboratory work was not an easy job: it required the instruction, standardization, and control of people and laboratory equipment; the logistics to enable a constant flow of material from laboratories all over the world to Geneva, and vice versa; and a coordinated program to centralize and control data collection.

The Creation of Translocal Laboratory Practices

Due to the HRP's policy of decentralizing the synthesis work, standardization came to be of crucial importance. Some aspects of the development of new contraceptives, such as the synthesis of steroid compounds, were spread over various laboratories and locations, whereas other aspects—that is, purification, formulation, and biological evaluation of the compounds—were centralized and synchronized in three central laboratories (see Figure 1).

It is obvious that WHO would only succeed in this ambitious program if it was able to transform the specific practices of local laboratories into a single,

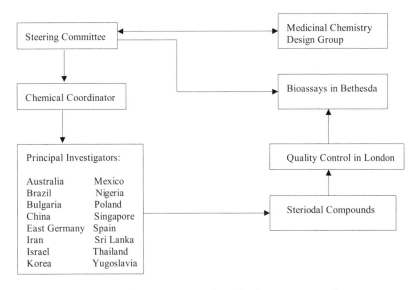

Figure 1. Structure of the WHO Steroid Synthesis Program (Matlin 1991: 5).

translocal research practice. The science studies literature on standardization outlines the problems that arise in creating uniform laboratory practices and emphasizes the tensions that exist between locally specific routines and universal standards imposed by centralized bodies. Recent studies of standardization practices (Bowker 1994; Galison 1987; Fujimura 1987) describe how difficult it is to create uniform research practices. Halffman (2002), drawing on Shapin and Schaffer's distinction between social, material, and literary technologies (1985: 25), suggests that we can understand standardization processes in terms of the control and routinization of people, objects, and texts. First, authority and control can be mainly delegated to people. In this case, standardization may be achieved by training and disciplining people and supervising their actions. Second, control and routinization can be delegated to objects: local laboratory cultures can be transformed into translocal research practices by applying standardized apparatus and materials. Third, standardization may be accomplished by texts: locally specific contingencies of laboratory work are diminished by the use of textual protocols or data report forms which contain highly detailed prescriptions for what needs to be done and what must be avoided. According to Halffman, all three categories are essential in stabilizing research activities among different laboratory settings.

At first glance, the HRP's steroid synthesis program seems to demonstrate all three control technologies. A closer look reveals a pattern of standardization in which literary technologies, and to an even greater extent material technologies, dominated the process. Supervision, assistance, and control of the chemists who participated in the steroid synthesis program were restricted to one or two face-to-face visits by the program's coordinator, Pierre Crabbé.

During the first three years of the program, the coordinator visited most laboratories at least once. The purpose of the site visits was

> to brief the investigators about the precise objectives of the program and its operating details, to offer appropriate scientific information and advice, to become familiar with the local research facilities, and to solve a number of administrative problems. Each center had difficulties, for example, inexperienced personnel, lack of sophisticated equipment and instruments, inclement weather conditions, or frequent power failures. . . . The coordinator acted as a general troubleshooter and was easily available to the various principal investigators. (Crabbé, Diczalusy, and Djerassi 1980: 993)

Direct feedback and control by WHO staff was thus very limited. This suggests that successful standardization does not necessarily require the presence of people who directly supervise and control the research activities. Nor does it require extensive communication among the participating laboratories: during the three years in which the program was carried out, only three meetings took place during which the coordinator and principal investigators discussed how the synthesis work was proceeding. This is not to say that these meetings did not have any impact. Stephen Matlin recalled that the meetings were characterized by a fair amount of peer group pressure: "There is nothing more shaming for a scientist than to go to a meeting to admit defeats" (Matlin interview 1994).

By contrast, literary technologies played a more extensive role in WHO's attempts to reduce the differences among the participating laboratories. The steroid synthesis program consisted of a predesigned procedure which left only a limited degree of freedom to the participating laboratory scientists. The design of the program, developed by the coordinator in consultation with the other leading steroid chemists, was clear and straightforward: each laboratory had to change the configuration of existing steroid compounds by inserting specific chemical compounds (acid chains) at specified locations in the molecule (position 17 of the steroid nucleus). A blueprint of the desired compounds (steroid esters) was made by the HRP team: they compiled a list of 16–20 ester structures which was sent to the participating laboratories. Each laboratory was requested to submit a research proposal "outlining how they intended to synthesize the acid chain to be introduced into the steroid molecule. The proposals were reviewed by the WHO secretariat, an outside referee, and the coordinator" (Crabbé 1980: 993).

These procedures reveal the highly predesigned and practical nature of the steroid synthesis program, in which literary technologies played a crucial role in controlling the actions of the participating laboratories. Texts were central in all the different phases of the steroid synthesis program. The WHO Secretariat in Geneva set up a control system to monitor all movement of material from Geneva to the various chemical laboratories, and from these laboratories to laboratories in London and Bethesda, and eventually back again to Geneva: "Every sample was followed by the WHO Secretariat and by the coordinator (appropriate forms were used at every stage of the program) until the biological results were returned"(Crabbé, Diczalusy, and Djerassi 1980: 993).

Up to that point, the participating scientists were allowed a certain degree of freedom. However, this freedom was restricted by the use of material technologies to standardize a variety of research practices. Most importantly, the WHO team provided the participating laboratories with standardized chemical reagents, small equipment items, and highly purified steroids that were to be used as "mother-compounds"—synthetic progestins (norethisterone and levonorgestrel) for the synthesis of compounds for female contraceptives and testosterone for the synthesis of compounds for male contraceptives. The only freedom allowed the chemists was to vary the length of the acid chain, the nature and degree of unsaturation, and the ring size: "The methods of preparing the side-chains were very much left to the principal investigators, and they were able to consult with Pierre Crabbé if they had a proposal, or if they were getting into difficulties, and they could contact him and ask for suggestions" (Matlin interview 1994; Crabbé, Diczalusy, and Djerassi 1980: 993). The only exception seems to have been that in some cases chemists had to synthesize new acids that were not previously described in the literature. This is the only phase in the synthesis work that was left to the expertise and creativity of the local laboratories. These research activities did not just consist of straightforward chemical work: "Some of these side-chains were very challenging and required very innovative chemistry and a high degree of skill; others were quite mundane, almost off-the-shelf chemicals, that had to be coupled together, but even the coupling methods used to join the side-chains to the steroid were not necessarily straightforward" (Matlin interview 1994).

This aspect of the steroid synthesis program thus shows that for a research program to be effective it is not necessary to lock all research activities into uniformly specified routines. Not all procedures and idiosyncratic practices need to be standardized, because the eventual results (in this case, chemical compounds with data sheets) can be monitored and controlled by textual and later testing procedures. In some phases of research a too strictly uniform approach might even be counterproductive, because it would fail to stimulate scientists to explore alternative routes. The steroid synthesis program thus illustrates that some phases in research can be left to the expertise and skills of individual laboratory scientists and do not require extensive direct control and supervision. Matlin again:

> I think there was very little standardization of chemical procedures be-tween the laboratories. They chose whatever methods and equipment they felt most suitable. Obviously, Crabbé visited each lab at least once so he could give advice, but by and large they were competent chemists who knew how to make compounds and they got on with the job. The stan-dardization was only in the context of the reasonable chemical pro-cedures for doing things, and that chemists by and large used the same kind of tools for investigating the purity of their products. . . . If you take a subject like synthetic organic chemistry and you give this task to people in different parts of the world they will be likely to come up with similar kinds of methods. (Matlin interview 1994; see aslo Crabbé, Diczalusy, and Djerassi 1980)

This suggests that in laboratory work, routine is an important part of the structuring activity, just as it is for medical work (Berg 1992).

This structuring role of routine acitivities does not imply that this part of the steroid synthesis program was left entirely to the dynamics of the local laboratories. This phase of the synthesis program exemplifies that locally specific routines were allowed only if they resulted in the desired end prod-ucts: "The laboratory working methods were [up to] the judgment of each competent scientist. They were asked to produce a product using good chemi-cal techniques. The target was in a sense to complete the appropriate form on which they could say: I have this product and it has this series of constants, of physical properties and has such and such a purity. And we acted as the final check on that" (Matlin interview 1994).

Moreover, data reports showing individual researcher's results were sent twice a year to the Steering Committee of the Task Force on Long-acting Contraceptives, and the participating laboratories had to report on their meth-ods and results at the three principal investigators' meetings that were orga-nized over the five-year period of the program. These reporting procedures had a tremendous impact, not only on standardizing the synthesizing activities but also on the productivity of the local laboratories. According to Matlin, there was a significant rise in the number of compounds submitted to his lab in London shortly before each Steering Committee meeting took place. Moreover, the quality of the compounds also improved due to these monitoring procedures (Matlin interview 1994).

Literary technologies, despite their decentralized mode of operation, thus defined to a great extent the "proper" activities that were expected from the participating laboratories.[11] However, the steroid synthesis program also shows that certain research activities cannot be organized in such a decentralized mode. As mentioned earlier, the compounds synthesized in the sixteen laboratories were eventually sent to three central laboratories for purification, formulation, and biological testing. The compounds were thus subjected to additional, highly centralized testing procedures. In this respect, the quality control lab in London seems to have played the most crucial role in standardizing research activities. To quote Matlin:

> The first real standardization step, I would say, was in my laboratory. Because everything came in whatever state of purity[12] and unless it was a complete disaster we did not go back to the synthetic chemist. . . . By the time things left our laboratory they were all analyzed by standard protocol, and they were all to a common level of purity. The quality control step was the sort of critical bringing together of everything. This had to be done in one laboratory and with an approved kind of protocol and continuity over a long period of time as well. Basically everything passed through my hands in terms of paper work and the analysis of results before it went out. Although over the period of six years I had a number of Ph.D. people working on it individually, I saw all the data they produced and I compiled the reports on that data myself. (Matlin interview 1994)

The chemical laboratory in London thus functioned to standardize the compounds produced by the other laboratories. Eventually, the compounds were sent for animal screening to the National Institute of Child Health and Human Development in Bethesda. These standardization efforts paid off. In 1981 the coordinator could report that the program, over a period of five years, had resulted in the synthesis of 380 steroids: approximately 310 progestin esters for female contraceptives and 70 androgen esters for male contraceptives (WHO/HRP 1981a).[13] A decade later, the WHO Annual Technical Report (1992) described the completion of two major phase III clinical trials on two monthly injectable contraceptives (progestins) for women, and one phase I study of a three-month injectable androgen for men, which, in combination with a long-acting progestagen, would be developed as a male contraceptive (WHO/HRP 1993: 10, 64; Waites interview 1994).[14]

Establishing a Position as Agent in Contraceptive Development

WHO's role in contraceptive R&D was not only restricted to institution build-ing and to the creation of new technical capacity in developing countries. Most importantly, WHO succeeded in redirecting contraceptive R&D to a specific type of product and markets. What actually happened was that an organiza-tion with no previous experience in drug development became active in an area that traditionally had been the exclusive domain of pharmaceutical firms. This created a situation in which tasks previously allocated to industry, such as the synthesis of compounds, the subsequent screening in animal tests, and eventual clinical trials, all shifted from the domain of industry to an inter-national public-sector agency. As a result, WHO occupied a challenging posi-tion. As a newcomer in the field of drug development, the agency had demon-strated that it was possible to do contraceptive R&D outside the control of industry. The WHO program thus illustrates how contraceptive R&D can be undertaken without the cooperation of industry, thereby providing a model that seems to be of particular relevance to the development of the so-called "orphan drugs": drugs for which there exists societal need, but which are not of sufficient interest to the pharmaceutical industry.[15] The steroid synthesis program showed that the pharmaceutical industry was not essential, at least during the early stages of drug development. In the late 1970s WHO gradually became aware of its changing position in the biomedical networks of drug development. Until then, it had been WHO policy to publish all results from its research projects without seeking to obtain patents. Its only concern was that relevant data should be accessible to a wide audience as soon as possible. Following its increased R&D efforts, WHO decided to change this policy. In 1982 the World Health Assembly endorsed a resolution that stated: "It shall be the policy of WHO to obtain patents, inventor's certificates or interests in pat-ents or patentable health technology developed through projects supported by WHO, where such rights and interests are necessary to ensure development of the new technology, and to promote its wide availability in the public interest" (Diczfalusy 1986). By changing its policy on patents, WHO established a much stronger position in its relations with industry. WHO now held the proprietary rights to the new products it developed.[16] Quoting Matlin again:

In the early days the policy was going to be that if WHO identified a new drug it would simply publish all the details so it could become public property. It was only in the early 1980s that they decided that the best way to protect the public interest was for WHO to file a patent. I think it came down to economic realism that if you just publish a drug which is going to be active and anybody can make it, you can no longer license the drug, you cannot control the conditions of manufacturing, and you cannot control the public price. WHO felt that their only way to entice the pharmaceutical company into collaborating would be if they could offer them an exclusive license.[17] (Matlin interview 1994)

WHO successfully applied for patents for three of the four new progesterone compounds, as well as the new androgen compound, that had been developed in the synthesis program (Diczfalusy 1986: 6; WHO/HRP 1986a: 26). In this manner, WHO became a potentially influential drug developer.

That dream could only be realized if WHO was also successful in attracting the interest of industry in the eventual large-scale manufacturing of its new products. It was at that point, however, that the WHO success story seems to have come to an abrupt halt. The final phase of drug development was outside the scope of WHO's capabilities: the organization possessed neither the facilities nor the capital needed for the manufacture and distribution of the products it was developing. To realize this crucial step, WHO would have needed to establish collaborative arrangements with the pharmaceutical firms. So it seemed as if the agency were back where it started: the development of new contraceptives still required the active involvement of industry. However, something crucial had changed. The very fact that WHO held the proprietary rights to potential contraceptives enabled the organization to negotiate with industry about what types of drugs would be manufactured and for which markets they would be produced. If WHO had not initiated contraceptive R&D projects, and if it had not decided subsequently to patent its products, it would never have gained such a position at all. Now, WHO approaches industrial partners for manufacturing and distributing its products and tries to negotiate agreements which guarantee that specific sectors of any potential market, notably the public sector, will be reserved for WHO. The private sector market generally remains within the domain of the pharmaceutical company. In this manner, WHO realizes the "cornerstone of the Program's relationship with industry": "the promotion and protection of the interests of the public sector with special emphasis on the needs of developing countries" (Diczfalusy 1986). By negotiating these agreements with industry, WHO ensures that the drugs will be manufactured and distributed to family planning organizations and other agencies in developing countries. Moreover, it uses its position as patent owner to negotiate a cheaper price for the public sector. These agreements also settle any questions of patents:

> Proprietary rights owned by the parties prior to the agreement remain the property of the originator, but are licensed to the other party. In the case of WHO, this may be on a royalty-bearing basis or the cost of the product to the public sector is reduced in proportion to the anticipated royalties. The company agrees to supply the public sector with the product, but in the event that it is unable, or unwilling to do so, it agrees to transfer the necessary technology and know-how to a mutually agreed third party with appropriate licensing arrangements, so that the public sector requirements can be met. (Diczfalusy 1986)

If WHO is successful in finding a suitable industrial partner, this results in regular mutual visits in which confidential data are exchanged and consultations take place with WHO's toxicology experts. Industrial representatives also attend relevant WHO meetings (Diczfalusy 1986; WHO/HRP 1983: 113). From 1971 to 1986 WHO reached more than thirty formal agreements with twenty-five companies in the United States, Europe, and Japan (Diczfalusy 1986). We thus may conclude that WHO has been quite successful in establishing its position within the contraceptive R&D market.

Nevertheless, WHO retains its dependency on industry. Willem Bergink was program manager of reproductive medicine of Organon in the early 1990s:

> There is a very active group at WHO and there are some researchers who collaborate with WHO in contraceptive research. This is very useful preparatory work. Look, it is very easy for them to do this preparatory work, but then they come up against a wall because they have no pharmaceutical units behind them that back them up. (Bergink interview 1993)

WHO thus still needs the cooperation of industry. The case of male contraceptive compounds, that is, long-acting androgen injections, shows that WHO faced serious problems in finding an industrial partner for the large-scale production of this novelty item. In 1985 WHO first approached two major pharmaceutical companies, Organon and Ortho Pharmaceuticals, both of whom declined the invitation to collaborate in producing the long-acting androgen 20 AET-I (WHO/HRP 1986a: 6). Acknowledging the difficulty of obtaining an industrial co-partner, WHO subsequently explored "alternative means of utilizing the expertise of the pharmaceutical industry in a consultative or advisory manner" (WHO/HRP 1987b: 19). Obviously, this strategy also failed, because in 1988 WHO made a second attempt to find industrial support. This time the organization approached five major companies, but once again in vain. They all declined for various reasons. One reason the pharmaceutical firms were reluctant to engage in the co-production of the long-acting androgen was the insecurity of WHO's patent position for 20 AET-1, which had not yet been legally confirmed at the time it approached the pharmaceutical firms (WHO/HRP 1991: 12–13).

Notwithstanding these disappointing negotiations, WHO was convinced of the attractiveness of its product. At one of the meetings of the steering committee of the Task Force for Male Fertility Regulation, in the fall of 1991, the members concluded: "WHO/NIH is offering any company a good deal in the form of a well established compound, pharmacological data, limited but increasing toxicological data and the capacity to do clinical trials to beyond Phase III. There is little risk and relatively small expense to the company" (WHO/HRP 1991: 26–27). The committee decided to make yet a third attempt to explore industry's interest in a collaborative effort for the development of 20 AET-1 and this time approached nine companies. The organization's persistence paid off: this time, it was more successful, receiving two positive responses, from Schering A.G. and from Jenafarm.[18] However, one of these firms was not deemed to be a suitable partner,[19] and the other firm would agree only tentatively to co-produce 20 AET-1. In this latter case, the firm agreed to support only limited clinical studies in a specific population (Caucasian men), "while reserving the right to withdraw at any time should the results prove unsatisfactory" (WHO/HRP 1992a: 28). The 1992 Annual Technical Report therefore concluded that "negotiations are continuing with industry for the collaborative development of this promising drug."

Conclusions

Reflecting on WHO's role in building an R&D network for contraceptive research outside traditional pharmaceutical industrial channels, we may conclude that WHO has been very successful in creating a protected space in this highly contested field. Since the early 1970s, nontraditional organizations such as WHO have become major actors in the development of contraceptive technologies, adopting activities that were traditionally assigned to industry. This shift from industry to public sector agencies has had a tremendous impact on contraceptive R&D. First, it has resulted in a reallocation of contraceptive research from Northern to Southern countries. We saw how WHO succeeded in creating a worldwide R&D network of chemical laboratories, most of which were located in developing countries. The steroid synthesis program functioned as an important mediator in transferring knowledge, skills, and equipment to laboratories in Southern countries. This reallocation of contraceptive R&D would never have happened if contraceptive R&D had remained within the domain of industry.

Second, the shift of contraceptive R&D from industrial laboratories to the WHO network of university laboratories reoriented contraceptive R&D toward other types of products and users—specifically, toward the development of long-acting injectables for both women and men in Southern countries. This development of contraceptives for women in Third World countries was a continuation of earlier research policies in the field of contraceptive development. For men, these developments heralded a revolutionary breakthrough in contraceptive R&D: previous research had been focused exclusively on women. Patents have played a crucial role in this process of path creation. As Bijker has suggested, patents are of interest in studying the dynamics of science and technology because they tell us something about power relations. Patents fix power relations: once established, they grant owners exclusive access to certain materials (Bijker 1994). This is clearly exemplified by what happened in contraceptive R&D. Until the 1970s industry was the sole entity holding proprietary rights to contraceptive compounds. This put constraints on the actions of newcomers in the field of contraceptive development, since most of the compounds that are of interest in making contraceptives are protected by patents owned by industry.[20] WHO was among the first to break this patent monopoly. The very fact that WHO succeeded in patenting its products enabled it to negotiate with industry about what types of drugs should be manufactured and also about the markets for these drugs.

The question that remains to be answered is whether alternative R&D networks such as those organized by WHO can replace the role of industry in contraceptive R&D. This chapter shows that, notwithstanding their success, newcomers in the contraceptive arena retained their dependency on industry. Most of these new organizations did not have enough venture capital to initiate the large-scale manufacturing of the products they developed. The development of contraceptives, from synthesis to animal and clinical testing and eventual large-scale manufacturing and distribution, requires long-term financial commitments that are beyond the capacities of non-profit organizations such as WHO (Mastroianni, Donaldson, and Kane 1990: 483). Although these new organizations can act as drug developers, they will never be able to replace industry.

Notwithstanding their dependence on industry, alternative R&D networks such as the WHO's steroid synthesis program played an important innovative role in contraceptive technologies, one which may best be understood in terms of its function as a "demonstration network." Demonstration networks are aimed at "demonstrating the feasibility of a new technical option for a collective good" (Laredo 1994: 2–4). The steroid synthesis program fits nicely into this typology of research networks. The demonstration of the feasibility of long-acting contraceptive compounds, particularly those for men, was a crucial goal of the entire endeavor. In Matlin's words:

> I think what is special with male contraceptives is the attitude of people. What has been fundamental has been the lack of any desire of almost everybody to engage in developing male contraceptives. Traditionally male contraception was always regarded as a non-starter by industry. There was a standing prejudice that men would not use a male contraceptive, and even if they did, women would not trust them to use it. WHO is getting quite advanced with their steroids, and I think this will help again to promote the idea of a viable male contraceptive. I don't know whether it is really an ideal drug, that remains to be seen. At least it will extend the public exposure to the idea of practical working methods. (Matlin interview 1994)

This strategic goal of the steroid synthesis program, to capture the interest of industry, seems to have had an impact. Despite industry's reluctance to invest in the technical and cultural novelty of male chemical contraceptives, it seems to have taken its first steps into the R&D of male contraceptives. In 1993 Organon decided to initiate a feasibility study to explore whether it could use some of its steroid products—which do not require long-term animal toxicology testing—to develop a male contraceptive (Kloosterboer interview 1993). WHO has clearly played an important role in clearing the atmosphere for industry to take an interest in R&D for male contraceptives, or to quote Willem Bergink:

> If you ask me why we are doing this [the feasibility study for a male contraceptive], it's simply because we are getting signals from WHO, from the researchers. We see the results, we review the literature. Then you get an idea how it works. They showed that it is scientifically and clinically doable. Well, to make up the economic picture is not so difficult. There will definitely be a market for it. (Bergink interview 1993)

The reallocation of R&D activities from industry to a non-traditional R&D network has had a tremendous impact on innovation in contraceptive R&D: without WHO, it is unlikely that long-acting contraceptives, particularly male hormonal contraceptives, would ever have been included in the contraceptive R&D agenda at all.

The other side of the coin, however, is that the shift of contraceptive development from the pharmaceutical industry to an alternative R&D network coordinated by a public sector agency has slowed down the pace of development of this technology. Although WHO has succeeded in creating a protected space for technological innovation in contraceptive development, the decentralized character of the network required extra time to standardize and synchronize the work of the participating laboratories, located all over the world. To reduce the extra time and work in accomplishing standardization, WHO mainly used texts and materials. We have seen how texts and materials, and not people, frequently traveled all over the world to create translocal research practices. Texts functioned as tools to create translocal research practices because they could be used to specify what work should or should not be done. Texts were also used to monitor all the phases of laboratory work. I have shown how WHO standardized the work of all participating laboratories by the use of protocols and data reports, which forced scientists to follow highly predesigned procedures and which enabled WHO to monitor what had happened to the locally produced compounds. Materials functioned as control technologies because they made scientists work with the same research materials (in this case, standardized chemical reagents and highly purified steroids to be used as "mother-compounds"). Moreover, materials could be subjected to centralized tests (O'Connell 1993). We have seen how the purification and formulation work and the animal testing of the locally produced compounds were centralized in three locations. Despite the fact that WHO has used mainly texts and materials instead of people as tools to accomplish standardization, the synthesis of new hormonal compounds has taken longer than it would have if this were being done in the laboratory of a large pharmaceutical firm. A similar dynamic existed for the clinical testing of hormonal contraceptives for men, which I will describe in the next chapter.

4

The Inaccessible Man: The Quest for
Male Trial Participants and Test Locations

· · · ·

Contraceptives are a very special type of drug. In contrast to other pharmaceuticals, contraceptive drugs are used by healthy and fertile adults rather than by people who suffer from a specific illness. The fact that contraceptives are not curative drugs creates specific constraints for the clinical testing of these pharmaceuticals. Whereas the testing of drugs to cure a specific disease relies on patients who can be assessed in clinical settings, the testing of contraceptives requires "healthy patients" who do not suffer from any particular disease and consequently do not belong to the clientele of a specific clinic. Consequently, contraceptive researchers need to develop specific procedures for gaining access to people who want to participate in clinical trials. When Gregory Pincus, who eventually became one of the "fathers" of the Pill, began testing hormones as contraceptives in 1951, he thus could not rely on the routines of other clinical testing. Moreover, the development of the first oral contraceptive for women took place during a period in which contraceptive research was highly constrained by political and moral taboos against contraception. In the United States, federal and state laws prohibited the dissemination of contraceptive information, including contraceptive devices, until well into the 1960s (Ward 1986: 6). The quest for "healthy patients" was eventually solved by removing the tests to a location outside the continental United States. Pincus found refuge in Puerto Rico, where laws prohibiting contraception did not exist at that time and the family planning movement had a widespread institutional base in the form of birth control programs and clinics (Ramirez de Arellano and Seipp 1983: 21, 29, 49, 94). This provided the required organizational infrastructure within which the testing of the Pill could take place.[1]

Since the 1970s, times have changed. Contraceptives have become part and parcel of our culture and the testing of contraceptives for women can nowadays easily follow the routines of other clinical testing. Clinical trials for new contraceptives for women usually take place in gynecological clinics and family-planning clinics, as happens with other drugs related to reproductive functions.[2] Given the changed attitudes toward contraceptives, one might expect that the enrollment of people for the testing of new contraceptives for men would no longer require any specific procedures. In this chapter I show, however, how the quest for "healthy patients"—if these "patients" are male—still could not follow the routines of other clinical testing. Contraceptive researchers seeking to develop new contraceptives for men could not rely on an established infrastructure specialized in male reproductive functions. Whereas researchers involved in female contraceptives could establish alliances and commitments with gynecological and family planning clinics all over the world, male contraceptive researchers had to start from scratch. As we saw in chapter 2, andrological clinics, those specializing in male reproductive functions, still led a marginal existence, and family planning clinics were still oriented to women as their major clients. In this chapter I will analyze how the male contraceptive research community that emerged in the late 1960s has tried to overcome these constraints. I describe the problems involved in locating male trial participants and then proceed to analyze the work involved in creating alternative infrastructures for clinical testing.

Problems with Access to Male Trial Participants

The clinical testing of hormonal contraceptives for men has a long history. For more than three decades a small research community has been involved in the testing of hormonal compounds for use as male contraceptives. The first publication to report the suppression of sperm production by hormones was published as early as 1939 (Heckel 1939). In the 1950s several small-scale trials were organized, among them one by Gregory Pincus, who eventually became one of the "fathers" of the first hormonal contraceptive pill in women. Pincus tested the same hormonal compound he used for his clinical trials with women (Enovid) on eight male mental patients and reported that it had a "definite sterilizing effect" (Vaughan 1972: 40). This was the first—and the last—time that Pincus included men in his trials. The men's mental disorders (they were classified as psychotics) made it difficult to collect semen to measure the effects of the hormonal compounds on sperm production (McLaughlin 1982: 120). Moreover, the men experienced side effects, such as shrunken testicles (Seaman and Seaman 1978: 84). Other American researchers, most notably Carl G. Heller, an endocrinologist at the University of Oregon Medical School, Warren O. Nelson, the medical director of the newly established Population Council (Zuckerman 1956: 58), and Alvin Paulsen, then at Wayne State University, performed several small-scale clinical trials with chemicals and hormonal compounds. Although most of these trials were designed to determine the effects of these substances on male infertility rather than to assess their contraceptive efficacy, they provided the first accounts of the possible use of these compounds as contraceptives (Briggs and Briggs 1974: 4). In the 1950s and 1960s, male contraceptive research remained limited to a very small number of researchers and clinical trials. A more continuous testing practice emerged in the early 1970s when several academic clinical centers in the United States and Europe initiated the testing of predominantly, but not exclusively, hormonal compounds as contraceptives among small groups of men ranging from four to thirty volunteers (database analysis). In the United States two major research groups were established: at the Department of Medicine of the University of Washington School of Medicine in Seattle, headed by C. Alvin Paulsen, an endocrinologist who had taken a predoctoral fellowship with Carl Heller, who had initiated the hormone trials in the 1950s (Paulsen interview 1994); and at the Harbor–UCLA Medical Center of the University of California at Los Angeles, headed by Ronald Swerdloff. Another important center for male contraceptive research emerged when the Population Council decided to include basic research into male reproductive functions (and, in a later phase, the clinical testing of male contraceptive compounds) on the research agenda of its laboratories in New York. In Europe two research groups were established: one in the U.K. at the Medical Research Council's Centre for Reproductive Biology in Edinburgh, headed by the endocrinologist John Aitken; and the other in Germany, at the Institute of Reproductive Medicine at the University of Münster, headed by Eberhard Nieschlag, who had specialized in internal medicine and endocrinology. As we saw in chapter 2, a major development for male contraceptive research occurred in 1972, when the World Health Organization (WHO) launched a new branch specifically devoted to reproductive research and training, the Human Reproduction Program (HRP), which included a specific task force on male contraceptives.

Male contraceptive research was, however, not restricted to the United States and Europe. Unnoticed for a long time by the Western academic community, China had already established an extensive clinical testing practice with Gossypol, a nonhormonal contraceptive prepared from cotton seed (Gossypol 1979). Although clinical trials with Gossypol had been going on since 1972, the news only reached the Western scientific press in the late 1970s.[3]

In the 1950s, 1960s, and 1970s researchers did not yet have problems gaining access to trial participants, although the type of men selected for the trials indicates the lack of an established infrastructure for testing hormonal compounds among men. As we have seen, Pincus had selected psychotic male patients. Heller and Nelson, and other researchers, recruited male prisoners (Zuckerman 1956: 58; Knight and Callahan 1989: 290). This was not an exceptional practice: in both the United States and Europe, prisoners were used as test subjects for the testing of all drugs until the 1980s. Other researchers tested hormonal compounds on their own patients. The practice of enrolling patients as trial participants continued well into the late 1980s. This was not only due to problems in gaining access to healthy men, but was also used as a strategy to obtain FDA approval for testing. Dr. Rosemary Thau, the manager of the Population Council, described how the choice of trial subjects was a result of negotiations with the FDA: "We are now testing the LHRH vaccine in men with prostate cancer in our clinic in Texas. The FDA, when we discussed it with them, advised fifty-fifty whether we should start with normal men or in cancer patients. At first they could not make up their mind, and then a month later they told us to start with the cancer patients" (Thau interview 1993).

Using patients as test subjects facilitated approval for clinical testing because researchers were allowed to perform toxicology tests on patients as part of their treatment for a specific disease. Such tests were not allowed among healthy people. Male reproductive researchers constructed a dual drug profile for hormonal compounds: the same compounds were tested both as contraceptives and as therapies for specific illnesses, which not only facilitated the process of gaining approval for testing but also functioned to attract the interest of pharmaceutical firms. Pharmaceutical companies that did not directly support research on male contraceptives seemed much more willing to collaborate on R&D projects aimed at the development of clinical applications, such as the treatment of hypogonadism and, especially, the treatment of cancer (WHO/HRP 1989: 38). Both WHO and the Population Council have used patients with a deficiency in androgen metabolism, or with prostate cancer, in trials of hormonal contraceptive compounds (WHO/HRP 1993: 10). Other researchers have selected osteoporosis patients to test hormones as contraceptives (Briggs and Briggs 1974: 586). Since the 1970s, however, most clinical trials have been performed on healthy men. This shift in the selection of men as trial participants is reflected in the rhetoric of the publications from these trials. In their descriptions of trial participants, researchers emphasize the contraceptive compounds have been tested on "healthy volunteers," "normal male volunteers," "normal men," or "young, healthy men" (Swerdloff 1985; Tom et al. 1992; Behre et al. 1992).

These early clinical trials included only a very limited number of trial participants, ranging from three to eighteen men per trial, with two exceptional cases of trials that included 46 and 116 men.[4] These so-called "phase I" trials, in which the biological activity, safety, and optimum dosages of drugs are tested on a small number of people, did not put too much constraint on gaining access to trial participants; men were typically recruited from among medical students and staff via the personal contacts of researchers and clinicians. Although researchers largely succeeded in recruiting the small numbers of men required, the lack of an adequate infrastructure nevertheless had a great impact on the clinical testing of male contraceptives. In "Birth Control after 1984," published in *Science* in 1970, Carl Djerassi, one of the pioneers in hormonal contraceptive research for women, suggested that the lack of an infrastructure for the testing of male contraceptives severely constrained progress in male contraceptive research:

> At present there appear to be available, in the entire United States, facilities for evaluating two drugs at a time. The complications would even be greater in phase II and phase III clinical studies. Women can easily be assembled for clinical studies through their association with Planned Parenthood clinics and individual obstetricians or gynecologists; there exists no simple mechanism for assembling similar groups of males for clinical experimentation. The prisons and armed forces are the only convenient sources, and results would have to be based largely on examination of masturbation sperm samples rather than on an evaluation of fertility control in an average population. (Djerassi 1970: 948)

Similar concerns were voiced by other researchers involved in clinical trials, as exemplified by Fred Wu, an endocrinologist who worked at the Medical Research Council's Reproductive Biology Unit in Edinburgh in the 1980s and later moved to the Department of Medicine at the University of Manchester:

> Recruitment for male contraceptive studies is actually very difficult. First of all, you want healthy young men, and these people usually don't go to see their doctor. Therefore you have to recruit to the general population, from the general community as opposed from the family-planning clin-

ics. Certainly in this country those people who go to family-planning clinics are usually female, and the men who go have already made up their mind to have vasectomy, and also very few husbands go along to the ante-natal clinic in the maternity hospital. So we initially tried recruitment in these places, thinking that these are the contact points for reproducing couples. We actually had very little success, and also relying on colleagues in hospital to try and recruit again was not very successful. (Wu interview 1994)

Due to this lack of infrastructure to gain access to volunteers, clinical testing remained for a long time restricted to a limited number of men, which hampered progress in male contraceptive research in the 1970s and 1980s. As Geoffrey Waites, the manager of the WHO Male Task Force from 1972 to 1995, put it: "The reason the field hasn't progressed as well since the 1970s was that most of the studies were done on ten to twenty men which gave us a little bit of an answer, but not a definite one" (Waites interview 1994).

The News Media as a Tool for Gaining
Access to Male Trial Participants

In the late 1980s recruitment of trial participants became a serious problem when clinicians began to organize phase II testing, which required many more male subjects than phase I testing. Phase II testing, designed to evaluate the efficacy and adverse effects of drugs, requires several hundred people per trial. Before moving to phase II trials, the toxicology and teratology of the compounds have to be tested in animals. Finally, phase III trials aim to test the drugs on even greater numbers of participants, in order to monitor rare side effects (Mintzes 1991). Clinicians involved in these trials first tried to recruit men through their contacts with gynecologists, in the hope that the doctors might be willing to cooperate by inviting the male partners of their female patients to participate in the clinical testing of the new contraceptive. For gynecologists, this could be a way to help women who complained of problems with existing contraceptives. However, the contacts with gynecologists turned out to be highly problematic. Clinicians who tried to enroll men through gynecological/obstetrical departments met with severe resistance from gynecologists. To quote T. Farley, a statistician involved in one of the first large-scale clinical trials organized by WHO in 1990:

For those investigators that worked and were used to working in obstetrics and gynecology departments, trying to recruit the couples for this study was quite difficult. They initially tried through those standard obstetrics and gynecology networks, but did not have much success, recruiting through those channels. There could be various reasons for this suspicion or mistrust by the GP's or the gynecologists. Obviously, they thought that this is not a reliable method, and she needs a reliable method and she shouldn't play around with these experimental methods. . . . The woman comes to the gynecologist wanting a review or a new contraceptive supply and of course the knee-jerk reaction is to give that to her, not to question: "By the way, what does your husband do, doesn't your husband think about giving you a rest?" It's just not the standard question in his repertoire, so it's not surprising in a way that that sort of channel doesn't work. (Farley interview 1994).

Fred Wu, who in the late 1980s and early 1990s was in charge of the center that participated in the multicenter clinical trials organized by WHO, had a similar experience: "Generally, they [gynecologists] have somewhat a protective attitude toward family planning. I think that they feel that this is the domain of obstetrics and gynecology, involved primarily with the regulation of the female reproductive function, and we are to some extent messing around with their field" (Wu interview 1994).

What seemed to be the problem was that the testing of male contraceptives interfered with the demarcation of boundaries between medical specialties. Gynecologists considered the development of contraceptives as within their domain of expertise. As all work on contraceptives prior to the 1970s was restricted to women, the gynecological profession had not come into competition with other medical specialties. This claim of authority was challenged when other clinicians took up the testing of male contraceptives. The above quotations illustrate the reluctant and defensive attitude of gynecologists: they responded to the requests of their colleagues by claiming contraception as their own exclusive domain. The organization of clinical trials for male contraceptives was considered threatening to their profession because it might possibly compete with their own clientele. If the contraceptive problems of women visiting the gynecological clinic could be solved by referring their male partners to male contraceptive trials, problems belonging to the domain of gynecology would be transferred to another specialty. This implied that the gynecologists might lose a part of their clientele.

Clinicians involved in male contraceptive testing thus had to find other ways to gain access to male trial participants. When gynecologists refused to cooperate, the clinicians tried to enroll men through other medical contacts.

The most likely specialty to approach was urology. Since urologists have a partly male clientele, they might, it was thought, be more willing to cooperate in the organization of clinical trials. However, this profession was also reluctant to assist in the recruitment of trial participants. Although urologists are partly specialized in the male body, those who are interested in reproduction focus mainly on infertility problems rather than on fertility control (Waites interview 1994; Weber interview 1993). Even andrology, the medical profession that specializes in male reproductive functions, could not solve the problem of finding volunteers for male contraceptive trials. Like urologists, most andrologists are mainly interested in infertility rather than fertility control (Waites interview 1994; Weber interview 1993). Scientists and clinicians working on male contraceptives thus faced a hostile medical community. The only practicioners willing to cooperate were general practitioners: they agreed to put up posters in their waiting rooms to attract men. This strategy was more successful; however, general practitioners have only been able to recruit small numbers of men.

Male contraceptive researchers, therefore, had to explore alternative routes to find participants for their trials. They decided to try their luck by going outside medical channels to the media: radio, television, and newspapers (Wu interview 1994; Farley interview 1994). This strategy turned out to be very successful. To quote Geoffrey Waites, the manager of the Male Task Force involved in the organization of two large-scale trials organized in the late 1980s and early 1990s by WHO: "In Finland and Australia, when the media was involved and a public statement was made by the investigator himself, both centers fulfilled their quota of thirty couples enrolled within one to two months after it, when they had spent nearly a year trying to get even one couple through their medical contacts" (Waites interview 1994).

The testing of male contraceptives thus depended largely on the creation of alliances with the news media. For most clinicians, "going public" was a completely new role. Alvin Paulsen, one of the pioneers in male contraceptive research, recalled his first contacts with the media: "I never used to call up the television and say 'Hey I'm working on such and such.' . . . You don't hold press conferences every day, so it was somewhat foreign to me to go public. . . . But they [the media] have been very useful" (Paulsen interview 1994).

Approaching the media to recruit men was obviously so delicate that it had to take place outside Paulsen's medical center in Seattle; Paulsen asked his secretary to contact the media using her private telephone phone number and to answer any phone calls at home. In the U.K., male contraceptive researchers had similar experiences. As Fred Wu recalled: "The media are very important. I don't like doing it though, because I didn't think I'm trained to deal with the media, but I'm forced to do it, because it's the only way I can get the recruitment" (Wu interview 1994).

Although scientists did not consider themselves experts in approaching the media, British scientists were nevertheless very successful in attracting media attention. In July 1993 Fred Wu and his colleagues at the public relations department of the University of Manchester drafted a press release and organized a special press conference. The press bulletin described the impending trial as "the most extensive trial of the 'male pill' ever carried out in the U.K." These attempts to interest the media were very successful. The press bulletin and the press briefing created a hype in the British newspapers. Within two days, more than forty news articles were published, in both the local and national press. The press coverage resulted in nearly 350 inquiries, whereas only thirty men were needed for the test. The Manchester clinicians thus demonstrated that they did not need their colleagues in the clinic: alliances with the news media gave them their long-sought access to participants for their trials. Despite their reluctance to go public, contact with the media has become part of the work of scientists in the field of male contraceptives. Since the late 1980s the enrollment of male trial participants through news media channels has become routine practice.

Creating New Infrastructures for Clinical Testing

Although the news media were a very useful tool for gaining access to trial participants, they were insufficient to recruit the large numbers of men required for phase II clinical testing. When WHO took up large-scale phase II testing, the number of men needed for these trials was estimated at more than four hundred: "Yes, the numbers are important when you want to count pregnancies that have occurred because the method has failed. And you can't get an answer out of a study involving ten men. So we have to advise statisticians right at the beginning who tell us, judging on the significance of the difference in the outcome, how many you need to enroll to get the answer you're looking for. And they came out with a figure of 450 or so couples" (Waites interview 1994).

The number of men to be reached was even much larger because of the high dropout rate during the selection procedure. Most researchers found that they had to perform one hundred interviews to create a test group of twenty men (Behre et al. 1992; Nieschlag, Lerch, and Nieschlag 1994: 42). This implied that one research group had to contact more than two thousand men to make a large enough test population, and this problem could not be solved by ads in the news media.

In the 1970s there was only one country in which the recruitment of men for clinical trials did not cause any problems: China. In "China Invents Male Birth Control Pill," published in the *American Journal of Chinese Medicine* in 1980, the authors reported that "China, famed for its historical inventions," had tested a contraceptive agent (Gossypol) among ten thousand men (Wen 1980: 195). Chinese researchers received cooperation from directories of industrial firms and local officials of the Communist Party. In the factories, men were addressed by megaphone to remind them to attend the clinics for the Gossypol trial. Consequently, factory workers made up the majority of trial participants, the rest consisting of peasants, Communist party cadres, and medical staff (Wen 1980: 197). The success of this recruitment strategy must be understood in the context of the authoritarian culture in China and its strict population control policy, whereby couples are allowed to have only one child.[5] Two decades later, Western researchers could take advantage of this efficient recruitment of trial participants in China, as exemplified by Geoffrey Waites's experiences with the recruitment of trial participants for the first WHO phase II trial by the participating center in China: "There was often a community feeling that the men should get together and volunteer, and so they got their cohorts of thirty in the space of a day or two. . . . So the outcome of all of our trials, not only for men but for women as well, is that the recruitment phase goes much more quickly and effectively in China. The way they do it has more to do with community recruitment and people responding in a community rather than asking individuals" (Waites interview 1994).

The historical scope of the problems with recruitment of men for contraceptive clinical trials in the Western industrialized world has been clearly articulated by Alvin Paulsen: "When you think about the fact, it's been over two hundred years since a male method was made available to the public— namely the condom, actually the rubber condom. When they learned how to vulcanize rubber, then they could mass produce condoms and that's when it was introduced to the public. But they didn't have any clinical trials on how effective it was or anything like that" (Paulsen interview 1994).

Given the almost complete absence of any institutionalized practice for the testing of contraceptives for men, male contraceptive researchers had to start from scratch: they had to build the infrastructures themselves. This was required not only to gain access to trial participants but also because the male contraceptive research community was too small to provide an adequate number of experts to perform trials with several hundred people. The only strategy available to researchers in the Western world was to join forces. If one institution could not provide the required number of trial participants and experts, a collaboration of several institutes might do the job. This strategy, simple though it may sound, was not easy to implement, because contraceptive researchers also faced the constraint of working in an area in which pharmaceutical firms do not play the role they usually do in drug development. Whereas pharmaceutical firms often control virtually all premarketing drug testing, including clinical trials (Abrahams 1994: 505), male contraceptive testing lacks the support of this key actor in drug development.

At that point in history, WHO became a crucial resource. As had happened in the phase of synthesizing male contraceptive compounds, WHO chose to fill the vacuum created by the absence of the pharmaceutical industry. In contrast to the individual research groups, in the late 1980s WHO had the organizational capacity and expertise to initiate and coordinate large-scale phase II testing. In the late 1970s, Alvin Paulsen, the first chairman of the steering committee of WHO's Male Task Force, and at that time a clinical investigator involved in the Contraceptive Development Branch of the National Institutes of Health in the United States, was asked to establish a network of research centers. As Paulsen recalled of this period:

> There wasn't a network of academic centers throughout the world dealing with the male. . . . And it was my duty to encourage and establish clinical trials. . . . Well then, I went around and visited Toronto, Seoul, South Korea, Hong Kong. We talked to people in Vancouver, B.C., and we talked to people in Copenhagen. We visited somebody in Nijmegen [The Netherlands] but they were not too interested. We approached centers who were working on male reproduction, not necessarily contraception, and tried to encourage them to participate in clinical trials. (Paulsen interview 1994)

To strengthen their commitment, after several years of cooperation some academic centers could receive the status of "WHO Collaborating Center for the Research of Human Reproduction" (Behre et al. 1992; Nieschlag, Lerch, and Nieschlag 1994: 37). Within the framework of such collaboration, researchers at the center participated in WHO/HRP activities such as the preparation of WHO reports, membership on committees, and the development and performance of research projects funded by, and on behalf of, WHO (Nieschlag, Lerch, and Nieschlag 1994). Eberhard Nieschlag, the director of the WHO Collaborating Center in Münster, Germany, and chair of the steering committee of the Male Task Force in the mid-1990s, described the importance of the WHO collaborating centers: "Clinical trials are extremely difficult. They are especially difficult in developing countries. And to have built up this network of centers in developing and developed countries as well is very important, because thereby you don't have to recruit companies and volunteers who may not be really interested but you have your long-standing relations" (Nieschlag interview 1995).

The Male Task Force was not the first to initiate multicenter clinical trials. The policy to establish collaborative centers was initiated by Dr. David Kessler, the first director of the Human Reproduction Program in the period between 1971 and 1983, to realize a central theme of WHO's agenda: the extension and strengthening of its networks for research and clinical testing with investigators in Southern countries.[6] Moreover, WHO's incentive to initiate multicenter trials was related to an awareness in the medical community that clinical testing should account for differences in physiological reactions and for the acceptability of contraceptives in different cultures.[7] What was new to the male contraceptive multicenter trial was that the network provided access to a sufficient number of men. To quote Christina Wang, an endocrinologist at the Division of Endocrinology and Metabolism and Reproductive Biology, Cedars-Sinai Medical Center in Los Angeles, and chairman of the steering committee of the Male Task Force in the early 1990s: "You always do multicenter trials because if it is done in one center you only have a certain number of subjects. In multicenter studies you are testing different populations from different social, economic or whatever backgrounds to know whether they are going to respond to the same matter equally, how it is acceptable, but also you need to do that to accumulate enough numbers" (Wang interview 1993).

Although Paulsen was successful in establishing an infrastructure for large-scale testing, it took yet another decade before WHO began to organize these trials. The major reason for this delay was ethical concerns within WHO. Efficacy trials of contraceptives imply a risk of pregnancy in the event the contraceptives fail. This is a problem for the testing of female contraceptives as well, and as such, not a new constraint on the clinical testing of contraceptives. A new aspect in the efficacy trials for male contraceptives was that this risk did not concern the bodies on which the contraceptives were tested. Although men were taking the contraceptives, women were at risk of pregnancy in case of contraceptive failure. Alvin Paulsen, who eventually succeeded in getting permission from WHO to approach academic centers all over the world to participate in the first large-scale trial, described the reluctance within WHO as follows: "It took us almost ten years to convince WHO to let us do this trial because of pregnancies: the woman is at risk, not the man. Well, they don't seem to understand that sometimes an unplanned pregnancy is very disturbing to the man. But it took us years to convince them. . . . If there's a female method they say they know the risk and the benefit ratio, and if it's a male method they say there is no risk to the male. But I'm saying that they are wrong. There is a risk to the male. . . . Well, we kept hammering at them" (Paulsen interview 1994).

The ethical concerns of the risk of pregnancy that constrained the initiation of male contraceptive efficacy trials had a highly political angle. By performing these trials, WHO not only had to take responsibility for diminishing the risks of pregnancy. The decision to initiate efficacy trials also implied that WHO would have to take responsibility for medical services to determine the un- wanted pregnancies of women whose partners participated in the trial in case the contraceptive failed. Since abortion has been, and still is, a highly con- tested issue, WHO encountered strong political resistance, most importantly among its member states. Ever since WHO had included contraceptive R&D on its agenda, several member states had systematically refused to give financial support to these activities. The United States, for example, had not figured among the donors of the WHO/HRP program until the Clinton administration finally challenged these anti-abortion policies in the late 1980s (Kammen 2000). WHO's reluctance to initiate efficacy trials can thus be understood in the context of abortion politics that constrained the financial support of con- traceptive research. Moreover, WHO also expected to meet with resistance from within the medical community, as exemplified by the experiences of the manager of the Male Task Force, Geoffrey Waites:

Some of it [the reluctant attitude and resistance of clinical centers to cooperate in the first large-scale efficacy trial] was related to attitudes to assisted abortion because in the protocol it says the partners are at risk of pregnancy. We think the risk is low, but nevertheless in the event of unwanted pregnancy, the couple will be advised on the outcome. It was left open whether they would continue with the pregnancy or not. If they elected to have an abortion, then it was implicit that the medical re- sources of the center would help them with that and all the medical treatment surrounding it. In certain national governments that was not acceptable, even though for the clinicians it would have been acceptable. And in certain countries that was unacceptable totally, both for gov- ernments and clinicians. I don't suppose that is different from female methods where there is a risk of pregnancy too. But the extra factor was that the method wasn't directly benefiting women, it was indirectly benefiting women through male acceptance. (Waites interview 1994)

WHO has an extensive procedure within the organization to approve clinical testing. First, a protocol for clinical testing is designed, which is usually done by the steering committee of the Task Force that wants to initiate the trials. This protocol has to go through the WHO toxicology panel to approve the drug that will be used in the trials. Then it has to be approved by the WHO Scientific Review Group, which evaluates the informed consent procedures. And then it goes through a third level of scrutiny called the Secretariat Committee for the Research of Human Subjects. Finally, there is a group of clinical staff members who take the advice of other WHO officials to evaluate whether the clinical trial meets WHO's standards for the conduct of clinical trials. Once the protocol has been approved by all these groups, the Task Force begins to enroll academic centers that are part of the network of collaborating centers. The clinical trial is then subjected to an external procedure, which may imply the approval of the minister of health of the government of the participating academic center, so the protocol often goes to a governmental office, which may look at it. If these procedures are passed, WHO provides the funding and sends the drug, which, if the drug is not yet in clinical use, also has to be approved by the national drug regulation authority (Waites interview 1994). These procedures can become very time-consuming, particularly when some of these groups disagree with specific aims or procedures of the clinical trial, as happened in the case of the protocol for the first multicenter clinical trials for male hormonal contraceptives, when ethical concerns were raised. The first multicenter trial therefore did not begin until the late 1980s, almost ten years after Paulsen had first contacted the academic clinical centers.

The first WHO multicenter trial consisted of a combined effort of ten clinical centers in seven countries in Asia, Australia, Europe, and the United States, and included 271 men. This trial was not only exceptional due to the number of trial participants, but also because it was the first trial in which the contraceptive efficacy of hormonal compounds was assessed on the basis of the incidence of pregnancy, which, as I described above, was initially considered unethical by WHO. In previous trials, contraceptive activity had been evaluated by sperm counts. The second WHO large-scale trial (which I will describe in chapter 9), a collaboration of fifteen centers in nine countries, included 399 men and was designed to redefine the criteria for assessing the efficacy of contraceptive compounds. The basic organizing principle for the multicenter clinical trials was that all centers should use the protocols designed by the steering committee of the Male Task Force, including the selection criteria for trial participants, instructions for informed consent procedures, and procedures for taking samples of semen and blood and giving injections (the administration mode used in these trials) (Farley interview 1994). To standardize data collection, the Male Task Force also designed the specific forms the principal investigator in each center had to work with, including forms for entry into the study, informed consent procedure, the identification of the trial participant, physical examination of the trial participant and the female partner, and semen and blood analysis (Waites interview 1994). To reduce differences in local clinical practice, WHO also provided training in the design of clinical trials, particularly to centers in Southern countries (Farley interview 1994).

The manual for semen analysis, first published in 1980, including a standard protocol, was initially introduced for Southern countries (Waites interview 1994). Due to the lack of experts in male reproduction in most Southern countries, semen analysis, which consisted of sperm counts to assess the suppression of sperm production by the contraceptive on trial, was often delegated to hematology laboratories: "When you talk to clinicians, they say we couldn't get a semen analysis properly assessed. It went to the hematology department, where people counted red cells. They did it on their afternoons off—they weren't really interested" (Waites interview 1994).

The manual, however, also fulfilled a role among clinicians in developed countries. When the manual was first published, it was ordered by many hospitals in Europe and North America (Waites interview 1994; Wang interview 1993). The manual thus functioned not only as a tool to standardize the local practices of centers participating in the multicenter trials, but was also instrumental in standardizing semen analyses in clinical practices unrelated to contraceptive trials. Members of the Male Task Force consider the production of the manual one of the task force's major achievements. Christina Wang:

In 1980 WHO published a standard manual of how to examine a man's semen, his ejaculate, and it was the first attempt to standardize semen analysis, which was wild before, everybody could do whatever he wanted, and since then this manual has gained enormous popularity. The second edition appeared in 1987, and the third in 1992 and this is one of the main contributions of the Male Task Force, that we brought the attention to people working in the field that you need a common method so that semen analysis of one lab can be compared to another lab, and obviously that was critical for the multicenter studies WHO does, or the clinical studies we have been doing. (Wang interview 1993; WHO/HRP 1992c)

The organization of multicenter clinical trials has not remained restricted to WHO. In the United States there exists the so-called "South to South network," a Rockefeller Foundation–funded research network that is mainly composed of Southern countries: Brazil, India, China, the Dominican Republic, and some African countries. This network has performed clinical trials on Gossypol. The Population Council has also established a network of clinical centers, with the prominent ones in Chile, the United States, Finland, Australia, and Japan (Thau interview 1993). Finally, in Europe, the Reproductive Biology Center in Edinburgh has established a collaboration with clinical centers in South Africa, Hong Kong, and Shanghai. The strategy to organize multicenter clinical trials has thus developed into an important tool for tackling the problems of securing adequate test locations and sufficient access to trial participants.

Conclusions

We can conclude that the organization of clinical trials for the testing of hormonal contraceptives for men required a great deal of extra work, compared to that required for the testing of other drugs. First, male contraceptive researchers had to put great effort into gaining access to male volunteers. The researchers involved in the trials of contraceptives for men could not easily follow the routines of other clinical testing. The quest for "healthy patients" could only be solved by approaching institutions outside the medical world, as had happened with the testing of the first hormonal contraceptives for women. There is, however, a difference between the testing of male and female contraceptives. Whereas the major constraint on the testing of hormonal contraceptives for women can be ascribed to political and moral taboos in the culture at large, the testing of male contraceptives was constrained by routine practices characteristic of the culture of the medical community itself. Attempts to find men for clinical trials did not succeed because male contraceptive research threatened to disrupt the boundaries between medical specialties, as was illustrated by the gynecologists' refusal to cooperate in the testing. Moreover, no profession was really interested in controlling the fertility of male subjects. Even family planning clinics, the escape route successfully used by Pincus in the testing of the first hormonal contraceptives for women, could not offer any help because their clientele was almost entirely female.[8] Faced with resistance and disinterest within the medical community, researchers had to explore alternative routes to enroll men: they had to engage in alliances with the news media to be able to begin testing hormonal compounds.

Second, male contraceptive researchers could not easily follow the routines of other testing because there was no available infrastructure for the organization of large-scale clinical trials in terms of laboratories, clinics, and the relevant expertise. This implied that male contraceptive researchers had to build the required infrastructure themselves, which was eventually realized in collaboration with public-sector agencies, most notably WHO. As with the synthesis of hormonal compounds, the advocates of new contraceptives for men had to create an alternative sociotechnical network for the clinical testing of the new technology in order to make up for the limited organizational capacity of the small male contraceptive research community and the lack of support from the pharmaceutical industry. Evaluating the efforts of this alternative network, we can conclude that the proponents of new contraceptives for men have been successful in overcoming the constraints and resistance they encountered in the clinical testing of male contraceptives. In the end, they succeeded in building the infrastructure required for the large-scale clinical testing of these contraceptives. The other side of the coin, however, is that the creation of alternative sociotechnical networks for clinical testing had a negative impact on the pace of the development of the new technology. It was only after two decades of scattered small-scale clinical testing that the advocates of male contraceptives eventually succeeded in establishing the required infrastructure for systematic large-scale clinical trials. This long period of testing is in sharp contrast to the testing of contraceptives for women, which usually required a period of approximately fifteen years, including phase III clinical trials and registration, activities which have not yet been initiated for male contraceptive testing.[9] We can thus conclude that the lack of the required infrastructure for clinical testing has seriously delayed the development of male contraceptives. To make things even more complicated, clinicians also faced other problems in the clinical testing of the new technology, which will be the subject of the next chapter.

5

The Co-construction of Technologies and Risks

· · · ·

The image of contraceptives as "drugs for healthy people" has made safety issues a major concern for all the actors involved in contraceptive development. A major aspect of the clinical testing of contraceptives, therefore, consists of trying to reduce the side-effects of the contraceptive on trial. As constructivist scholars have suggested, side-effects are not intrinsic properties of contraceptive compounds that are unambiguously revealed during testing. This is not to deny that compounds may exert specific effects on physiological functions. There is, however, more to say about the processes by which certain compounds come to be defined as carrying specific health risks. First, experiments generate an infinite number of signals. A major part of the work that goes into testing therefore consists of simplifying these signals to create order in the complexity of data. During testing, and clinical trials are one specific type of testing, scientists make explicit or implicit choices of what should be foregrounded and what should be considered as less important in assessing health risks (Law 1988; Latour 1987). Second, scientists decide what signals are relevant to include as indicators of potential health risks. One of the arguments in this chapter is that this choice is not necessarily related to claims about linkages between the artifact and side-effects established in previous contraceptive clinical trials, but draws on claims that are made in contexts unrelated to the compound on trial. Third, processes in which observations of adverse effects are transformed into claims of health risks are ultimately social processes in which scientists and other actors negotiate to reach consensus. Evelleen Richards, for example, has described how the assessment of therapeutic treatments is shaped by the professional interests of the assessors and by wider social concerns, that is, by consumer choice and market forces (Richards 1988). John Abrahams has analyzed the role of pharmaceutical companies in assessments of drug safety and concludes that the commercial interests of these firms profoundly shape the assessment of health risks (Abrahams 1994; Abrahams and Sheppard 1999). Steve Shapin has described the constitution of risks in terms of the interaction between science and politics. He has shown how the tacit rhetorical constructions of the social order help constitute risk, trust, and knowledge, and how this knowledge helps in turn to shape social order (Shapin 1994). In sum, there is broad agreement that risks are sociotechnical and political constructs.

This chapter tries to unravel how those involved in the clinical testing of hormonal contraceptives for men have constructed the health risks of the technology-in-the-making. As we saw in the previous chapter, the clinical testing of hormonal contraceptives for men has a long history. Whereas clinical testing of contraceptives for women usually takes place over a period of some fifteen years, clinical trials for male contraceptives have been conducted for more than three decades and have yet to result in a final product. This extensive testing period makes it possible to study in detail how specific compounds come to be considered as risky or not. At first glance, one would be inclined to think that extensive testing should result in a reduction of the complexity of signals and eventually lead to a stabilization of claims about the relationship between the compounds and their supposed side-effects. If testing covers a long period of time, chances increase that the actors involved in the assessment of health risks will eventually reach consensus about the safety of the drug. In this chapter, I will argue that lengthy clinical testing did not necessarily result in closure, but may instead have led to an increasing complexity and multiplication of claims about the linkages between side-effects and the artifact on trial. Based on an analysis of reports of clinical trials of contraceptives for men in the period from 1958 to 1996, this chapter will show how the number of indicators to assess the health risks of contraceptive compounds, and the health risks associated with these compounds, gradually increased. I continue by describing the ways in which scientists tried to cope with risk factors. Finally, I will discuss the factors that have contributed to a destabilization of the results of the clinical testing.

What Is at Risk?

Clinical Trials in the 1950s and 1970s

A report on one of the first clinical trials specifically designed to assess the effects of hormonal compounds on the reproductive functions of men appeared in the *Annals of the New York Academy of Science* in 1958. A group of four American endocrinologists at the University of Oregon Medical School and the Rockefeller Institute for Medical Research in New York, including Carl G. Heller, one of the pioneers in research on hormones and male reproduction, and Warren O. Nelson, medical director of the recently established Population Council (Zuckerman 1956: 58), reported the results of a clinical trial among twenty "healthy adult males," all prisoners at the Oregon State Penitentiary, in which three types of steroids were tested: two testosterone preparations and one progesterone compound (Enovid, developed by Gregory Pincus as an oral contraceptive for women). Although this trial was designed to determine the effects of the new steroids because of their expected "widespread clinical use," rather than to assess their contraceptive efficacy, the paper has become one of the referential texts in reviews of male contraceptive research (Briggs and Briggs 1974: 4).[1] The paper included a short list of indicators to assess the effects of the compounds on reproductive functions in men. In this early trial, scientists monitored ten topics: mean sperm count, testicular size, body weight, changes in breasts (gynecomastia), sexual desire (libido), ability for erections and the production of seminal fluid (potency), hormone excretion patterns, sperm motility, testicular morphology, and emotional well-being. Although the trial was not presented as an experiment to test the contraceptive effects of the compounds, the results section of the paper nevertheless opened with a description of the hormonal effects on sperm production, which was reported as reduction to zero sperm (Heller et al. 1958: 650). The report also mentioned that all subjects had lost their sexual desire and had difficulties with erections and the production of seminal fluid. A reference to this text in 1989 ironically concluded that "loss of libido and the inability to attain erection would obviously constitute an effective birth control measure" (Knight and Callahan 1989: 289). Since then, the interference of hormones with sexual function has become a dominant concern in the clinical testing of hormonal compounds as contraceptives (Reddy and Roo 1972; Briggs and Briggs 1974; Skoglund and Paulson 1973).

The results of the first trial in which hormonal compounds were tested explicitly for contraceptive purposes were published in *Contraception* in 1972 (Reddy and Roo 1972). Reports of subsequent, small-scale trials appeared in the same journal in 1973, and in *Nature* and the *International Planned Parenthood Federation Medical Bulletin* in 1977.[2] The results of a trial that included the testing of two testosterone compounds as contraceptives among larger numbers of men (eighty-eight subjects instead of the usual number of between five and fifty subjects, as was the case in the previous trials) were published in 1976 (Spilman, Kirton, and Kirton 1976: 197–209). This trial was performed by C. Alvin Paulsen, who had initiated the hormone trials in the 1950s. In this particular trial, he collaborated with John M. Leonard, clinician at the Division of Endocrinology at the USPH's hospital in Seattle. The report of this trial illustrates the type of indicators used to assess health risks in clinical trials in the mid-1970s: seminal fluid volume, sperm concentration, germ cell morphology, hormone levels in the blood, liver function, renal function, serum electrolytes, hematology, blood pressure, body weight, gynecomastia, libido, potency, testicular size, and testicular tenderness. Although these fifteen indicators show similarities with those used in the clinical trials in the 1950s, eight new features had been added, including seminal fluid volume, germ cell morphology, liver function, renal function, serum electrolytes, hematology, blood pressure, and testicular tenderness (Spilman, Kirton, and Kirton 1976: 198). Some indicators used in the 1950 trials, such as sperm motility, testicular morphology, and emotional well-being, were no longer included in this trial. Since this trial was designed to assess the contraceptive activity of the steroids, the indicators were divided into two categories: indicators to assess the effects of hormones on sperm production (desired effects, including seminal fluid volume, sperm concentration, and germ cell morphology); and "adverse reactions" (undesired effects, including the other twelve parameters). A clinical trial at the Medical Center at the University of California in Los Angeles, performed by Ronald Swerdloff, another pioneer in male contraceptive research, testing a testosterone compound among thirty-nine adult men and published in 1979, added five new indicators. Whereas two parameters used in Paulsen's trial (blood pressure and testicular tenderness) were not included, Swerdloff tested for skin problems (oiliness of skin and acne), glucose metabolism, vital signs, hair growth, and prostatic size (Swerdloff et al. 1979: 663, 667). We can conclude that the parameters considered relevant for assessing the adverse effects of hormonal compounds in contraceptive trials had doubled by the end of the 1970s. Whereas the clinical trials in the 1950s mentioned seven indicators to assess effects other than those concerning sperm production, the mid-1970 trials included a list of fifteen indicators.

As in the 1950s publications, the adverse effects on sexual function were foregrounded in most reports that appeared in the 1970s. Compared to the 1950s, breast changes (gynecomastia) had become less central. In the 1970 trials, scientists no longer used estrogenic compounds to diminish these adverse effects. Using different compounds, or chemical manipulation of the compounds, has been employed as a strategy to reduce adverse effects, as I will describe later. Although the same strategy was used to solve the problems associated with impairment of sexual function, sexuality remained a central topic in the 1970s trials. A review presenting the state of the art in this field, written for WHO, which had just expanded its program to include male contraceptive development, is illustrative of this foregrounding of sexuality. The introduction to this review begins: "The ultimate aim in the regulation of fertility in the male is the development of suitable methods which reversibly interfere with his fertilizing capacity without compromising libido and potency" (Kretser 1974: 562).

Other review articles published in the 1970s contained a similar message. In "Towards a Pill for Men," published in 1976, libido and potency were the central topics in the evaluation of different approaches in male contraceptive research (Briggs and Briggs 1974).[3]

Clinical Trials in the 1980s

The clinical trials organized in the 1980s showed a list of indicators to assess the adverse effects of hormonal contraceptives similar to those used in the 1970s, except for three major changes. First, there was a standardization of methods to measure effects on sexuality and well-being. Whereas in the 1950s and 1970s the assessment of adverse effects on sexual function was based on short interviews, the protocols of many 1980 trials included extensive questionnaires dealing with changes in sexuality.[4] The protocol of a clinical trial published in Contraception in 1980 described a "Sexual Problem Checklist" that had to be answered by men participating in the trial every two weeks during the fifteen-month period of testing (Bain et al. 1980: 367). A protocol of another trial (1985) described an even more extensive technique for monitoring changes in sexual function: the use of a "Daily Protocol of Sexuality" (Michel et al. 1985: 665). The first multicenter trial organized by WHO, involving research centers in Bangkok, London, Santiago, Seoul, Toronto, and Hong Kong, included a questionnaire on the impact of the hormonal compounds on trial on sexual desire, feelings, and behavior, including thirty indicators to monitor changes during this trial. The results were published separately from the biomedical results in Studies in Family Planning (WHO/HRP 1982). This publication illustrates the reframing of sexuality that took place in the early 1980s. Whereas in the 1970s reports on sexual function were presented solely as indicators of adverse effects, in the 1980s sexual function was framed in terms of criteria to assess the acceptability of male contraceptives, as is exemplified in the WHO report:

In addition to extensive agreement on the need for new male contraceptives there is also consensus that noninterference with sexual functioning ("libido" and "potentia") is an important aspect of acceptability and must be taken into account along with other criteria such as safety, effectiveness, and reversibility. Because theoretical and clinical evidence suggests that steroid hormones alter the secretion of testosterone and thus may affect sexual interest and performances, it is important to examine new preparations for male fertility regulations to assess their effects on male sexuality. (WHO/HRP 1982: 32)

The standardization of monitoring techniques to assess changes in sexual function severely changed the representation of sexuality in clinical trial reports. Although the 1980 trials reported fewer negative changes in sexual functioning (one report even described positive changes; see Michel et al. 1985: 670), the use of standardized questionnaires led to a situation in which the interference of hormonal contraceptive compounds with sexuality became more fully articulated than in the previous trials. Whereas in the 1950s and 1970s the changes in sexual function were represented in just two categories (libido and potency), the 1980s reports show a multiplication of parameters to assess sexual function. Something similar happened with well-being, or "psychological functions." In the 1950s and 1970s, "emotional well-being" (1950s) and "psychological complaints" (1970s) were, if they were included at all, monitored by occasional observations or short interviews. In the mid-1980s, the protocols of clinical trials began to include extensive questionnaires and psychometric tests as tools to monitor changes in emotionality, mood, and personality, such as the Freiburg Personality Inventory, the Emotional Inventory, the Scale of Mood (Michel et al. 1985: 665), and the Freiburger Complaints Lists (Behre et al. 1985: 816). Again, the introduction of these new representation techniques, including more parameters and tests, increased the visibility of adverse effects.

What was new in the 1980s as well were studies specifically designed to assess the acceptability of male hormonal contraceptives. The first acceptability study was organized by the WHO Task Force on Acceptability of Fertility Regulating Methods as part of their multicenter clinical trials published in 1980 and 1982. The protocol for these studies was designed in 1976 and included eight objectives—five related to the acceptability of the contraceptive on trial, two related to sexuality, and one concerning the development of specific instruments and strategies "to facilitate collaboration with biomedical scientists in future clinical trials" (WHO/HRP 1976: 2). The introduction of acceptability studies implied the involvement of a new group of actors in male contraceptive clinical testing: social scientists.[5]

Finally, the 1980 trials show the emergence of significant new indicators to assess the adverse effects and new health risks that became associated with male hormonal contraceptives, which resulted in an increasing complexity, reflected both in terms of this assessment of the adverse effects and in the organization of the trials. In 1982 Alvin Paulsen, John Leonard, and William Bremner, who had joined Paulsen's research group in Seattle, published a review of male hormonal contraceptive clinical trials in which they concluded that the results of clinical trials with androgens indicated a general lack of adverse effects. This did not imply, however, that all problems had been solved. On the contrary, the authors warned the reader of new complications related to the use of androgens as contraceptives, most notably the risk of thrombosis: "Nevertheless, there are many potentially toxic effects of androgens, including effects on thrombosis and platelet aggregation. It is quite possible that important effects of this type would not have been appreciated in the small number of men studied to date" (Paulsen, Bremner, and Leonard 1982: 161).

Other review articles in the early 1980s show a similar concern for the potential risk of thrombosis for men taking androgens. In "Evolution of Steroids as Contraceptives for Men" (1983), the authors emphasized that the assessment of health risks of hormonal contraceptives for men should include an evaluation of thromboembolic risk factors (Foegh 1983: 9). Moreover, the 1980 clinical trials show the inclusion of yet another health risk: the suppression of HDL cholesterol, which may lead to the development of coronary heart disease (Guerin 1988: 192). Things became even more complicated when American reproductive scientists articulated a third potential serious health risk: prostate cancer (Knight and Callahan 1989; Wu 1988). In "Male Contraception Involving Testosterone Supplementation: Possible Increased Risks of Prostate Cancer?" published in The Lancet in 1987, the authors expressed their concern that long-term use of testosterone in methods of contraception might lead to an increase in prostate cancer (Schally and Comura-Schally 1987: 448).

This increasing complexity also affected the organization of clinical trials. The evaluation of potential risks of cardiovascular diseases and prostate cancer required other expertise beyond that needed in the previous trials. Whereas the 1970 trials typically consisted of clinical chemistry methods, hormone assays, and sperm evaluation tests, the mid-1980 trials also required expertise in blood coagulation studies (platelet aggregation studies and studies of fibrinolytic activity and capacity to assess risks of thrombosis), lipid chemistry evaluation (to evaluate the risks of coronary heart disease),[6] and rectal palpation (to assess the risks of prostate cancer). In order to organize a clinical trial, researchers thus had to put more effort into enrolling and coordinating the expertise of a much wider variety of laboratories. A clinical trial in Denmark (1985) described the collaboration of six different departments and laboratories.[7]

Clinical Trials in the 1990s

In the 1990s the major change in the clinical testing of hormonal contraceptives consisted of a change in scale. Whereas the trials in the previous two decades included only relatively small numbers of men, the 1990s witnessed the emergence of clinical trials with several hundreds of trial participants, most notably the organization of two large-scale, phase II clinical trials organized by WHO and published in 1990 and 1996 (WHO/HRP 1996). Since the 1970s, the three-phase testing model had become standard practice in the medical community and in drug regulatory policy. In phase I trials, the biological activity, safety, and optimum dosages of drugs are tested on a small number of subjects, usually between 20 and 50 participants. Before moving to phase II trials, the toxicology and teratology of the compounds have to be tested in animals. Phase II trials include a larger number of people (100–200) and are designed to evaluate the efficacy and adverse effects of drugs. Finally, phase III trials aim to test the drugs on an even larger number of participants in order to monitor rare side-effects (Mintzes 1991). The first WHO trial consisted of a combined effort of ten clinical centers in seven countries in Asia, Australia, Europe, and the United States and included 271 men. This trial was not only exceptional, due to the number of trial participants, but also because it was the first trial in which the contraceptive efficacy of hormonal compounds was assessed on the basis of the incidence of pregnancy. In previous trials, contraceptive activity had been evaluated in terms of sperm counts. The second WHO large-scale trial, a collaboration of fifteen centers in nine countries involving 399 men, was designed to redefine the criteria to assess the efficacy of contraceptive compounds (WHO/HRP 1996). These trials illustrate the increased complexity of clinical testing of hormonal compounds in the 1990s, not only with respect to the increase in indicators but also in terms of scale. The fact that these large-scale trials took place in ten or even fifteen different clinical centers all over the world increased the need for standardization. As we saw in chapter 2, WHO played a crucial role by providing a manual to standardize methods for semen analysis, by distributing reagents for the radio immunoassay of hormones, and by designing protocols and data forms. WHO also contributed to the standardization of test procedures in male contraceptive research. In *Guidelines for the Use of Androgens in Men*, WHO included guidelines for mandatory and optional tests for male contraceptive trials (WHO/HRP 1992b). The design of the protocol, the coordination, and the data collection and analysis took place at WHO headquarters in Geneva (WHO 1990b: 957). These trials illustrate all the work that goes into adjusting differences between local clinical and laboratory practices. Even routine laboratory methods were not used in a uniform way, a problem that was tackled by applying specific statistics.[8]

Most importantly, both WHO trials are illustrative of the wide range of indicators and tests that have become routine practice in the clinical testing of hormonal contraceptive compounds in the 1990s: semen analysis (sperm concentration, motility, and form); analysis of biochemical parameters; analysis of hematological parameters; hormone assays of semen and blood; analysis of urine; cholesterol assays; blood pressure measurements; liver function tests; occurrence of acne and gynecomastia; physical examinations (including rectal palpation of the prostate and estimation of testicular size, and body weight measurements); structured standardized questionnaires; and focus group discussions to assess changes in sexual function and psychological changes and the acceptability of the methods (including evaluation of subjective motivation, side-effects, and sexuality). A new element in these trials was the use of focus group discussions with participants in the clinical trials to evaluate their "subjective" experiences. The acceptability studies of the mid-1990s also included questionnaires for the female partners of the trial participants as a new tool to monitor changes in sexuality and psychological reactions (Suppression of spermatogenesis 1997). As in the trials of the 1980s, the long-term safety of the use of hormonal compounds, and particularly the risks of cardiovascular and prostatic diseases, were foregrounded as major concerns in the 1990 trials (Handelsman 1991; Wallace and Wu 1990: 63, 65; WHO/HRP 1996: 828).

In sum, three decades of clinical testing of hormonal contraceptives for men have resulted in an increase in the number of indicators considered as relevant to assessing adverse effects, as well as an increase in the health risks associated with hormonal contraceptive compounds. The clinical testing of male hormonal contraceptives is exceptional not only because it covers such an extensive period. Compared to other drugs, the testing of hormonal contraceptives for men also shows a remarkable gap between the organization of phase I testing and phase II testing. Whereas the time period between phase I and phase II testing is usually three to four years, it took more than a decade before phase II trials to evaluate the efficacy and safety of hormonal compounds among large numbers of men were initiated.[9] The basic concept of the hormonal regimen selected for use in the two WHO trials in the 1990s, testosterone enanthate, had already been established by 1978 (Paulsen et al. 1978: 959). Or, to quote Alvin Paulsen, the first chair of the steering committee of the WHO Male Task Force, who was involved in the organization of the phase II trials: "In 1978 we knew already that we wanted testosterone by itself because it was the least complicated. It had been on the market for thirty some years, so it was known and there had been enough small studies to know that we could suppress spermatogenesis. . . . So there was a lot of information available" (Paulsen interview 1994).

As we saw in the previous chapter, the major reason for this delay was ethical concerns within WHO about the risk of pregnancy to the female partners of the trial participants in case the contraceptive on trial failed. This delay had enormous consequences for male contraceptive testing. In the period between 1978 and the late 1980s, the wider environment of male contraceptive research changed in some important respects, which destabilized the field. In the first place, the environment changed due to an increased public awareness of heart disease as a major health threat for men. In the early 1980s, reports were published in which medical scientists claimed that changes in plasma lipids, particularly in high-density lipoprotein cholesterol (HDL cholesterol), might have a deleterious effect on the cardiovascular system (Wallace and Wu 1990; Babiak and Rudel 1987). Despite the uncertainties surrounding this claim, these reports resulted in a "cholesterol scare," particularly in the United States, where the government launched the National Lipid Education Program to inform patients how they could reduce the risk of coronary disease. The increased attention to lipids as a cause of cardiovascular disease did not leave male contraceptive research untouched. In the words of William Bremner:

> There has been a lot of attention paid to measuring lipids. Since the National Lipid Education Program there is a lot of screening going on and everyone is aware of their cholesterol. . . . With this sort of national program going on and an awareness of lipids in general, anything that affects it adversely, any medication, any contraceptive, even though there is no evidence that it really does have any impact, is suspect. We felt obliged to measure lipids. . . . Even though the clinical significance of that is unknown, with the national awareness and the awareness by

funding groups, the general thought is that that is going to be unacceptable if there is any effect on good cholesterol. (Bremner interview 1994)

Although the interference of androgens with plasma lipids had been known since the late 1950s (Foegh 1983: 31) and had been described in a male hormonal contraceptive trial as early as 1973, this adverse effect became foregrounded only in the mid-1980s (Skoglund and Paulson 1973: 363), due to the widespread concern about heart disease. Whereas researchers doubt the clinical significance of the negative interference of hormones with HDL cholesterol for the development of coronary disease, a major part of clinical testing in the 1990s was still focused on finding alternative modes of administration or lower doses of hormones in order to avoid any suppression of HDL cholesterol (Bremner interview 1994; Matsumoto interview 1994; Handelsman 1991: 232). To quote Matsumoto, a former student and then a colleague of Bremner at the research group in Seattle: "It's a concern, I don't think it's that much of a problem. As long as it is a concern to somebody or a lot of folks, it's going to be a concern to us" (Matsumoto interview 1994). Ever since then, lipid measurement has become a major indicator to assess the safety of male contraceptives, and male contraceptive compounds have become associated with a new potential health risk: coronary heart disease (Pavlou et al. 1991; WHO/HRP 1996; WHO/HRP 1990b; Tom et al. 1992).

A second major change in the environment of male contraceptive research took place when physicians, women's health advocates, and consumer organizations caused some alarm when they informed the public that the contraceptive pill for women was suspected of increasing the risk of thrombosis. Although the first reports describing this health risk had already been published in the mid-1970s, this claim became a major public concern in the 1980s (Seaman and Seaman 1978). Since male contraceptive researchers used basically the same hormones as were contained in the compounds of the Pill for women, they had to include yet another indicator in their tests: the measurement of coagulation factors. The report of the first clinical trial that included this indicator explicitly referred to the problems with the Pill for women: "A natural concern from experience with the female oral contraceptive is the possibility of an increased risk of thromboembolic events, especially since males already have a higher incidence of these diseases than women. For these reasons, evaluation of thromboembolic risk factors is mandatory" (Foegh 1983: 9). Since the early 1980s specific measurements to assess the risk of thrombosis have become routine practice in male contraceptive testing (WHO/HRP 1996; Bhasin, Handelsman, and Swerdloff 1992; Behre et al. 1992).

A third potential risk that became foregrounded in the early 1990s was a hormone-induced increase in aggression. Again, the impetus to foreground this risk did not emerge from the results of previous male contraceptive testing but came from elsewhere. In the early 1990s, the media paid a lot of attention to the abuse of anabolic steroids by sportsmen, which resulted in a growing concern for the influence of androgens on mood changes, particularly aggression. Geoffrey Waites described this event:

> I think that current concerns are much more to do with mood change. . . .
> It has come up in the media much more strongly recently and that has
> influenced drug regulatory policies somewhat too, especially in Sweden,
> where there exists a concern around the abuse of anabolic steroids, and
> these have often been androgens. And so one is left in a climate explain-
> ing that the drugs we use are given at doses that are much less damaging
> to normal, adult people. Some of my investigators have been called as
> expert witnesses in cases where litigation is based on change of behav-
> ior as a consequence of drugs. But we are trying to address all those
> changes. We have protocols to look at changes in aggression, changes in
> behavior, in our multicenter trials. (Waites interview 1994)

WHO considered the alleged association between androgens and aggression important enough to initiate a clinical study in 1994 specifically designed to address this issue (WHO/HRP 1994: 2)

The long period between phase I and phase II clinical trials thus facilitated a situation in which male contraceptive compounds became associated with two new health risks (coronary heart disease and thrombosis) and one new psychological risk (aggression), which resulted in a destabilization of the field. Most importantly, this destabilization resulted from debates on health concerns unrelated to male contraceptive testing, rather than from the dynamics of the field itself.

Strategies to Cope with Risk Factors

How have scientists tried to reduce the increased complexities resulting from the long period of testing? Although scholars in social studies of science have paid attention to the dynamics of clinical trials,[10] the question of how scientists try to cope with adverse effects has not been addressed systematically. Studies of the strategies designers use to devise solutions in cases of conflicting user representations in the design of technical systems provide a useful means to analyze the dynamics of reducing complexities in clinical testing. As

Akrich has described, one of these strategies consists of relying on the technical system itself. Designers change the physical features of technical artifacts in such a way that the object assumes all the required functions (Akrich 1995: 178). A similar strategy can be observed in the clinical testing of male hormonal contraceptives. In the past three decades, manipulation of the artifact has been a major strategy to cope with adverse effects. In the 1970s and 1980s, numerous attempts were made to diminish the negative interference of hormonal contraceptive compounds with sexual function. The reports of the clinical trials in the 1950s and early 1970s foregrounded loss of sexual desire (libido) and problems with erections and seminal fluid production (potency) as major adverse effects. The hormonal compounds used in these trials depressed sperm production but simultaneously lowered the production of testosterone, the steroid described as important for regulating male sexuality.

One way in which scientists tried to solve the problem of hormonal interference with sexual function consisted of the development of combined hormonal compounds instead of single compound contraceptives. In "Successful Inhibition of Spermatogenesis in Man without Loss of Libido: A Potential New Approach to Male Contraception," published in *Contraception* in 1973, two Brazilian researchers claimed that they had solved problems with libido by giving supplementary androgens to the trial participants: "One of the reasons for the unavailability of a male contraceptive pill based on the same biological principles as the female pill lies in the difficulties of achieving suppression of fertility in the male without interfering with his sexual drive and potency. . . . In the present report, preliminary clinical trials are described in which progestin induced suppression of spermatogenesis is achieved without loss of libido and potency in healthy men implanted with long-acting testosterone Silastic capsules" (Coutinho 1973: 208).

Remarkably, the subdermal testosterone capsules used in this trial had not been developed for this purpose, but were originally designed as testosterone replacement therapy for hypogonadal men: men who suffer from endocrine dysfunctions of the testes (Coutinho and Melo 1973: 208). Other researchers adopted a similar approach, introducing other methods of administration of testosterone such as subcutaneous injections (Bhasin, Handelsman, and Swerdloff 1985). Since the 1980s, the use of combined hormonal compounds has developed as one of the dominant approaches in male contraceptive research (Bain et al. 1980; Swerdloff and Heber 1983; Foegh 1983; Belkien et al. 1984). Manipulation of the artifact by combining different hormonal compounds has also been used as a strategy for coping with other adverse effects such as interference with lipoprotein metabolism (Kretser 1974; Skoglund and Paulson 1973: 365).

Although this strategy was successful in reducing the complexities concerning adverse effects, it simultaneously increased the complexities of designing a contraceptive that would be easy to use. Most of the combination contraceptive agents consist of two different modes of administration, combining pills with injections or implants or plasters, or injections with implants, which complicates the acceptability of the contraceptive.[11] Strategies used to diminish adverse effects thus run the risk of creating "technological monsters": artifacts that are "extremely sophisticated but finally quite ineffectual because they are unable to attract the users for whom it was intended" (Akrich 1995: 179).

A second strategy to solve health-risk problems consisted of delegating the risks to women. The use of androgens to restore sexual function not only complicated the mode of administration, but also decreased the efficacy of the contraceptive-in-the-making. Ironically, the supplementary androgens applied to prevent adverse effects caused another side-effect: they supported spermatogenesis, the process that had to be suppressed rather than stimulated. This created a serious threat to the whole trajectory of developing male hormonal contraceptives (Akhtar et al. 1985; Bouchard and Garcia 1987; Guerin 1988; Bhasin et al. 1985). Similar problems emerged in clinical trials with single agents, such as the testosterone enanthate used by WHO. Even with the most effective hormonal compounds, complete suppression of sperm production (azoospermia) could only be induced in 50 percent to 70 percent of the participants (Aitken and Wu 1989: 691).[12] Whereas the major research activities in the 1970s and early 1980s consisted of tinkering with the artifact to reduce side-effects, problems with efficacy dominated research from the early 1980s to the mid-1990s. A review article in 1994 described these constraints as follows: "The failure to obtain complete suppression of spermatogenesis in all men with these hormonal regimens and the consequent concerns about contraceptive failure acted for many years as a deterrent to more extensive efforts" (Matlin 1994b: 855).

Several research groups tried to address the problem by manipulating the artifact (Knuth, Yeung, and Nieschlag 1989). The major strategy consisted, however, in trying to redefine the criteria for assessing the contraceptive efficacy of contraceptives for men. Until that time, hormonal compounds were considered effective only if they could switch off sperm production completely. The rationale underlying this criterion was that one could only conclude that a man was no longer able to fertilize his partner in the case of azoospermia, the term that is used when sperm concentrations in the semen are reduced to zero or undetectable levels. In the mid-1980s, scientists concluded that if azoospermia remained the target to assess contraceptive efficacy, hormonal compounds could never be made into effective contraceptives (Waites interview 1994). For the Population Council, one of the important organizations involved in male hormonal contraceptive research in the 1970s and early 1980s, the failure to achieve zero sperm level with hormonal compounds was such a serious problem that the organization decided to stop its research activities in this area.[13] As Rosemary Thau, director of the Population Council's Contraceptive Development Program in the early 1990s, put it: "Hormonally you cannot really do much about the male system. . . . If you have a group of one hundred men the percentage who respond with azoospermia is simply too small. And even the ones who do don't maintain azoospermia. So we just stopped it. We decided it is not worth our time" (Thau interview 1994).

In the mid-1980s scientists suggested that this crisis in male hormonal contraceptive development could only be won over by changing the target from zero sperm (azoospermia) to low sperm concentrations (oligospermia). This suggestion triggered an intensive debate and controversies on the question of the extent to which it could be guaranteed that men with low sperm counts could really be considered incapable of fertilizing their partners (Knuth and Nieschlag 1987: 126–27). The advocates of changing the criteria for hormonally induced infertility suggested that "azoospermia may not be the absolute prerequisite for effective fertility suppression in men" (Wu 1988: 458), but their opponents argued that "the only true test of infertility is azoospermia" (Crabbé, Diszalusy, and Djerassi 1980: 207) and adhered to the opinion that azoospermia was an absolute requirement for safe male contraception (Guille et al. 1989: 118; Foegh 1983: 35; Bialy and Patanelli 1981: 103). They suggested that, "although the chance of pregnancy is significantly reduced at very low sperm levels, fertilization is still theoretically possible if few sperm are present" (Bain et al. 1980: 376). At the heart of the controversy were differences in the assessments of the degree of protection from unwanted pregnancy that could be guaranteed if oligospermia were to be accepted as the criterion for contraceptive efficacy. At that time, the fertility of men who produced only a small number of sperm had not yet been subjected to any clinical testing (Wu 1988: 457). The contraceptive efficacy of hormonal compounds had been assessed by semen analysis rather than by protection against pregnancy. Participants in male contraceptive trials were expected to use other contraceptives than the one on trial to avoid the risk of unwanted pregnancies. Assessment of the fertility of men with low sperm concentrations, however, required participants to practice unprotected sex during the trial.

One way to circumvent this problem was to assess the fertility of men with low sperm levels by the application of an in vitro test. In the mid 1980s, several laboratories used the so-called zone-free hamster oocyte penetration test, introduced in 1976 to diagnose the fertilization potential of lowsperm levels in men with fertility problems (Aitken 1986; Matsumoto 1988: 324). Initially, WHO considered this test unethical because it implied crossing species boundaries: human sperm were used to fertilize hamster ova (Waites interview 1994). Given the widespread use of this test, WHO changed its initial resistance and convened a workshop in 1985 to reach consensus about a standardized protocol for performing the sperm penetration assay (Aitken 1986: 145). The use of laboratory-only methods provided a temporary solution, because male contraceptive researchers insisted that "the precise extent of the risk [of unwanted pregnancies] can only be assessed accurately by a formal clinical efficacy trial (Aitken, Wallace, and Wu 1992: 422; Bhasin et al. 1985: 456).

In the early 1990s WHO therefore instigated the first large-scale clinical trial to examine the effectiveness of hormonal contraceptives in men who practiced unprotected sex. Initially, the protocol of this trial allowed men with a sperm concentration of less than five million sperm per milliliter to have unprotected coitus with their female partners (Bhasin et al. 1985: 456). The choice of this threshold had triggered intense debates within WHO: "The question is what is the threshold. You can include men to five million per ml, but that's a lot: a lot of sperm and a lot of debate, since subfertile men with five million per ml often are shown to be fertile and they father a child. So there was intense debate on whether one should let normal men suppressed by drugs to the level of five million per ml have unprotected intercourse. Was the risk too great? We wouldn't know until we tried, so we started at five million per ml" (Waites interview 1994).

Indeed, the risk turned out to be too great. During the trial, WHO lowered the threshold to three million per ml because a couple of pregnancies had occurred among the female partners of men whose sperm concentrations had been reduced to a level between three and five million per ml (Bremner interview 1994). The coordinating center in Geneva had developed special procedures to monitor what happened in the ten centers participating in the trial. Farley, the statistician in charge of data collection and analysis at WHO's headquarters in Geneva, described the results:

In the male trial there was a lot of concern about pregnancies, so we were notified by fax of them and we also had contacts by telex or telephone whenever a pregnancy occurred. There was major concern when the trials started that there might be a high pregnancy rate, as is very standard in trials. There are procedures for stopping the trial if things are going wrong, so there were criteria in the protocol that, whenever a pregnancy occurred, we should review the data and calculate the pregnancy rate. If it was unacceptably high (there was a definition of what was unacceptably high) then we should consider either stopping the trial or stopping just that center, or something else. But this is pretty standard in any trial. . . . What was unusual about this study was that the end point which we were mainly interested in was pregnancy, which was also the reason for stopping the trial. (Farley interview 1994)

The protocol of this trial mentioned that the trial should be stopped if the estimated pregnancy rate should exceed "12 pregnancies per 100 person-years." The reference used to legitimize this criterion was the incidence of pregnancies in the first year of condom use (WHO/HRP 1996: 823). Because the number of pregnancies exceeded the failure rate of condoms, WHO had to lower the threshold from five to three million sperm per milliliter. In this manner, WHO managed to reduce the incidence of unwanted pregnancies from the four pregnancies that had occurred among the four hundred couples participating in the trial. This outcome enabled WHO to find a much more favorable reference to legitimize its decision to take the risk to test hormonal contraceptive compounds among couples who practiced unprotected sex.[14] In the final publication of the trial, the authors compared the contraceptive effectiveness of the male hormonal contraceptive with the effectiveness of the Pill for women (WHO Office of Information 1996). Moreover, the publication indicated that WHO's strategy to optimize response rates had been very successful. Whereas in previous trials with zero sperm concentrations as a target, only 50 percent to 70 percent of the men were considered incapable of fertilizing their partner, the change in target from zero to low sperm levels resulted in a success rate of 98 percent (WHO/HRP 1996: 827).

This strategy to solve the problems of the efficacy and adverse effects of male hormonal contraceptive compounds, however, implied a gendered redistribution of risks. The revised criteria to assess the contraceptive efficacy of male hormonal contraceptive methods allowed for higher risks of pregnancy than in the case of the previous criteria of azoospermia. Consequently, the problems of efficacy and the risk of sexual dysfunction for men became transformed into a problem of risk for women, that is, an increased risk of unwanted pregnancy. Although this risk turned out to be much lower than had been expected, the principle is nevertheless the same. The risks of male contraceptives were delegated to women rather than men.

A third strategy used by male contraceptive researchers to cope with adverse effects is a very drastic one, namely, to stop all further development of the compounds. This has happened in the case of several non-hormonal compounds, such as bis-dichloroacetyl diamines (disturbed liver metabolism) (Matlin 1994b: 857); cyproterone acetate (interference with sexuality, adrenocortical function, and intratesticular changes) (Kretser 1978: 857); and Nitrofurans (toxic side effects) (Kretser 1978: 356; Jackson 1975: 655; Knuth and Nieschlag 1987: 117). Those hormonal compounds for which clinical testing has been discontinued due to adverse effects include estrogens (sexual dysfunctions, weight gain, and changes in breasts) (Davis 1977: 361; Paulsen 1977: 460; Kretser 1974: 569; Jackson 1975: 655) and oral testosterone compounds (liver damage) (Kretser 1978: 355; Matlin interview 1994). Finally, Gossypol, a drug derived from the cotton plant that was first tested by Chinese researchers in the mid-1970s, illustrates the locally specific nature of the assessment and acceptability of adverse effects of male contraceptives. Although Chinese researchers initially concluded that clinical testing on more than ten thousand volunteers, the largest test population in the history of male contraceptive development, had shown no "appreciably harmful side effects" (Wen 1980: 195), Western scientists warned against the irreversibility of the method, genetic damage, and long-term toxic effects on heart and liver (Gossypol prospects 1984: 1109; Gombe 1983: 207). Nevertheless, the Western world showed great interest in this promising new lead in male contraceptive research. During the 1970s and 1980s, numerous derivatives and analogues of Gossypol were synthesized in order to reduce the adverse effects. Until the late 1980s, WHO was involved in coordinating animal testing, standardization, purification, and synthesis work on Gossypol in seventeen countries (Gossypol prospects 1984: 1109). Based on a major review of these studies, involving researchers from China, Europe, and the United States, WHO finally decided in 1986 to discontinue its involvement with Gossypol because it did not meet their standards of safety and reversibility (Matlin 1994b: 858; Waites, Wang, and Griffin 1998). Remarkably, not all Western scientists share this opinion. Currently, the Population Council is still working on Gossypol, including the clinical testing of new Gossypol compounds (Waites interview 1994; Nieschlag interview 1995).

The fourth strategy adopted to solve problems of adverse effects was the suggestion to postpone further research of potential risks to the post-marketing phase. This tactic has been used for drugs with long-term risks such as those of cardiovascular diseases and prostatic cancer, as is illustrated in the report of the second WHO large-scale multicenter trial in 1996: "Any long-term effects of such regimens notably on prostate or cardiovascular disease can be determined only by appropriate long-term surveillance when such methods are widely used in the community, as for female hormonal methods" (WHO/HRP 1996: 828–29). Again, hormonal contraceptives for women were used as a reference to legitimize policies in male contraceptive research.

The mid-1990s saw the emergence of yet another strategy, which consisted of the introduction of a new model of risk assessment. Instead of focusing solely on risks, WHO and several male contraceptive researchers suggested that the benefits of hormones should be included in the assessments of contraceptive compounds (WHO/HRP 1996: 828; Wu interview 1994). The conclusion section of the report of the first large-scale WHO trial, where the authors discussed cardiovascular and prostatic risks, exemplifies this strategy: "These hypothetical risks must be balanced against the non-contraceptive benefits on bone, muscle and blood-forming marrow which may protect against age-related osteoporosis, debility and anemia" (Handelsman 1991: 232).

Dependencies, Gender Bias, and Risk Models

The history of the development of hormonal contraceptives for men thus suggests that lengthy testing does not necessarily lead to a stabilization of the field in terms of final decisions regarding the safety of specific products. In contrast to traditional views of clinical testing, which emphasize the autonomy of the scientific community and the importance of scientific standards in shaping decisions in clinical testing, the case of male contraceptives shows how the standards used to evaluate the safety of compounds in terms of acceptability of adverse effects are not solely in the hands of scientific experts but depend on assessments by other major actors and norms in the culture at large.[15] The most important, but invisible, actor is the pharmaceutical industry. Although pharmaceutical firms have been, and still are, largely absent from the actual testing of male hormonal contraceptives, they are nevertheless major agents in shaping standards to evaluate safety. As I learned in the interviews with some of the major investigators in clinical testing, most researchers are well informed and fully aware of the safety standards adopted by pharmaceutical firms. Alvin Paulsen: "Risks are minor. . . . The dropout in our clinical trials is low with male methods, compared to female methods. The men feel good, they don't feel sick, they don't have headaches, all the problems that women experience with even low-dose pills—or some women do. . . . But people are so nervous about male methods. I'm talking about drug regulatory agencies, the policymakers, pharmaceutical firms, because they have been sued up to their eyeballs on the pill" (Paulsen interview 1994).

Fred Wu also noted the crucial role of the industry as a gatekeeper to assess safety: "People in industry are also concerned about long-term safety, obviously from the medical-legal point of view as well. And unless we can produce good information in short and long-term safety, I think that it would be very difficult to convince some of the establishment or large companies to participate in this kind of development" (Wu interview 1994). Finally, as Eberhard Nieschlag, the chairman of the WHO Male Task Force from 1985 to 1991, put it: "Side effects may be minor, but even minor effects, if millions of people are taking it, can mean great financial risks. That's why the pharmaceutical industries say: no, no interest. They are not interested because of liability problems" (Nieschlag interview 1995).

To be sure, the fact that pharmaceutical firms are important actors in the assessment of the safety of drugs is not specific to male contraceptive development but also applies to other drugs. There is, however, one major difference. As John Abrahams has described for risk assessments of benoxaprofen, a drug used to treat arthritis, pharmaceutical companies usually underplay the side-effects. Lynn has described a similar process in the assessment of environmental risks (Lynn 1986). In male contraceptive risk assessment, the opposite happens. Here, the pharmaceutical firms tend to overplay the health risks.

The safety standards set by pharmaceutical firms don't stand on their own, of course. Ever since the increased public demand for reduced health risks of contraceptives, which emerged in the late 1960s as a result of criticism from women's health advocates of the serious health risks of the Pill and the IUD, pharmaceutical firms have had to operate within a climate characterized by a high risk of liability suits. Due to a dramatic increase in lawsuits for oral contraceptives in the 1980s, liability costs in the field of contraceptives are higher than for any other drug category (Djerassi 1989: 357). Consequently, the debates on the risks of contraceptives have shifted gears. The assessment of side-effects is no longer framed exclusively in terms of a concern for health risks to contraceptive users, but has been transformed into an assessment of financial risks, as described in the quotes above. In this respect, we may conclude that the development of male hormonal contraceptives has been a matter of bad timing. As Nieschlag said: "It [the constraints on the development of male contraceptives] has got worse. If we had had this long-acting testosterone in the early seventies, everybody would be using it today. The restrictions were not as bad as it is today" (Nieschlag interview 1995). The safety of contraceptives is thus not an inherent, universal quality of the artifact defined by autonomous scientists, but rather the result of historically specific circumstances.

The assessment of health risks is shaped not only by historically specific notions and practices regarding contraceptives, but is also constrained by previous experiences with steroids. Since the first "Pill scare" in the late 1960s, steroids have been portrayed as risky drugs, as exemplified by Matsumoto's experiences in this field:

> The history of contraceptive development has a big impact on what any individual investigator is pursuing. I think it has a big impact on us now because we are hormonally based. . . . Once the female birth control pill was released and they started having side effects, there was a big negative steroid image that built up that steroids were bad. They can give you heart disease and strokes. So that early history, what was going on in female contraception and the side-effects of the Pill, were indirectly affecting male contraception. If it happens in the female, it can happen in the male. All these things have gone on in parallel and have affected the development of male contraceptives. (Matsumoto interview 1994)

Again, safety standards for male contraceptives are not the result of autonomous decisions based on evaluations of the compounds on trial, but depend also on images of risks developed in previous comparable settings. Since the late 1960s, all work on steroids has been constrained and shaped by the controversies and debates surrounding the use of the female contraceptive Pill.

The dependency of the male contraceptive community on standards and norms developed by other actors or in previous settings has yet another component. Scientists and clinicians not only face problems because they work on contraceptives or hormones, they are also constrained by the fact that they work on hormonal contraceptives for men. The debates on the assessment of health risks of male contraceptives reveal the structuring role of gender norms in constructing standards of safety. During the three decades of testing, the risk of interference of contraceptives with sexual function has been the most hotly debated side-effect. This concern reflects a cultural preoccupation with norms of masculinity that can best be summarized as "no tinkering with male sexuality." By choosing hormonal approaches to male contraceptives, scientists and clinicians who took up the testing of the compounds entered a high-risk zone: the suppression of sperm production by hormones resulted in a lower production of testosterone, an androgen described preeminently as the sex hormone because it regulates sexual function. Although this problem had been solved in the early 1970s by reorienting contraceptive R&D toward combined hormonal contraceptives, which consisted of a contraceptive component and supplementary androgens to restore sexual function, the fear that a hormonal contraceptive for men might affect libido continues to dominate the field. Most publications in the scientific and journalistic press covering the clinical testing of male hormonal contraceptives in the last two decades have emphasized that the hormones on trial did not have a negative impact on male sexuality. Even in the late 1990s, the image of hormonal contraceptives as a threat to male sexuality was still very much alive, as shown by the view of one representative of a pharmaceutical firm, Driek Vergouwen, the director of R&D at Organon, a Dutch company that had become involved in the clinical testing of male contraceptives in the late 1990s: "The Pill for men inhibits libido. This might be considered as an advantage—refraining from sex constitutes a perfect contraceptive—but men don't take the Pill to refrain from sex" (Brand and Schwartz 1999).[16]

This concern with sexuality in contraceptive research shows a definite gender bias. Since the introduction of the female contraceptive pill in the early 1960s, women taking the Pill have complained about loss of sexual desire (Diller and Hembree 1977: 1275; Seaman and Seaman 1978: 325).[17] Although oral hormonal contraceptives for women operate by a mechanism similar to that of hormonal contraceptives for men, problems with sexuality were only acknowledged in the mid-1990s, when researchers first initiated studies to investigate the impact of the Pill on female sexual behavior. John Bancroft, the endocrinologist in charge of these studies and director of the Kinsey Institute for Research on Sex, Gender, and Reproduction, in Indiana, has described this structuring role of gender norms as follows: "The evidence that oral contraceptives [for women] can influence sexuality may be more firm. It is interesting that when steroidal contraception recently began to be developed for men, right at the top of the research agenda from the outset was concern about what effects it might have on men's sexual behaviors. But, for the female Pill, here we are forty years down the road doing work that should have been done decades ago" (Bancroft, cited in Check 1999: 21).[18]

Gender differences in the assessment of risks are apparently not restricted to sexuality. The experiences of researchers involved in the testing of hormonal contraceptives indicate a tendency in risk assessment to give more weight to the side-effects of male contraceptives than to those of female methods. According to Geoffrey Waites, reflecting on his experiences as manager of the WHO Male Task Force: "I can still remember putting out the table of the side-effects of one of our studies. There was one case of discontinuation because of lipid changes. This led to an outcry, a lot of comments coming from obstetricians and gynecologists who were on the committee. It didn't help me by saying that none of the partners had menstrual disorders, which is a reason for discontinuation in female trials. Thirty to forty percent of women can't tolerate these side effects. It didn't help me at all to say that" (Waites interview 1994).

Fred Wu, the endocrinologist in charge of male clinical contraceptive trials at the University of Manchester, had similar experiences. People who reacted to his work often suggested that the use of hormones was more risky for men than for women (Wu interview 1994). Finally, a review article published in *Contraception* in 1974 indicated a similar imbalance in risk assessment for male methods compared to female methods. Discussing the early clinical trials with estrogens, the author concluded: "The occurrence of symptomatic gynecomastia and other metabolic side-effects such as demonstrated in women receiving oral contraceptive preparations, make it unlikely that estrogens will be accepted in formulations to interrupt male fertility" (Kretser 1974: 569). The construction of standards to assess the side-effects of contraceptives thus also depends on gendered cultural norms regarding the acceptability of risks.

Finally, the practices of three decades of clinical testing of male hormonal contraceptives reflect a preference for a specific risk model. Given the explicit emphasis on sharing risks, an argument frequently used since the 1960s to legitimize the need for new male contraceptives, one would expect that the assessment of health risks would include an evaluation of the differential risks of the couple. This is, however, not the case. To the contrary: in publications covering male contraceptive clinical testing in the last three decades, there was only one report describing this model. In "Bridging the gender gap in contraception: Another hurdle cleared," the author concluded: "The health implications of male contraception must balance the risks and benefits in both the user and his spouse" (Handelsman 1991: 232).

As illustrated in the quotation above, Geoffrey Waites has tried in vain to introduce this model into WHO. The implication of this shared risk model would be that the risks for men, for example, the risk of altered cholesterol levels, would be weighed against the benefits to the female partner, for example, the absence of irregular menstruation (a side-effect of hormonal contraceptive implants such as Norplant) or the reduced risk of thrombosis (a side-effect of hormonal contraceptive pills). This type of risk assessment is completely absent from the reports of male contraceptive trials. The representation techniques for risks in the reports of clinical trials include only the health risks for men, which reflects an individual risk model. Although this model is also dominant in female contraceptive research, there is a striking difference. In the individual risk model for men, the health risks of contraceptives are compared with the conditions of untreated, healthy men. For women, the health risks of contraceptives are calculated against the risk of pregnancy, including maternal mortality and morbidity, health risks related to abortion, and psychological and social problems related to unwanted pregnancies (Foegh 1983: 9; Matlin interview 1994).[19] This gendered individual risk model tends to minimize the health risks for women and enlarge the risks for men. Taking the condition of healthy men as a reference ultimately transforms any side-effect into an unwanted aberration. The use of this gendered individual risk model also complicates the evaluation of health risks in terms of the time scale. Some authors claim that safety is more difficult to establish for men than for women because of the longer reproductive lifespan of men. In a shared-risk model this problem would not exist, because one would take into account the period when female partners are using contraceptives.

Conclusions

Summarizing the practices of three decades of male contraceptive testing, I conclude that the dominance of the individual risk model and the low acceptance of risks in the male contraceptive community and in the culture at large,[20] particularly where men are concerned, accounts for the lengthy period of testing. Due to these constraints, the clinical testing of male hormonal contraceptives has culminated in a quest for zero risk. The aim of clinical testing has been transformed from evaluating the clinical relevance of changes in indicators induced by the compounds on trial to showing that these compounds do not affect any of the indicators selected to assess safety, even those whose clinical significance is unknown (Bremner interview 1994).

> But I think we're getting a little bit closer, we're getting to realize that we know a lot more than even five years ago about what is required to induce reversible contraception. . . . Now it's refinement of the technique which needs to be done and the development of practical methods of administration and then making absolutely sure that it is safe, even to the point

where we use a laboratory value like serum lipid levels to actually make sure that there aren't any adverse effects of any of the parameters that we know are affected by androgens or progestins or whatever. (Matumoto interview 1994)

Needless to say, the quest for zero risk can never be realized because all drugs cause side-effects (Mastroianni, Donaldson, and Kane 1990: 102).

Most strikingly, the assessment of health risks of male contraceptives shows a structuring role of gender norms in constructing standards of safety.[21] During the three decades of testing, the risks of interference of hormonal contraceptive compounds with sexual functions has been the most debated side-effect. This concern reflects a cultural preoccupation with norms of masculinity that can best be summarized as "no tinkering with male sexuality." Contraceptive researchers reiterated and sustained conventionalized performances of masculinity which emphasize heterosexuality as the core of masculine identities (Connell 1987; 1995). The clinical testing of male contraceptives has been severely delimited by this hegemonic masculinity. This chapter thus shows how technologies that are at odds with hegemonic masculinity have a hard time coming into existence. This conclusion underscores my theoretical argument that technological innovation can only be understood if we include the creation of alignments between technologies, users, and identities in theorizing technological development.

PART II

. . . .

Configuring the User:

Articulating and

Performing

Masculinities

6

The Politics of Language: Changing Family Planning Discourse to Include Men

. . . .

The development of radical new technologies is hard work. In the first part of this book we have seen how including men in the contraceptive R&D agenda required a drastic transformation of firmly entrenched sociotechnical networks and related vested interests of reproductive scientists, clinicians, and pharmaceutical firms that had focused for a long time on women rather than men. Technological innovation in male contraceptive technologies, however, requires more than changing previously established sociotechnical networks, and more than a conceptualization of technological change solely in terms of such networks. To understand the gender dynamics of technological innovation, we need a conceptualization of technological change that acknowledges the cultural embeddedness of technology. Technology should be viewed not only in terms of networks of techniques, materials, knowledge, institutions, experts, and social groups, but also as including the relationships between technologies and identities. Technologies can only become successful if actors, both inside and outside of the scientific community, articulate and transform the identities of the prospective users of a technology. Technological change requires the mutual adjustment of technologies and identities.

This is particularly so for male contraceptive innovation. The predominance of female contraceptives has shaped gender identities of both women and men in such a way that the use of contraceptives has become largely a woman's job. In the second half of the twentieth century, contraception came to be excluded from hegemonic masculinity. The following chapters aim to trace the cultural work involved in destabilizing these conventionalized performances in gender identities. This is a crucial part of technological innovation: if the advocates of new contraceptives for men fail to revise cultural preconceptions, it is very likely that the technology will fail altogether. Although reproductive scientists play an important role in configuring the user of new male contraceptive technologies, they are not the only actors involved in constructing a context of use. To make visible the cultural work involved in male contraceptive innovation, we will have to travel to locations other than just laboratories and medical clinics. In contraceptive technologies, the world of family planning is an important location for understanding the processes involved in the mutual adjustment of technologies and the identities of prospective users. The history of the development and implementation of contraceptives for women demonstrates the importance of family planning clinics for these technologies. Family planning clinics function not only as locations for testing new contraceptives, they are also important sources for creating and reaching audiences for the new technologies. The next two chapters therefore extend the analysis to the world of family planning. A naive visitor to this world might be surprised to learn that this realm has been—and still is—predominantly inhabited by female clients and female service providers. Prior to the 1980s, family planning clinics and other services were primarily oriented toward women, which is largely due to the gender asymmetry in available contraceptives for women and men. Not only are there fewer male than female contraceptives, but there are also different modes of administration. Two of the three contraceptive methods available for men do not require a family planning clinic for distribution: withdrawal needs no program services at all, and condoms are widely available in many countries through a large number of commercial outlets. The only male method that needs a medical provision is vasectomy. In Western countries, most vasectomies are performed by physicians and are not restricted to family planning clinics (Gordon and DeMarco 1984). In contrast to male methods, most modern contraceptives for women are provider-dependent. The IUD (intrauterine device), the Pill, hormonal implants, and injections all require medical prescriptions or interventions. Although the Pill, like other methods, is also distributed by physicians, the availability of these methods, particularly the Pill, has led to an increase in the number of family planning clinics and has directed service delivery almost exclusively to women (Stycos 1996; Gordon and DeMarco 1984). Given this background, it is evident that the absence of family planning services for men has been, and still is, a serious constraint for the development of new contraceptives for men. However, times are changing. In the last two decades family planning discourse has shifted toward including men in family planning.[1]

This chapter aims to describe the strategies men and family planning advocates have used to change family planning discourse toward including men and the barriers they have faced in their endeavor. I will show how family planning researchers, feminists, and family planning organizations have become increasingly involved in counteracting and transforming the dominant cultural narratives on masculinity, male sexuality, and birth control embedded in family planning research traditions and the policies of national and international family planning organizations and women's health organizations, in an effort to overcome the barriers to changing family planning discourse toward including men. I shall then describe how men and family planning advocates have changed the objectives and vocabularies of family planning discourse. I shall conclude by describing the strategies that men and family planning advocates have adopted thus far to begin to reconcile the conflicts of interest among themselves and with women's health advocates.

Traces of Change

The debate on the need to include men in family planning can be traced back to the early 1960s. One of the first criticisms of the selective attention to women in family planning was published in *Research in Family Planning* in 1962. In "A Critique of the Traditional Planned Parenthood Approach in Developing Areas," J. Mayone Stycos (presently Professor of Population and Development Studies at Cornell University, then affiliated with Princeton University) argued that the ideology of the international family planning and population establishment was guilty of several "biases" that resulted in a neglect of men in family planning.[2] The author recommended a greater emphasis on men in family planning services that could be realized by "much greater utilization of male employees . . . greater reliance on male contraceptive techniques, emphasis on the economic and social rationale for birth control rather than on health, and greater utilization of mass media" (Stycos 1962: 500 in Stycos 1996). I discovered Stycos's paper because a revised version was reprinted in the newsletter *Men and Family Planning*, launched by the Population Council in October 1996. Stycos's paper thus has lived two lives: one in the early 1960s and one in the late 1990s. The reactions to this publication show, in a nutshell, the change in perspective that has taken place in the world of family planning over the last thirty-five years. Whereas in 1962 Stycos's paper met with the "consternation and scorn of many of his peers," the Population Council's newsletter praised Stycos's arguments because they represented "the new perspective being taken seriously today by the mainstream in the post-Cairo area" (Population Council 1997: 1).[3]

This shift toward including men in family planning discourse is clearly reflected in the family planning research literature. In the early 1960s family planning articles focused exclusively on women. Publications on men and family planning first appeared after the mid-1960s. In the following years, the number of published articles on women and men seemed to reach an equal number of about 700 per year for both sexes. In the late 1960s, however, the number of published articles on women continued to grow to about 2,500 per year. On the other hand, the number of published articles on men declined to 600 in the late 1980s, increasing again to 900 by 1993. Moreover, there has been an increase in the number of publications with both "women" and "men" or "couple" as keywords, which shows a pattern similar to that of the references to publications on men (Stycos 1996: 5).[4]

Other signs of change can be found in the tools used by family planning organizations and researchers to collect data on family planning, particularly the large-scale demographic surveys that have been carried out since the establishment of birth control programs in the 1950s and 1960s. During the 1970s and early 1980s, the World Fertility Survey (WFS)—the first worldwide program to collect statistics on fertility, particularly in Southern countries, and in that time the principal source of information concerning family planning and contraceptives—largely ignored men. Men were interviewed in only four of the 42 surveys (Hulton and Falkingham 1996: 90). The WFS standard questionnaire only included questions for women about their husbands' occupations and education. In the early 1980s, the WFS intended to develop a special questionnaire for "husband surveys." Although a draft was prepared, it was never developed into a final questionnaire (Singh 1987: 89). In the thousand-page report of the WFS, men are made invisible once again; the index of that volume does not contain a single item on men (Cleland and Scott 1987).

The two large-scale surveys that followed the WFS in the mid-1980s, the Demographic and Health Survey (DHS) and the Family Planning Survey (FPS), initially showed a similar almost exclusive attention to women. Since 1984 these two survey programs have interviewed more than 300,000 women in more than forty Southern countries (Robey et al. 1992: 1). As a result, a country's fertility rate has been, and still is, measured as the average fertility rate of women (Sachs 1994: 15).[5] Compared to the WFS, the DHS questionnaire included more questions about women's partners. In this survey program, women were asked questions about their partner's attitudes toward family planning, number of children, and communication on matters of sex and reproduction. Although the DHS thus provided more information on male attitudes toward family planning, this information was still based on experiences reported by female respondents. The first surveys in which men were interviewed as individuals were initiated in 1987 in Mali by the DHS and in 1993 in Jamaica by the FPS (Robey et al. 1992: 38–39).

Since 1985 "young adults" have also come to be included in demographic surveys, particularly in Latin America and the Caribbean. In these surveys, married and unmarried young people (men and women) were interviewed to collect information about their sexual experience and contraceptive use (Robey et al. 1992: 28). The name of this survey, "The Young Adult Reproductive Health Survey" (ARHS), indicates its specific focus. Whereas the DHS and the FPS were designed to monitor and control the growth or decline of populations, the ARHS aimed to collect data to address the problems of teenage pregnancy and sexually transmitted disease (Robey et al. 1992: 29). The decision to include men in these surveys thus stems from a concern with public health rather than an effort to lower population growth rates. Although men were gradually included in family planning research and demographic surveys in the 1980s, one reviewer of the family planning literature concluded as late as 1996 that men are "as yet a little understood group" (Hulton and Falkingham 1996: 98).

Agents of Change

As happened with contraceptive R&D, women's health advocates have been important actors in changing the status quo in family planning. Over the last two decades, feminist activists, both inside and outside family planning organizations, have lobbied extensively to change family planning policy to include men in family planning as an important tool to improve women's health. Since the early 1980s, women's health groups worldwide have collaborated to advocate a shift toward shared responsibility between women and men in matters relating to reproduction, sexual behavior, and health. One major strategy adopted by feminists in their campaign to include men in family planning has been to try to change the policy agenda of the U.N. International Conference on Population and Development, organized once every decade. The U.N. conference in Mexico in 1984 was the first conference to mention the importance of including men in family planning. The action program that was developed at the Mexico conference emphasized the need for new male contraceptives as well as better information and education to stimulate men to participate in family planning (U.N. 1984). Due to the activism of women's health organizations and family planning organizations—most notably the international, U.S.-based, non-governmental organization Access to Voluntary and Safe Contraception (AVSC) and the Population Council—the issue of men and family planning became even more central during the U.N. conference in Cairo in 1994 (U.N. ICPD 1994a). At that conference, 183 nations signed a program of action calling for an expansion of programs to "enable men to share more equally in family planning," and emphasizing the need to develop new male contraceptives (U.N. ICPD 1994a). The affirmation that family planning activities should reach out to men fitted neatly into the change in perspective first put forward in Cairo toward recognizing "individual reproductive rights" rather than demographic concerns as the goal of family planning programs (Harper 1994: 6; Hulton and Falkingham 1996: 98). The program of action adopted at the Cairo conference defined reproductive rights as "the rights of men and women to be informed and to have access to safe, effective, affordable and acceptable methods of fertility regulation of their choice" (U.N. ICPD 1994b: para. 7.2).[6]

In the years following the Cairo conference, international and national family planning and population agencies strengthened their policies to include men in their programs. In 1994 the AVSC initiated a specific family planning program to "increase the international family planning community's awareness of and commitment to male involvement in family planning" (Jezowski 1994: 8; Population Council 1997:10). In February 1995 the Population Council started the newsletter *Men and Families*, published in Spanish and English and distributed throughout Latin America and the Caribbean. The Population Council also launched a newsletter in 1996, entitled *Toward a New Partnership: Encouraging the Positive Involvement of Men as Supportive Partners in Reproductive Health*, with the aim to "share information among our network on partnership that includes Council staff working regionally and in New York [the Population Council's headquarters] as well as staff from collegial organizations that have also begun to focus on this topic" (Population Council 1996: 1).

Over the last couple of years, these newsletters have reported on a small but growing number of family planning organizations and programs that have initiated special activities to focus on men in countries in Africa, Latin America, the Caribbean, the U.K., and the United States. These initiatives include holding workshops to involve policymakers and local religious leaders, adapting family planning services in the clinic to serve men, hiring and training male family planning workers, and campaigning to change the attitudes of men toward family planning, including "discussion groups, lectures, drop-in centers, counseling, 'Fathers Clubs,' videos, etc." (Jezowski 1994: 8; Sachs 1994: 19; Gallen, Liskin, and Kok 1986; Danforth and Green 1997).[7] These changes in family planning are also visible in national family planning policy programs. Kenya and Mexico have formulated policies to enhance men's responsibilities in family planning (Hardon and Hayes 1997: 19). The strategies of women's health groups and family planning organizations to include men in family planning policies have been successful, particularly on the international level.[8] In the late 1990s men were no longer the "forgotten 50 percent of family planning" (Potts 1976).

Counteracting Hegemonic Representations of Men and Masculinity

Given the almost exclusive focus on women that dominated the family planning community in the 1950s, 1960s, and 1970s, the change in perspective toward including men in family planning has not been easy to achieve. The problem was not just that men were absent from family planning discourse, which could have been solved simply by adding men as a new target group in family planning. In the eyes of the advocates of male participation, one of the major barriers was the existence of what they called widely held "myths" about men's attitudes toward family planning. A closer look at the family planning research literature identifies the images of men which the advocates of men's involvement in family planning considered problematic for their endeavor.

The most troubling image of men, as perceived by Stycos and other key actors such as WHO, was "the commonly held notion that men in developing countries are against family planning" (Male participation 1995: 3). To counteract this representation of men, social scientists conducted several surveys to show that men had a very positive attitude toward family planning. Based on surveys in the 1960s, social scientists pointed to the fact that "an overwhelming majority of males approve of family planning" (Mishra 1967: 208). Studies conducted in India revealed that men even tended to be "more receptive to adopting new ideas [about family planning methods] than females" (Mishra 1967: 163). Men and family planning advocates thus tried to replace hegemonic representations of men with representations that were easier to reconcile with their own endeavors. However, the introduction of these contrasting representations did not easily convince the research community and policymakers of the positive attitude of men toward family planning. Even in the 1990s men and family planning advocates thought it necessary to repeat the same message, as exemplified by a report of WHO. In 1995 WHO presented survey data and concluded that "75% of the men approved the use of family planning" (Male participation 1995). In a similar vein, Population Communication Services concluded in 1994 that "surveys conducted in several countries show that—contrary to popular beliefs—men want much more information about family planning" (Jezowski 1994: 8). Obviously, the representation of men as opponents of family planning is a very persistent image in the culture at large.

Another image of men that advocates of men's involvement in family planning tried to counteract was the idea that men want more children than women. In the 1996 version of his paper, Stycos criticized American family planning researchers, in particular the Population Reference Bureau, for keeping this "myth" alive "despite the overwhelming evidence that male attitudes are so close to female ones" (Stycos 1996: 6). Stycos criticized this organization for a misreading of the data of a DHS survey on male attitudes toward family planning. Whereas the Population Reference Bureau had presented its analysis of the DHS data under the headline "African Men Want More Children than Their Wives" (Ebin 1996), Stycos suggested that this conclusion was only valid for "five or six West African nations" and not for the ten countries in East Africa, North Africa, and Asia that had participated in these surveys (Stycos 1996: 6).

The idea that men want more children than women has been a very dominant representation of men, particularly non-white men. When Stycos started his research on human fertility in the 1950s in Puerto Rico, he expected to find support for his hypothesis that "machismo was producing sex crazed males anxious to demonstrate their fertility," but he found little evidence to support this claim. Instead, he found that "gender differences in desired family size were small, that machismo was not a major factor in fertility goals" (Stycos 1996: 2). Similar conclusions were reported in surveys conducted in Chicago in the early 1960s, where the authors concluded that "there is no evidence whatever that Negroes' high fertility arises from a desire for larger families or from high fertility attitudes and values. Instead, Negro fertility attitudes are very similar to those of the white population" (Mishra 1967: 162–63). The Chicago surveys were initiated to examine "a number of often heard accusations that the low socio-economic status men [such as the Negro population] want larger families; that they do not approve of family planning; that they do not foresee the dangers of rapid population growth as it concerns themselves, their community, and the nation, and that males, in general, are indifferent to family planning matters" (Mishra 1967: 266). These studies illustrate how family planning researchers in the 1960s tried to come to terms with the then dominant representation of lower-class men of color as the "other," as the scapegoats of "overpopulation." As late as 1972, a British social scientist concluded from a survey among "lower class males" in Britain that "any attempted reeducation process [in family planning] must take into account the lower-class male's fear of emasculation" (Balswick 1972: 195).[9]

The machismo view of men identified by family planning researchers not only emphasized gender and class differences in desired family size, but also contained a strong emphasis on the higher fertility of men "because they stay fertile much longer than women do, and because they tend to be more pro-miscuous" (Sachs 1994: 13). A publication by the Worldwatch Institute in 1994 exemplifies this representation of men and fertility. In "Men, Sex, and Parent-hood," the authors told the story of a Moroccan emperor who had fathered "more than 1,000 children by the time he turned 50" (Sachs 1994: 14). Al-though the authors mentioned briefly that male attitudes had changed in the previous two decades, they used this example to argue that many men, par-ticularly in sub-Saharan African countries, "have continued to have large families, in part because large families serve as cultural symbols of a man's virility and wealth" (Sachs 1994: 14). Although the image that "the typical man wants a large family to prove his masculinity" no longer dominates family planning discourse, this representation is thus still alive. A different version of this representation, this time addressing Western men, can also be found in feminist discourse in the 1980s, where women claimed that gender differ-ences in contraceptive use "can be understood partly by recognizing that virility is tied to fertility in Western industrial society" (Kinnon 1985, in Laird 1994: 459).

The intriguing thing is that a representation of men that portrays (high) fertility as an essential part of masculinity can also be found among the advocates of male involvement in family planning, although they use it in a different way. For advocates such as Stycos, who want to dismiss the macho image as a myth, this representation constrains both the larger effort to legitimize the feasibility of involving men in family planning and the need to develop new male contraceptives. If men do not want to control their fertility, advocacy of a focus on men in family planning will remain an uphill battle that can never be won (Stycos 1996: 2). Other advocates, such as the Worldwatch Institute, however, use this representation as a rhetorical device to argue that family planning organizations should make a greater effort to reach men because "their higher fertility levels contribute disproportionately to population growth." If people continue to dismiss these "facts," they argue, the effort to reduce the rate of population growth is likely to fail (Sachs 1994).

The cultural work of men and family planning advocates has not been restricted to articulating non-hegemonic representations of men. A major part of the work consists of redefining what should be considered as the major constraints on involving men in family planning. Pioneers such as Stycos redefined the problem as one of communication between partners, rather than of male opposition to family planning. Based on his field studies in Puerto Rico, Stycos concluded that "husbands and wives often failed to communicate on mundane matters, but especially on matters of sex and reproduction" (Stycos 1996: 2). Since the 1980s, decision making in matters of family planning and contraception has become a major issue in family planning research.[10]

Another redefinition of the problem of involving men in family planning put forward by men and family planning advocates is that family planning services are not accessible to men. These advocates suggest that "only theoretically have men been always 'welcome' in family planning clinics." In practice, family planning clinics were set up "by and for women to focus on women's sexual health needs" (Seex 1996). This would explain the fact that less than 3 percent of service users are men (Seex 1996: 111). In a recent survey among USAID-funded family planning agencies, the woman-centered focus of family planning clinics and programs was mentioned as one of the most important constraints to involving men in family planning (Danforth and Green 1997: vii). Some men in family planning have reformulated the problem in terms of a resistance among service providers to considering men as potential clients of family planning clinics (Jezowski 1994: 9).

A third way of redefining the problem of men and family planning, put forward by male involvement advocates, does not define the problem as one of unwilling men or family planning clinics but as one of the availability of contraceptive technologies for men. The marginal role of men in family planning is ascribed to the introduction of new contraceptives for women and the scarcity of contraceptives available for men. Here, the advocates refer to studies showing that the introduction of the IUD and the oral contraceptive pill in the 1960s resulted in a decrease in the use of male contraceptives (Seex 1996; Stokes 1980: 6). The view that the major constraint in including men in family planning is the lack of choice in contraceptive methods for men is articulated particularly by WHO (Male participation 1995: 3). This redefinition of the problem is an important rhetorical device for articulating and legitimating the need for the development of new contraceptives for men, a project in which WHO plays an important role.

Changing the Objectives and Vocabulary of Family Planning

An important strategy in the advocacy of male involvement in family planning has thus consisted of counteracting the dominant cultural narratives on men and family planning. This was only a first step in changing family planning discourse toward the inclusion of men. Another equally, or maybe even more, important part of the cultural work of men and family planning advocates consisted of changing the objectives and vocabulary of family planning. An impression of these changes can be derived from the titles of the literature on men and family planning published between 1983 and 1996.[11] A large part of this literature consists of what I call traditional family planning discourse, that is, a discourse in which population control and limiting family size are articulated as the major objectives of family planning. But there is one important difference: men, rather than women, are the targets of research and family planning. In this literature the authors simply adopt the same language that has long been used in the traditional family planning literature on women. Key terms frequently used include "male fertility trends," "male knowledge of contraception," "male attitudes toward family limitation," "men's role in family planning," and so on. Most published reports relate information on national surveys or specific case-studies in Southern countries. A second variation on the traditional family planning discourse, which also includes a large part of the published reports on men and family planning, is a focus on couples and decision-making in family planning, a trend I mentioned in the previous section of this chapter. Titles that exemplify this approach are "Couples' Decision-making Process Regarding Fertility" (Beckman 1978b); "Family Planning Communication between Spouses in Sri Lanka" (Kane and Sivasubramaniam 1989); "The Role of Interspousal Communication in Adoption of Family Planning Methods" (Shah 1974); and "Who Decides? Determinants of Couple Cooperation and Agreement in United States Fertility" (Williams 1992). These trends represent the least drastic changes in focus in family planning discourse. They required only a change in research subjects. Instead of women, family planning researchers focused on men and couples. A clear departure from the objectives of traditional family planning is visible in the family planning literature which focuses on male adolescents in Northern countries, particularly the United States. Whereas the objectives of traditional family planning are framed in terms of controlling populations or limiting family size, this literature addresses the problem of so-called "single parent families," under titles such as "Fatherless America: Confronting Our Most Urgent Social Problem" (1995), "Good Dads—Bad Dads: Two Faces of Fatherhood: The Changing American Family" (1988), and "Fertility and Commitment: Bringing Men Back into Fertility in the United States" (1996). This literature reflects the growing concern in the United States that emerged in the late 1980s regarding teenage pregnancy and its social effects on families. Here, we see the first indications of a change in discourse. Since the late 1980s, the vocabulary of family planning research has been enriched with words such as "commitment" and "responsible fatherhood." Another departure from the objectives of traditional family planning is visible in the literature which links family planning to reproductive health issues. Due to the increase in sexually transmitted diseases, particularly HIV, sexual behavior is not only of interest in regulating fertility but also in preventing sex-related diseases. As a result, terms such as "safer sex," "prevention of sexually transmitted diseases," and "reproductive health" have been introduced into the vocabulary of family planning literature.

Last, but not least, the appearance of men in family planning literature reflects a third change in the objectives of family planning. In this literature, the focus is not so much on single-parent families or sexually transmitted disease as on gender equality. Indicative of this shift are publications with titles such as: "Does the Responsibility for Family Planning Rest Primarily with Women? (1983)," "Of Patriarchy Born: The Political Economy of Fertility Decisions" (1983), "Male Responsibility for Family Planning" (1984), "Achieving Gender Equality in Families: The Role of Males" (1995), "The Misunderstood Gender: Male Involvement in the Family and in Reproductive and Sexual Health in Latin America and the Caribbean" (1996), and "Notes on Rethinking Masculinities" (1996). Here, we see a drastic change in vocabulary that can be ascribed to the advocacy of the women's health movement in the 1980s and 1990s. Key terms in this grouping of literature include "gender equality," "sharing responsibilities," "power relations in the family," "autonomy of women," "male involvement," and "masculinities"—all terms that were completely absent from family planning discourse prior to the 1980s.

The incorporation of a feminist-inspired vocabulary is also reflected explicitly in the reports of the U.N. International Conference on Population and Development held in Cairo in 1994. The program of action of this conference devoted an entire chapter, entitled "Gender Equality, Equity, and Empowerment of Women," to feminist concerns. The chapter contained a special paragraph on "Male Responsibilities and Participation": "The objective is to promote gender equality in all spheres of life, including family and community life, and to encourage and enable men to take responsibility for their sexual and reproductive behavior and their social and family roles" (U.N. ICPD 1994b: par. 4.25).

The action program also specified the areas of men's shared responsibility: "parenthood, sexual and reproductive health and behavior, including family planning; prenatal, maternal and child health; prevention of sexually transmitted diseases, including HIV; prevention of unwanted and high-risk pregnancies; shared control and contribution of family income, children's education, health and nutrition; and promotion of the equal value of children of both sexes" (U.N. ICPD 1994b: par. 4.27).

The U.N. Fourth World Conference on Women held in Beijing in 1995 showed a similar shift in discourse. At this conference the terms of debate were explicitly redefined by framing men's participation in family planning as an important tool for improving women's health and rights. The plan of action stressed the importance of including men in reproductive health programs: "Shared responsibility between men and women in matters related to reproductive and sexual behavior is essential to improving women's health" (quoted in Danforth and Green 1997: 3).

The U.N. documents thus exemplify the wide variety of concerns that underlie the change in family planning discourse toward including men. Whereas the objectives of the family planning community prior to the 1980s were largely framed in terms of lowering population growth rates, the last two decades have witnessed an enormous broadening of the agenda toward increasing equality between men and women and preventing diseases, especially sexually transmitted infections. This change is also reflected in a change in terminology: the documents of the U.N. conferences and policy programs of family planning organizations are increasingly framed in terms of reproductive health rather than family planning.

The Contested Nature of Vocabularies

The analysis presented thus far may have given the impression that changing the objectives and vocabulary of family planning has been a smooth process. However, appearances are deceptive. In texts such as bibliographies, words that hide worlds of difference can peacefully coexist. Published articles that appeared in the mid-1990s indicate that different vocabularies can hide more than worlds of difference; they can also hide severe conflicts and struggles. Terminology became a contested zone in the world of family planning in the mid-1990s. The very use of words such as "male involvement" has become a risky practice. I learned this when I contacted the Population Council to obtain more information on their work to involve men in family planning. In response to my request, I was told that the Population Council preferred the term "men as partners" in discussions about how to involve men in family planning: "The Council is very actively moving forward in the area of what we are calling 'Partnership' issues. We prefer this term of 'male involvement' because we like to see greater involvement of men that does not in any way impede women's autonomy in terms of sexuality and reproductive health— something that still is far from being a fact in many cultural settings" (e-mail from Ann Leonard, Population Council, 6 August 1997). Or, as one of the participants at the Beijing conference in 1995 formulated it: "Raise the subject of male involvement in reproductive health, and you raise hackles" (Steele Verme, Wegner, and Jerzowski 1996: 10).

An analysis of two feminist journals may give more insight into the potential conflicts hidden behind apparently neutral, dispassionate terms like "male involvement." In May 1996 *Reproductive Health Matters*, a British journal with an editorial policy to publish papers that "offer women-centered perspectives and take gender issues into account," devoted a special issue to men and family planning, laconically entitled "Men." The introduction to this special issue clearly demonstrates the highly political and contested nature of the cultural work to include men in family planning. In the first section, entitled "Why Men? Why Now?" Marge Berer, the editor of the journal, voiced her concerns as follows:

> Now, just as women's specific problems are finally getting some attention on the world stage, and well before those problems have been adequately addressed, it seems that focusing only on women is no longer acceptable. Arising from the International Conference on Population and Development (Cairo, 1994) there have been calls for men to work for and support the empowerment of women. Yet in an apparently unnoticed transformation of intent, a growing chorus of voices in the field have turned this into a call for male involvement and male participation in reproductive health—in some cases with any reference to women muted or even missing. (Berer 1996: 7)

To support her argument that women are in many ways subordinated to men, Berer went on to describe the dominant role men play in the world of family planning, not as users of contraceptives or clients of family planning services, but as "researchers, clinicians, senior-medical staff, policymakers, law makers and funders." The editor also warned the reader that despite the gradual changes in power relations between men and women, "this is a dangerous moment for both men and women in the history of gender relations, because men's self-definition as well as women's growing sense of independence and autonomy are both at stake" (Frykman 1996: 11). Referring to differences between men and women in matters of reproductive health—men do not die or suffer from complications of pregnancy and childbirth—Berer concluded that "involvement of men in the few areas where women have achieved or desperately need autonomy may end up empowering men even more, that is to say, disempowering women even further and not the other way around" (Berer 1996: 8, 10).

The introduction to the special issue of *Reproductive Health Matters* thus illustrates the major reservations of some feminist critics regarding attempts to include men in family planning. A change in focus toward men is considered by these critics to be a serious threat to the still fragile achievements of the women's health movement to make family planning policies congruent with policies to increase women's autonomy and to decrease gender inequalities. By articulating this criticism, feminists tried to intervene in family planning policies by putting power relations between men and women back on the agenda. This intervention can be understood in the context of the declining support for feminist concerns in society at large in the mid-1990s. In a period in which *The Economist* devoted a leading article, entitled "Men: Tomorrow's Second Sex," to the decreasing dominance of men in the labor market and at home in Northern countries, policies that explicitly call for changes to include men are easily understood by feminists as a "backlash" (*The Economist*, 28 September 1996). In *Reproductive Health Matters*, the editor explicitly situated the issue of male involvement in family planning in the context of this wider debate by including two papers that focused on changes in men's positions in society. In "Men: The Most Powerful 'Minority' Ever," the author described tendencies among men in England in the 1990s to claim an identity as "victim[s] of virtually every force in modern society," as if to conclude that if men succeeded in becoming acknowledged as victims, "women [would] have a lot to lose because men could become 'the most powerful minority ever created' " (Wilkinson 1996: 157). And in "Space for a Man: The Transformation of Masculinity in Twentieth-Century Culture," the author reached a similar conclusion when he described a trend in Swedish society where men have begun to profile themselves against women to try to reconquer positions they have lost (Frykman 1996: 12, 16). As these papers were reprints of previously published papers in journals for a different audience, the authors did not discuss the problems that might arise by including men in family planning.

These feminist interventions illustrate the ambivalence of the women's health movement toward involving men in family planning. On the one hand, feminists figure as advocates of making men responsible for family planning; on the other hand, feminists figure as major critics of the shift in focus in family planning toward including men. Some feminists even articulated a strong opposition to the entire endeavor, particularly if family planning services for men competed with reproductive health services for women. This position is most clearly voiced by the editor of *Reproductive Health Matters*:

> Women carry a far greater burden of reproductive morbidity and mortality, and of physical and social responsibility for fertility and its consequences, than men. These are matters of life and death for women, yet in many countries "need" has not been translated into comprehensive, accessible information, support or services for all women. Why then should it do so for men? Furthermore, who will pay? It may well be women who have to pay—in decreasing funding for services for women. On the grounds of need alone, in a world of scarce resources for women and women's health, services for women must come first. (Berer 1996: 10)

The editor concluded the Introduction by accusing organizations that had been working for women's health for decades of jumping on the bandwagon of focusing on men to get extra funding. One of these organizations, the International Planned Parenthood Federation (IPPF), also figures as a contributor to the special issue on men. In the mid-1980s, this organization launched poster campaigns that explicitly addressed men's sexual attitudes to encourage them to empathize with women in matters of family planning. In her contribution to *Reproductive Health Matters*, Judith Frye Helzner, Director of Program Coordination of the IPPF, largely endorsed the criticism voiced by the editor that a focus on men might increase inequalities between women and men: "As more agencies in the field begin to take on this issue, a critical view is called for, to avoid the potential for worsening current inequalities in female–male power dynamics, not only at the level of individual contraceptive users, but also in program design and management" (Frye Helzner 1996: 146). Helzner thus extended feminist criticism to include the gender dynamics between women and men in family planning organizations. Helzner's and Berer's contributions show the volatile, political issues at stake in changing family planning discourse toward including men.

The IPPF's contribution to the special issue of *Reproductive Health Matters* shows that feminists have been very successful in convincing family planning organizations of their concerns. In her paper, Helzner explicitly adopted feminist concerns regarding women's autonomy as a reference to evaluate the developments in the field of men and family planning over the last twenty years and concluded: "Family planning organizations deploy very different approaches towards including men in family planning. Not all of these are created equal—those which would increase or even just maintain male power at the expense of women should not be considered advances in the field" (Frye Helzner 1996: 146). Moreover, Helzner did not hesitate to criticize some of her colleagues in the field of family planning: "In some work on the involvement of men as contraceptors and as male program staff in the field, there are studies which note in a neutral way, or ignore, the broader context of inequality between men and women in society and in the workplace. There is something unsettling about these so-called gender-blind or gender-neutral analyses" (Frye Helzner 1996: 148B).

To illustrate her concern, Helzner pointed to family planning campaigns in Guatemala and Zimbabwe, where the staff had encouraged men to take control over their female partners' use of contraceptives, and she described the negative impact such campaigns would have on the power relations between men and women "in a situation where men are already making decisions about almost everything" (Frye Helzner: 148). The family planning literature shows similar examples of family planning programs that promote the counseling of husbands about new contraceptive methods used by their partners, as is exemplified in titles like "Effect of Husband Counseling on Norplant Contraceptive Acceptability" and "Oral Contraception in Bangladesh: Social Marketing and the Importance of Husbands" (Frye Helzner 1996: 148).

Another feminist journal that exemplifies the conflicts underlying the advocacy of involving men in family planning is *Arrows for Change: Women and Gender Perspectives in Health Policies and Programs*. This Malaysian-based journal, funded by the Swedish International Development Authority, specifically addresses audiences in the Asian Pacific region, including "decisionmakers in health, population, and family planning, and women's organizations" (Men's roles 1996 : 2). The May 1996 issue of this journal opened with an editorial entitled "Men's Roles and Responsibilities in Reproduction." Although the editor of this journal reached a conclusion similar to that of her colleague at *Reproductive Health Matters*, she approached the problem from a different angle. Evaluating the attempts that have been made since the early 1980s to increase male participation in family planning programs, the editor concluded that the use of contraception by men had not increased significantly in this period. In contrast to many biomedical researchers and WHO, she did not ascribe this failure to the lack of appropriate contraception for men but to the demographic objectives of many family planning programs that do not address "the underlying beliefs and attitudes on the roles of women and men in reproduction" (Men's roles 1996 : 1). Referring to the U.N. conferences in Cairo and Beijing, the editor of *Arrows for Change* concluded: "The old concept of male participation needs to be recast to focus on reproductive responsibilities towards the long-term goal of recognition of the equal rights and responsibilities of women and men (gender equality) in the family and society" (Men's roles 1996: 2).

The red line that runs through these feminist criticisms can thus be summarized as a warning that policies designed to include men in family planning run the risk of increasing gender inequalities if they fail to acknowledge the current power relations between women and men. For feminists, any policy in the field of family planning, including those concerning the role of men, should be directed toward increasing women's reproductive health and rights. So, instead of focusing on the needs of men in matters of reproduction, family planning policies should be oriented toward involving men in a more "women-supportive" and "constructive way" (Berer 1996: 9). This view is articulated most explicitly by the editor of *Reproductive Health Matters*: "If empowering women is to remain the end point of the exercise, then policies for change that involve men must also be grounded in a women-centered and gender-sensitive perspective, not just taking men's perspectives or needs into account" (Berer 1996: 9).

Although the editors of the two feminist journals and the program director of IPPF voiced very similar criticisms, they did not offer the same solutions. Whereas the editor of *Reproductive Health Matters* concluded that women's reproductive health services should come first in times of scarce resources (which in the present situation of limited funding for family planning implies a withdrawal from involving men in family planning activities), the editor of *Arrows for Change* and the director of the IPPF called for a critical reflection on the terminology used in family planning policies concerning men in an effort to develop a gender awareness among policymakers and the staff of family planning organizations. Or, to quote Helzner: "There is as yet no generally accepted understanding of what men's involvement actually means. . . . The seemingly simple phrase 'male involvement' still hides a variety of different meanings and philosophies. . . . In this post-Cairo, post-Beijing age, we need to reach a new consensus on the meanings of these terms, and on when these concepts are appropriate" (Frye Helzner 1996: 146).

Inventing a New Language

In the mid-1990s, changing the very words in which family planning policies involving men are framed became an important strategy for negotiating the acknowledgment of women's autonomy and reproductive health as an integral part of family planning policies. To realize this, feminists chose two influential arenas: the U.N. International Conference on Population and Development, held in Cairo in 1994, and the U.N. Fourth Conference on Women, held in Beijing in 1995. The articles in *Reproductive Health Matters* and *Arrows for Change* are a reflection of discussions initiated during these conferences. A closer look at the debates that took place during the U.N. conference in Cairo allows us to analyze these negotiations in more detail.

During the Cairo conference, the question of how to increase men's participation in family planning was one of many issues under debate, both during the official meetings of the conference, where the member nations had to reach agreement on a program of action, and in the meetings of the NGO Forum, a conference organized by non-governmental organizations and held in conjunction with the U.N. conference. The NGO Forum is of particular interest here because women's health organizations are non-governmental organizations and therefore not allowed to participate in U.N. conferences. The NGO Forum devoted three workshops to the subject "Men, Family Planning, and Reproductive Health," organized and sponsored by AVSC and attended by policymakers, family planning managers, women's health advocates, male contraceptive researchers, and family planning service providers. In "The Language of Male Involvement: What Do You Mean?," a paper published in the November 1996 issue of *Populi*, the U.N. Population Fund magazine, three directors and managers of the Association for Voluntary and Safe Contraception (AVSC) vividly described the atmosphere of the debates in Cairo:

> The current language of male involvement raises more questions than it answers. The 1994 International Conference on Population and Development and the 1995 Fourth World Conference on Women are two cases in point. In preparatory meetings for both conferences, participants endured the heat and humming fluorescent lights of the U.N.'s basement conference rooms and argued back and forth for hours about what was and what was not implied by certain words pertaining to the concept of

male involvement. Consensus was reached eventually, denoting, if nothing else, that it is important to acknowledge male involvement in reproductive health. But what is meant by involving men and the words with which to describe their involvement—let alone the question of how to get them involved—remain contentious issues. (Steele Verme, Wegner, and Jerzowski 1996: 10)

The AVSC not only facilitated these debates by organizing and sponsoring workshops on this issue, it also adopted the role of trying to create consensus about which terms were acceptable in formulating policies to increase men's participation in family planning. The debates among women's health advocates and family planning organizations in Cairo indicate that the then current terminology to describe men's roles in family planning elicited various interpretations and reactions among both parties. This debate focused particularly on three commonly used terms: "men's involvement," "men's programs," and "men's responsibility." "Men's involvement" was considered problematic because it implies that men are not yet involved in family planning and that involvement is necessarily a constructive act. This term turned out to be unacceptable for those feminists who argue that "men are already too involved in reproductive health as policy makers, service providers, or husbands" (Steele Verme, Wegner, and Jerzowski 1996: x). We have seen this type of argument voiced by the editor of *Reproductive Health Matters*. The term "men's program" has turned out to be equally problematic for women's health advocates. The AVSC summarized the criticisms evoked by this term as follows: " 'Men's programs' portends an oppositional force to women's programs that is alienating or threatening to many women's health advocates. Won't men's programs simply compete for or siphon off resources now devoted to women's health? Just as men's interests dominate politics and health care, won't that happen with men's programs in reproductive health? Will women's concerns in reproductive health, long fought and hard won, be sidelined again?" (Steele Verme, Wegner, and Jerzowski 1996: 11).

Compared to the terms "men's involvement" and "men's programs," the term "men's responsibility" was considered less problematic because the term "responsibility" has positive connotations and is closely linked to feminist concerns with family planning. Women's health advocates have used this term to argue that men should share the burden of contraception and to participate more actively in childrearing and family life. The AVSC, however, considered this term problematic because of its negative normative connotation for men. According to the AVSC, the term can be read as a judgment that men are irresponsible in nature. Moreover, the term does not speak to the interests of men in relating to their own partner's reproductive health. Because none of the existing terms seemed to be acceptable to both parties, the AVSC opted to introduce a new term, "men as partners": "By running into these linguistic pitfalls and testing a number of alternatives, we have come to propose language for our work that describes men as partners, a concept we hope evokes more balanced roles and acknowledges that women's reproductive health, whether we like it or not, is influenced by their partners (and vice versa)" (Steele Verme, Wegner, and Jerzowski 1996: 11).

By introducing this term, the AVSC did not try to meet all criticisms put forward by women's health advocates. The conclusions of "The Language of Male Involvement: What Do You Mean?" show an explicit departure from radical feminist views that prioritize women's reproductive health at the cost of men's reproductive health: "Just as we have fought for recognition of women's many roles, needs and interests in reproductive, productive and sexual life, so we feel that it is important to address these for men. When discussing men's participation in reproductive health, we should not walk backwards down the road we have traveled in advocacy for women's reproductive health: let's stop classifying clients' needs and behaviors by gender and avoid such stereotyping in the words we use and hear" (Steele Verme, Wegner, and Jerzowski 1996: 12). "Men as partners" thus became the new term meant to consolidate the conflicts of interest between the presence of men in family planning initiatives and the less radical women's health advocates.

It is not a coincidence that the AVSC adopted this role of bridging the worlds of women's health advocates and advocates of men in family planning. In contrast to other family planning organizations, the AVSC already had a long-standing tradition of focusing on men and family planning policies. Initially founded in 1943 as the Association for Voluntary Surgical Contraception, the AVSC had been involved with sterilization services based on free and informed choice for both women and men. Due to its policy to extend the AVSC's activities to contraceptives other than surgical methods, the AVSC changed its name to the Association for Voluntary and Safe Contraception in 1991. The AVSC was among the first family planning organizations to launch a special program to address men's roles in family planning. In the AVSC News of October 1991, the organization announced its initiative, initially named the AVSC Men's Program, as follows: "Constituting about half of the world's population, men represent the last great untapped market for family planning information and services. Although the AVSC and the agencies with which it works have made significant progress in introducing vasectomy to men around the world, a good deal more remains to be done. Consequently, AVSC has launched a special male initiative both to expand male sterilization services and to involve men more in contraceptive decision-making" (Harper and Jezowski 1991: 7).

The AVSC claimed a leadership in integrating men's programs into existing family planning programs: "AVSC will serve as a leading resource in addressing technical issues related to men's involvement in family planning. AVSC will continue to be a leader in addressing men's medical issues and in advancing understanding of the information and counseling needs of men" (Men's programs series 1994: 6). In the first years, articles in the AVSC News dealing with the Men's Program were largely framed in terms of "sharing responsibility" and "men's needs," stressing the need for "men's programs." The AVSC's attempts to reach consensus on the terminology can thus be understood as a strategy to diminish feminist resistance to its own program activities. In January 1996 the AVSC realized its advocacy of a new terminology by renaming its "Men's Program" the "Men as Partners in Reproductive Health" project.

Since 1996 this term has been adopted by other major actors in the world of family planning, most notably the Population Council. As mentioned earlier, the Population Council has included men on its agenda since the mid-1990s. Whereas the AVSC's decision to focus on men fitted seamlessly into the organization's long-standing tradition to implement vasectomy services for men, the Population Council's change in focus can be understood in the context of the organization's involvement in R&D for new contraceptives for men. In the memo in which the Population Council announced its policy to focus on men, the authors referred explicitly to this role of the Population Council. The paragraph in which the Population Council claimed a role for family planning organizations in changing gender roles is followed immediately by a paragraph describing the active involvement of the Population Council in contraceptive R&D: "In addition to our leading role in the development of male contraceptives across divisions, a number of Council staff are already beginning to explore the territory—an important precursor to the printing of maps!" (Leonard and Moore 1996: 4).

Whereas the AVSC defined the problem of the restricted role of men in family planning as a problem of limited access to family planning services, the Population Council defined the problem in terms of a lack of choice in male contraceptives (Chikamata 1997: 7). The Population Council's Center for Biomedical Research is currently involved in R&D and the clinical testing of two new male contraceptives methods: immunological methods and Gossypol

(Johansson interview 1996). The Population Council thus plays a dual role in the field of men and family planning. Like the AVSC, the Population Council is an important mediator between the world of women's health advocates and family planning initiatives involving men. In addition, the Population Council is an important actor in bridging the world of male contraceptive R&D and the world of family planning. In this respect, the Population Council is a typically hybrid organization that incorporates two worlds in one organization: contraceptive R&D (prior to the 1960s, mainly the domain of university and industrial laboratories) and family planning services. By combining so-called "hardware" and "software" approaches to family planning, the Population Council plays a pivotal role in changing family planning discourse toward including men. The name of the Population Council's newsletter specifically addressed to issues of the role of men in family planning, *Towards a New Partnership: Encouraging the Positive Involvement of Men as Supportive Partners in Reproductive Health*, exemplifies the effort of the Population Council to adopt a new language designed to reconcile the potentially conflicting interests of women's health advocates and family planning initiatives for men. The terms "new partnership," "positive involvement," and "supportive partners" are explicitly chosen to avoid any chance of misreading the objectives of the Population Council. In "MEN —What Are We Going to Do About Them?," a memo distributed by the Population Council among its staff members in February 1996 to assess their interest in including a focus on men in the work of the Population Council, the authors explicitly referred to and positioned themselves in the debate initiated by women's health advocates:

> It has been a long and hard fight—and one that is far from over—to even affirm that women have a right to control their own sexuality. Therefore, the process of integrating men into the reproductive health equation needs to be weighed carefully against the embryonic, and still precarious, rights of women to control their bodies, especially their reproductive functions. We need to find ways to involve men as supportive partners and not simply make them another "target" audience—possibly at the risk of their partners' well-being. (Leonard and Moore 1996: 3)

The debates over which words should be used to address the role of men in family planning show how the same terminology can have completely different meanings for different groups. Whereas "male involvement" has a positive connotation for advocates of men in family planning, because it is a useful term to express the need to share responsibilities for family planning between the sexes, women's health advocates read the term as a threat

Table 1

Terminology Appropriate to Emphasize the Individual Reproductive
Rights of Women and Men

Women	Men
Reproductive rights of women	Reproductive rights of men
Autonomy	Men's needs
Empowerment of women	

to women's autonomy in matters of contraception. The reverse happened
with the term "men's responsibility." This term has positive connotations for
women's health advocates, who argue that men should share the risks of
contraceptives. Advocates of family planning for men, however, interpret this
term as a judgment that men are intrinsically irresponsible. The debate over
terminology thus shows that words are not neutral. Language may exert hidden power. What is at stake in this debate is "who controls whose fertility"
(Steele Verme, Wegner, and Jerzowski 1996: 10). The AVSC clearly acknowledged these political aspects of language. By introducing the term "men as
partners," they intervened in a debate that, without intervention, could have
led to a further polarization between women's health advocates and family
planning initiatives for men. The term "men as partners" implies a drastic
change in perspective. Whereas terms such as "male involvement" and "male
responsibility" take men as the referent and address the moral qualities of
individual men, the term "men as partners" is a relational term defined from
the perspective of women (as family planning is practiced by heterosexual
partners). Or as AVSC's president Amy Pollack has formulated it: "Men's and
women's health are not isolated. As informed partners, we're stronger together" (Wegner 1997: 2). In this approach, family planning becomes a relational rather than an individual issue. Most importantly, the term is defined
from the perspective of women and can therefore be more easily reconciled
with issues of women's autonomy. "Men as partners" can thus be considered
a powerful metaphor because it brings together worlds that were in danger of
drifting apart.[12] If we adopt the view that "power is about whose metaphor
brings worlds together," as Leigh Star has suggested, we can conclude that
the advocates of family planning for men, and most notably the AVSC, have
been very successful in negotiating their interests. As I previously showed, the
term "men as partners" has become accepted as the dominant terminology in
the world of family planning. Women's health advocates, at least the less
radical organizations, have also been successful in negotiating their interests,

Table 2
Terminology Accepted during the U.N. International Conference
on Population and Development, Cairo, 1994

Women	Men
Reproductive rights of women	Men's responsibility
Autonomy	Men as partners
Empowerment of women	

particularly in securing reproductive rights and autonomy for women. Without their advocacy of women's reproductive health, the AVSC would not have managed to create consensus on terminology for family planning policies involving men. It is very likely that without this debate, the Cairo action program would have been framed in completely different terms. Given the change in focus toward recognizing individual reproductive rights rather than demographic concerns as the goal of reproductive health programs, the Cairo conference might well have had the outcome that appears in table 1. The terminology used for men would have become a mirror image of the terminology for women. Due to the intervention of women's health advocates, family planning policies and programs have adopted a strikingly different discourse for men, as shown in table 2. Women's health advocates have thus been very successful in changing the terms of the debate, and in creating a discourse and family planning for men that acknowledges feminist concerns.

Conclusions

Men have come to be included in family planning discourse. Changing family planning discourse toward including men, however, did not consist simply in adding men as a new target group: it required drastic changes in the objectives of family planning. Whereas the objectives of family planning prior to the 1970s consisted of controlling population growth and limiting family size, the 1980s witnessed a change toward a more diverse set of objectives, including concerns to reduce single-parent families, prevent sexually transmitted diseases, and enhance gender equality. This transformation was not a smooth process. Like the advocates for including men in contraceptive R&D, advocates of family planning for men faced severe constraints. Changing the family planning discourse toward including men required counteracting the dominant cultural narratives that portrayed men as being against family planning and as wanting more children than women. The dominant representation underlying these images was that fertility is an essential part of masculinity. As we have seen in this chapter, advocates of men and family planning for men have tried to overcome these barriers by trying to replace the hegemonic representations of men and masculinity with images that are more easily reconciled with their endeavors. To do so, they initiated qualitative research and surveys that showed that a large proportion of men approved of family planning. These studies articulated that the machismo image of men that equates masculinity with fertility is in decline.

The changes in family planning discourse toward men can largely be credited to the activism of women's health advocates, several family planning organizations (most notably the AVSC and the Population Council), and several social scientists in the field of family planning research.[13] Although women's health activists have been important agents of change, the role of this social movement shows a peculiar pattern. Feminists advocated making men more responsible for family planning, but they also acted as major opponents of including men in family planning. These contradictory activities can be understood if we take into account that the women's health movement is broad and diverse. Over the last two decades, women's health advocates and groups have articulated different views about which strategies are most effective for improving women's reproductive health and empowering women (Kammen 2000: 90–91). As we have seen, women's health advocates had different views of the eventual effects of including men in family planning. Whereas one group of women's health advocates considered men and family planning activities as competing with reproductive health services for women, another group considered the change toward including men in family planning as compatible with their interests. They suggested that sharing responsibilities between women and men in matters of reproduction and sexual behavior is essential to improving women's reproductive health.

These two conflicting assessments not only gave rise to heated debates among women's health advocates and groups, they also shaped the discourse about family planning for men. The radical feminist view provided another constraint on the emerging family planning programs involving men. It was therefore no coincidence that the family planning organizations involved in these activities put quite an effort into diminishing feminist resistance to their programs. The AVSC has played an important role in bridging the world of women's health activists and the world of family planning services for men. Here, we have seen how language can be an important tool in overcoming resistance. The term "men as partners," initiated by the AVSC, has functioned as such a tool in bringing both these worlds together. This reconciliation between the interests of both groups has been of crucial importance for the endeavor to transform family planning discourse toward including men. Women's health groups and advocates of family planning for men constitute important nodes in the sociotechnical networks around male contraceptive innovation. As the history of contraceptive development teaches, the women's health movement has been a major actor in demanding the development of new contraceptives and in lobbying against the introduction of specific methods. If organizations involved in family planning for men had paid no attention to feminist criticism, they would have run the risk that the critical voices of feminists would have gained momentum and eventually hindered the implementation of family planning incentives for men in the U.N. policies concerning family planning.

Most importantly, the reconciliation of the interests of advocates of men's involvement in family planning and women's health activists resulted in the transformation of family planning from an individual issue, in which women's interests are opposed to those of men, to a relational issue which emphasizes the common interests of women and men in matters of family planning. Consequently, policies involving men have come to be framed in completely different terms than the rhetorics used for women. Family planning policies for men are formulated not in terms of "men's needs" or "men's reproductive rights," which would have been the counterpart of the language adopted for women. Instead, they are framed in terms of "men's responsibilities" and "men as partners." Feminist interventions in the debate on men and family planning thus resulted in a situation in which representations of men in terms of autonomy and control of reproduction were prevented from gaining cultural articulation. Inventing new language thus played a major role in promoting the involvement of men in family planning discourse.

But now that the words are in place, what about the practices? It goes without saying that changing discourse requires more than just changing the terms of the debate. Discourse-building involves material interventions to put the words into practice. The next chapter therefore focuses on the material work that was required to change family planning discourse toward including men.

7

Making Room for Men: Configuring Men as Clients of Family Planning Clinics

. . . .

After having three children, my wife went on the Pill for her contraception because we could no longer afford an accident with the natural methods we were using. Her blood pressure immediately shot up, and she was advised to discontinue. She tried other methods but they had complications, too. I felt I was being unfair and it was my duty too, to take part in family planning. One morning we went together to our local family planning clinic. I will never forget how embarrassed I felt. There was not even a single man there, just queues of women and their babies. This was a woman's world and I felt totally lost.—Male visitor to family planning clinic, 1995

In the last two decades, men have come to be included in family planning discourse. A closer look at the practices of family planning services reveals, however, that there exists a huge gap between the rhetoric of promoting the involvement of men in family planning and the daily practices of family planning clinics. Today, most family planning clinics are still almost exclusively women's spaces (Leonard and Moore 1996: 3; Berer 1996: 6). In a typical family planning clinic we find waiting rooms crowded with women, a largely female staff, medical professionals specialized in female reproductive functions, opening hours in the daytime, and furnishings designed for women and babies. Most clinics have no facilities for men, not even a place for them to sit (Leonard and Moore 1996: 3). In the United States only 6 percent of all clients of publicly funded family planning clinics are men (Schulte and Sonensteinn 1995: 212). In the U.K. this proportion is even lower: in 1994 men constituted less than 3 percent of service users (Seex 1996). Other countries show a similar picture. The fact that family planning clinics are designed for women is also visible in the work practices of the clinics. Most clinics use clinic-record forms that have no space to record male visits for counseling (UNFPA 1995: 35). Donor agencies measure the success of family planning services only in terms of female-oriented services (Danforth and Green 1997: 1). Outreach workers of family planning clinics usually receive credit only for the number of women they have visited; visits to men are not counted (UNFPA 1995: 35). Giving attention to male clients is thus not considered part of the everyday responsibilities or the contractual requirements of family planning practitioners, nor as a relevant component of performance indicators of family planning programs.

The gap between the rhetoric and the practices of family planning is dramatically shown in a sign on the entrance to a family planning clinic in India that reads: "NO ENTRANCE FOR MEN" (AVSC 1997e). Changing family planning discourse to include men thus literally means making room for men. The incorporation of men as a clientele in the world of family planning depends not only on changing the objectives and rhetoric of family planning, but also requires a lot of material work. In this chapter, I want to explore two important aspects of this work. First, I will focus on the reorganization of the infrastructure of family planning clinics, particularly on changes in the organization of spaces and work. Second, I will analyze the material work involved in enrolling men as visitors to family planning clinics. The chapter concludes by showing how configuring men as clients of family planning clinics has led to the creation of a new category of patient.[1]

Whose Space Is It? Demarcating Spaces, Budgets, and Tasks

Where should men, the "new patients" of family planning clinics, be accommodated? This basic question has been asked ever since the need to introduce family planning programs and services for men was first articulated (Harper 1994: 9). Since clinics specializing in reproductive health care for men did not exist, there were two available options: either create new infrastructures for men, or integrate services for men into existing family planning clinics and primary health care clinics.[2] Most of the countries that have developed policies to include men in family planning have adopted the integrated approach. In the United States, male programs are primarily integrated into existing family planning clinics, hospital-based clinics for teenagers, and school-based clinics (Schulte and Sonensteinn 1995: 213). Similar situations exist in Latin America, Africa, Asia, and Europe. A 1997 survey of activities funded by the U.S. Agency for International Development (USAID) involving men in these regions indicated that most agencies preferred to integrate services for men into existing projects rather than to establish a separate new infrastructure for men (Danforth and Green 1997: viii).[3] The same survey suggested that only a few agencies actually promoted activities for men. Most USAID cooperating agencies have adapted services to provide for couples rather than targeting men separately (Danforth and Green 1997: 25). The U.N. Population Fund (UNFPA), another important sponsor of family planning programs, has reported similar experiences. A review of the literature on projects involving men indicates that most family planning clinics seem to give low priority to providing services for men (UNFPA 1995: 38). In the United States only 2 percent of publicly funded services focus on men (AVSC 1997c: B-1). Although most organizations and agencies favor an integrated approach, they do not seem to have much success in implementing that policy. The major constraint seems to be a lack of sufficient funding. A survey of publicly funded family planning clinics in the United States conducted by the Urban Institute in 1993 concluded that many clinics received no funding to cover services for men (Schulte and Sonensteinn 1995: 216). Other resources, such as the federal government's Title X program, a reimbursement program for users of family planning services, do not count men, "although they are not precluded from services funded by the program" (Schulte and Sonensteinn 1995: 216). Vasectomies, one of the services offered to men, are severely underfunded. The only exception is funding for STD and HIV services, although most clinics reported that these funds were insufficient as well (Schulte and Sonensteinn 1995: 216). Moreover, U.S. clinics report a lack of continuity in funding for male programs. Projects receiving temporary or startup funding are "often not refunded after the initial money is spent, regardless of the programs' efficacy" (Schulte and Sonensteinn 1995: 225).

Due to these funding limitations, agencies that have initiated services for men in the United States, Latin America, Asia, and Europe do not plan to increase their male involvement programs in the near future (Danforth and Green 1997: vii). The problem of scarce resources is even more precarious because of severe political pressure by women's health advocates who argue that services for men should not divert funds from women's programs (Danforth and Green 1997: 19). In Programming for Male Involvement in Reproductive Health: A Practical Guide for Managers, distributed by AVSC International in 1997, program managers were instructed that "it is essential that the inclusion of men's services not compromise resources for women" (AVSC 1997a: 2).

Since resources for programs and services for men are so scarce, most clinics give very limited space to men. Some clinics have established a separate waiting area or a separate entrance for men. Other clinics have changed their decor to look less women-centered (UNFPA 1995: 2; Ketting 1993; Schulte and Sonensteinn 1995: 216). Such changes require only minor adaptations and low-cost alterations in the existing infrastructure. This demarcation of spaces for female and male clients is not always unproblematic. One family planning clinic in London became a site of serious conflict when a male service provider appropriated a part of the waiting room by making a small circle of chairs to demonstrate different types of condoms to young men visiting the clinic. The male service provider described the conflict that ensued:

> At the team meeting after that day's clinic, one of the staff said that she was unhappy with me setting up an inner circle to talk to young men within the waiting room. She felt this was very exclusive and possibly unnerving for the young women sitting there, who might wonder what we were talking about. Similarly I felt uncomfortable working in this way as I felt very exposed: the space seemed unsafe both for me and the young men. I was wary about what language to use and how to respond to young men's banter as, in the past, female workers have accused male workers of colluding with young men's sexism. (Seex 1996: 112)

This conflict succinctly demonstrates the potential for conflict in allocating spaces to men in the predominantly female world of family planning clinics. Waiting rooms and staff meetings have become an arena for renegotiating gender relations concerning sexuality, both among staff and patients. Allocating space to men is thus not simply a question of logistics. It also entails a careful reconsideration of how men and women can share space in a culture with gendered cultural norms and attitudes toward sexuality. In the case of the clinic in London, the real location of space created a sharp competition among the staff. The experiences of one male staff member illustrate the highly politicized nature of sharing space: "The meeting was very tense. It felt as if we were fighting for possession of the supposedly shared space of the waiting room. Whose space was it? I felt that there was an unspoken feeling that young women were the priority in the clinic and the young men had to fit around them. Similarly, I as the male worker had to 'sort out' the young men without impinging on the rest of the clinic or the other staff" (Seex 1996: 112).

The conflict in the clinic in London could only be solved by a clear-cut spatial demarcation of facilities for male and female clients and staff. Initially, young men visiting the clinic were asked to avoid the waiting room and to use chairs specially set up for them in the corridor. In this manner the staff tried to prevent the young men (aged 12–18 years), who arrived in small groups and "were often quite noisy," from disrupting the quiet and orderly atmosphere of the clinic. The space in the corridor, however, turned out to be insufficient to accommodate the newcomers, because they appropriated the corridor as a place where they could banter and flirt with the young women who were visiting the clinic. Finally, the staff could solve the problem only by reserving a separate room for their male clients (Seex 1996: 113).

A handful of clinics in other countries have adopted similar spatial strategies to demarcate the boundaries between services for women and men. Thanks to the initiatives of family planning organizations in Brazil, Kenya, the United States, and Colombia, family planning programs have been enriched with a new infrastructure: the men-only clinic. The first segregated family planning clinic for men was opened in São Paulo, Brazil, in 1981. This clinic, run by Pro-Pater (Promocão da Paternidade Responsavel) provides vasectomies, urology services, and treatment for sexual problems and infertility, and has led to an increase in vasectomy prevalence from 0.2 percent in 1981 to 6 percent in 1990 (UNFPA 1995: 49). The mid-1980s witnessed the emergence of other men's clinics as well. In New York City a family planning clinic took the initiative to establish the Young Men's Clinic. Since its inception in 1986, this clinic has provided reproductive and general health care to between approximately four hundred and five hundred male teenagers (AVSC 1997c: 33). It has chosen to spread its services for women and men over time rather than space: on Monday evenings and Friday afternoons, male clients use the same facilities that are used by women during the rest of the week. The clinic was started after the staff of the family planning clinic realized that only 1 percent of the clinic's clients were men, and that the few men who attended the clinic appeared very uncomfortable to be there (AVSC 1997c: 15).[4] In contrast to the clinic in London, the major impetus to provide separate services for men was not to protect services for female clients but to improve services for men. Since 1993, five "Male-Only Centers" have been opened in Kenya, providing low-cost family planning services for men. The center in Nairobi provides vasectomy services; counseling on infertility, sexually transmitted diseases, and sexual problems; information on family planning methods; and a free supply of condoms to its male clients (AVSC 1997b: 19). The clinics in Kenya have a history similar to that of the men's clinic in New York City. One of the major incentives was to create an environment where men would feel comfortable (AVSC 1997b: 19).

The most extensive network of male clinics, however, is operated in Colombia by Profamilia (Asociación Pro-Bienestar de la Familia Colombiana), the leading private non-profit family planning association in Colombia. In 1985 Profamilia opened two Clinicas para Hombres (Clinics for Men), one in Bogotá, the capital, and one in Medellín, Colombia's second largest city (UNFPA 1995: 49; Plata 1996: 171). Even before opening its first clinics for men, Profamilia already had experience in offering services to men. This family planning organization had been carrying out vasectomies for fifteen years (AVSC 1997b: 9).[5] The clinic in Medellín is located physically within the main Profamilia clinic serving women, but has a separate entrance, a separate waiting area, and a special cashier for men. The clinic in Bogotá began in a similar way, but since 1994 it has become completely separated from the main clinic (AVSC 1997f: 20). The clinics in Bogotá and Medellín were so successful in generating income that Profamilia has expanded its services to include seven male clinics.[6] The experience in Colombia thus illustrates that creating separate infrastructures for men works quite well. Nevertheless, the Colombian model has been adopted by only a handful of clinics worldwide, mainly because of the extra costs of creating separate facilities for men and the number of male clients required to make these services cost-effective. Due to cost considerations, Profamilia does not plan to expand its sex-segregated services for men; separate clinics for men are only feasible in large cities, where they can attract a large enough clientele who can afford to pay for the services (AVSC 1997f: 41; AVSC 1997f: 19). Attempts to create men's clinics in Mexico and Ecuador failed because they did not attract enough male clients to make the clinics self-sufficient (UNFPA 1995: 49).

Resources are thus a major constraint on establishing men's clinics, not only because of the need to build separate facilities but also because operating a men's clinic requires hiring specialized staff. Creating separate facilities is a one-time investment that can often be realized by attracting special funds from donor agencies that want to promote men's involvement in family planning. Hiring specialized staff, however, is a recurring cost for a clinic which eventually needs to become cost-efficient. The staff of the clinic in Bogotá, for example, consists of six urologists, two general practitioners, two sex therapists, one general surgeon, one plastic surgeon, four lab technicians, one records assistant, three counselors, one receptionist, and three nurses (AVSC 1997b: 21). Although most other clinics have a smaller staff because they offer a more limited array of services, providing medical services for men requires a staff with a specialization different from that of women's programs. This is particularly so for clinics that offer vasectomies, urology services, and surgical circumcision.

Establishing men's clinics involves not only hiring staff with specializations other than those found in the traditional clinics, but may also mean hiring male staff. Since family planning clinics have traditionally focused almost exclusively on women, most clinics have a predominantly female staff: receptionists, nurses, and doctors are usually female (Schulte and Sonensteinn 1995: 212; Seex 1996: 111). The extent to which men need male service providers has been, and still is, a contested issue. Debates about staffing men's clinics illustrate the gendered nature of the boundary work between service providers specialized in services for women, who claim to be experienced enough to serve the new patients, and newcomers in the field who challenge this claim by suggesting that male clients need new, male experts. Advocates of the "men-need-men approach" suggest that family planning clinics fail to attract men because the overwhelmingly female clientele and staff reinforce the image of these clinics as organizations for women only (Danforth and Green 1997: 36; Schulte and Sonensteinn 1995: 216). Current service providers, it is argued, are poorly informed regarding male contraceptive methods and sometimes share the same misconceptions as their clients (UNFPA 1995: 3). The AVSC has described these experiences in terms of "provider bias against male involvement": "Providers assume that men are not interested in taking responsibility for family planning, and this assumption becomes a self-fulfilling prophecy. . . . Providers may not offer male methods or may provide inadequate information about them, may present them in a negative light and may make men feel uncomfortable visiting clinics and asking questions about family planning" (UNFPA 1995: 43). The USAID survey in 1997 also mentioned the lack of trained service providers for men as a serious constraint on involving men in family planning (Danforth and Green 1997: 20). Moreover, proponents of the men-need-men approach emphasize that men prefer to receive medical services and information from other men.[7] Clinics in Mexico, for example, found that male service providers were more effective in distributing condoms. Female outreach workers, staff members who visit potential clients in workplaces and schools, turned out to be less successful in reaching men, because male clients did not take female workers seriously (UNFPA 1995: 46).

The gender of the provider is not only considered relevant for serving clients, but also for the providers, as is exemplified by the experience of a family planning clinic in Pakistan. The Family Planning Association of Pakistan had to hire male staff to be able to provide contraceptive services to men. As Dr. Mobeen Afzal, the medical director of this clinic, explained: "[In the beginning] one major drawback is that nearly all doctors employed by FPAP were women. From the point of view of service providers we [women doctors] are reluctant to attend to men. There is an inherent shyness we have. It happens with paramedic staff as well. . . . As far as I am concerned, I can talk to a male client. But there may be questions I cannot answer satisfactorily. I am not sure how far I can go" (AVSC 1997g: 23).

The practice of this clinic is that, for medical services only, women work with women and men with men. For counseling, the gendered organization of work is less rigid. In this case, age is an important factor: older female service providers can talk to younger male clients, and older male staff can talk to younger female clients (AVSC 1997g: 23). In the U.K., male staff were required for yet another reason. Following an incident in a clinic in London where young men knocked down a female receptionist to take condoms, the staff decided to hire a male service provider (Seex 1996: 111–12).

Opponents of the men-need-men approach, however, question the importance of the gender of services providers. Referring to the experiences of clinics in Colombia, Uganda, and the United States, they suggest that in most cases it makes no difference whether the staff is male or female (Wegner 1997; AVSC 1997b: 21). They emphasize that the gender of the service provider is less important than qualities such as honesty, competence, and a respectful attitude (Wegner 1997; AVSC 1997b: 32). However, both advocates and opponents of the men-need-men approach seem to agree that in some cultures male clients indeed prefer male providers, particularly for specific medical services, such as genital and urethral exams (Wegner 1997; AVSC 1997b: 21). Debates on the question of whether male clients need male staff thus show how the demarcations of boundaries between who should and should not be considered qualified to serve the new client develops along the lines of gender, age, and body parts. In some cultures, tensions and potential conflicts can be solved by reallocating tasks between female and male staff, or between older and younger female staff. In this real location of tasks, some male body parts are constructed as needing special male care, whereas others are represented as objects that can stand the gaze of both male and female service providers.

The introduction of male clients not only challenged specific gender routines and norms in provider–client relations, it also disrupted the gendered pattern in work relations that characterized the world of family planning prior to the emergence of the new client. For decades, most family planning clinics were staffed almost exclusively by women. The introduction of male staff to serve the new clients thus challenged the status of the family planning service providers as a predominantly female profession. Many female staff members considered the opening of "their" profession to men as a potential threat to the careers of women. Men can become serious competitors in times of job scarcity (Danforth and Green 1997: 10). Moreover, the introduction of male staff members was perceived as a threat to the established working styles of female service providers. In a clinic in San Francisco, for example, female clinicians had difficulties in adjusting to men's different working styles and were jealous about the publicity given to the male program. The male staff faced similar problems because they felt they had to compete with the existing, very successful women's program (Gordon and DeMarco 1984: 46). In one clinic in London, female staff members felt that men colluded with the male clients' sexism (Seex 1996: 112). Profamilia's clinics in Colombia also reported problems between the staffs of its men's and women's clinics. In Bogotá, for example, a rivalry arose between the staffs at the men's and women's clinics because the men's clinic had moved into a newer, more modern building, and because that clinic turned out to be financially profitable. In addition, this clinic encountered rivalry between urologists, who work with men, and gynecologists, who work exclusively with women. Urologists, the newcomers in the Profamilia clinics, preferred to have a separate director to "maintain their autonomy and fight for their particular interests." The staff serving women, however, was opposed to having a urologist as director of the clinic because "they worry about what will happen to women's services" (AVSC 1997b: 35).

Finally, the debates on staffing family planning clinics to adjust services to accommodate male clients illustrate how traditionally female professions continue to be valued less than male professions. Clinics in the United States have faced difficulties in hiring male staff because male clinicians preferred other medical settings (Schulte and Sonensteinn 1995: 216). Working in a family planning clinic is perceived as a low-status job for men. On the one hand, there is little room for professional advancement. On the other hand, family planning clinics seem to have low social prestige, at least among men, as illustrated by the experiences of a male service provider in a family planning clinic in San Francisco: "When I go to a party and people ask me what I do, I get an excited reaction from women, who think it's wonderful. But from the men, its just 'Oh.' I just don't fit into their frame of reference. . . . I feel invalidated by other men" (Gordon and DeMarco 1984: 46). Or, as one of the directors of the male program of this clinic concluded: "We feel like the women of the program. It's as if the roles had all been reversed" (Gordon and DeMarco 1984: 46). This experience is different from that of other medical professions where men have entered traditionally female jobs. Male nurses, for example, have not encountered serious problems in obtaining social prestige (Otten 1985).

The debates on space, budgets, and staff thus show how the introduction of men as new clients into family planning clinics has been, and still is, a contested issue that requires a transformation of traditional gender structures and norms in provider–client relations, as well as in the relations among various medical professions.

How to Attract Men

Men's clinics are peculiar phenomena not only because they challenge existing gender norms and practices. They are also interesting because they challenge the standard view of how clinics come into existence. The major incentive to make special clinics for men was not that the waiting rooms of existing family planning clinics were overcrowded with men desperately seeking professional help for reproductive or sexual problems. To the contrary, in most clinics male clients could be counted on the fingers of one hand. The need for male reproductive services was not articulated by the client, nor by a consumer or health movement for men, nor by the medical profession, as happened with services for women. Although family planning clinics for women originated from population-control incentives, rather than from a mandate to serve the needs of women, individual women (and since the 1980s, women's health advocates) have always been important in articulating the need for good reproductive health services for women (Kammen 1998; Gordon and DeMarco 1984: 45). As we have seen, the need for family planning and reproductive health services for men has been articulated only by women's health advocates; non-profit public-sector agencies such as the United Nations, WHO, and the Population Council; and national private family planning policy organizations like AVSC. This top-down approach creates specific constraints on men's clinics. Now that clinics are able to include men, are men willing to go to the facilities created especially for them?

In this section, I want to explore the strategies used to configure men as clients of the men's clinics. How do family planning organizations operating segregated clinics for men try to enroll their new male clients? In order to answer this question, I will focus particularly on the recruiting strategies and services provided by two clinics: the Clinica para Hombres in Bogotá and the Young Men's Clinic in New York City. To what extent are men as clients treated differently from the traditional clients of family planning clinics, that is, from women?

Transgressing the Boundaries between the Public and the Private

At first sight, one would not expect to find the most extensive network of men's clinics in Colombia, a country where the culture of machismo is still alive.

Colombia consists of a mixture of about ten originally Latin-Mediterranean cultures with a tradition of machismo characterized by rigid norms and customs about the roles and responsibilities of men and women. In these cultures men and women have their own well-defined spheres of influence. The public sphere, including the street, the pubs, workplaces, and related activities, is considered a strictly male domain. The private sphere, including the home and all activities that take place there, such as taking care of children, food, and the health of the family, is considered to be the woman's domain. In addition, machismo cultures have strict norms and double standards for the sexual behavior of men and women. Whereas men are allowed and expected to have numerous sexual partners and to have children with more than one woman, women are expected to practice sexual and reproductive fidelity.[8] In Colombia, as elsewhere, times are changing. In recent decades, urbanization and education have led Colombian society to reevaluate these dualistic gender roles. Women from all social classes have appropriated the public sphere by entering both lower- and higher-paid jobs, whereas men are fathering fewer children with fewer women. Important cultural gatekeepers, such as the Catholic Church, have urged men to become more involved in fathering. As a result of the women's movement's advocacy for women's rights, equality between the sexes and the prohibition of discrimination against women has been written into the 1991 Constitution (AVSC 1997b: 6–7). Colombia has also made important changes in its public health system. In 1992 the Colombian government adopted a National Plan for Sex Education, with a federal mandate that obliged schools to include sex education in their curricula, covering such topics as gender roles and teenage pregnancy, HIV/AIDS prevention, and reproductive health rights (AVSC 1997b: 5). Moreover, Colombia adopted a new national health insurance plan which allows individuals "to choose their health care provider from an array of registered health maintenance organizations, which in turn are reimbursed by the government according to pre-established rates. The law specifically mentions family planning as a service which all individuals have the right to receive" (AVSC 1997: 5–6).

These developments indicate that traditional values about the roles of women and men are changing, and that there exists a growing awareness of reproductive health issues in Colombia. Nevertheless, family planning organizations such as Profamilia have to work within the legacy of machismo. A nice illustration of how this legacy still affects men's attitudes is the way in which a client of one of Profamilia's family planning clinics legitimated his decision to have a vasectomy: "Why should it be her who uses family planning, why not me? I am older than her. She is only 26. You never know what might happen.

These days you hope that a marriage lasts, but you never have any guarantees. I hope that nothing happens . . . but she might want to have children with someone else. I am content with the number of children I have. And the other thing is, you know, this [getting a vasectomy] is a way to know if she is unfaithful to me. I'll know if she has been with someone else" (AVSC 1997b: 26).

Establishing men's clinics in a culture in which men's virility has been measured for centuries by the number of their children sets specific constraints on operating these clinics. What strategies do family planning service providers use to attract men to the traditionally female, private domain of the family planning clinic?

The practices of Profamilia's men's clinics in Bogotá, Medellín, and Cartagena[9] indicate that the clinic's staff has to put great effort into enrolling male clients. First, they devote a considerable amount of their time to so-called outreach activities. This is a common practice in many family planning programs because service providers have learned that people are more likely to visit a clinic for services if the staff has first visited potential clients in a location outside the clinic (Population Reference Bureau 1995: 7). However, Profamilia's usual outreach programs did not reach men because they were mostly organized in a community center during daytime hours. Neither the location nor the time were convenient for men because they don't frequent community centers and are usually working during the day (AVSC 1997b: 16). Consequently, the staff at the men's clinics had to adapt their outreach activities to accommodate men. They decided to go directly to the places frequented by men. The clinic in Cartagena, for example, approached taxi drivers as a means to recruit men. In Medellín, staff members gave talks at companies that had contracts with Profamilia. During some of these visits, counselors were accompanied by doctors who performed pelvic, genital, or prostate exams (AVSC 1997b: 16) Initially, the clinics in Bogotá and Medellín had a separate coordinator to plan these outreach activities and other organizational tasks designed to adapt services to the new clients. Currently, this work is integrated into the work of the counseling staff, who have to devote part of their time to outreach activities (AVSC 1997b: 31).

A second tactic used by the staff to recruit men involved radio and television campaigns. At the opening of the new clinic in Bogotá, Profamilia launched a press release to advertise its new services. On other occasions Profamilia has used radio and television to encourage the media to feature stories about the clinics. Television turned out to be an excellent tool for reaching men. Almost every time television advertising was used, the number of men visiting the clinic increased. Due to cost considerations, however, this recruitment tool was not used very often (AVSC 1997b: 17). Instead, the staff put great effort into participating in radio and television talk shows, for which they did not have to pay (AVSC 1997b: 31). In its publicity campaigns, Profamilia has promoted the image that the clinics are spaces for men. In the words of Dr. Jaime Perez, a urologist at the men's clinic in Bogotá: "One of the things that puts men at ease in terms of coming to the clinic is the way the clinic is presented as a clinic for men. The publicity around the clinic has promoted this image. . . . The mere fact of being a clinic specifically for men gives the clients a sense of calm" (AVSC 1997b: 31).

A third recruitment strategy for attracting men is the development and distribution of educational material. Profamilia has produced brochures specifically for men on gender roles, vasectomy, male involvement in family planning, and condom usage (AVSC 1997b: 17). Outreach activities, media advertisements, and educational efforts are thus important tools for recruiting the new client.

Outreach programs and media campaigns are only a first step toward encouraging men to visit a clinic that they see as typically a women's world. These traditionally feminine spaces need to be adapted to the preferences and needs of men. In this respect, the fact that many clinics for men have separate entrances speaks volumes. Separate entrances can be seen as both symbolic and material passageways between the public domain outside the clinic, where men traditionally dominate life, and the private domain inside the clinic, where men are newcomers. Separate entrances are intriguing spaces because they facilitate crossing the boundaries between these traditionally male and female worlds. Separate waiting rooms have a similar symbolic and material function: men remain separated from the female domain, although they are physically present within this domain. Thus, men are less conscious of being in a traditionally female space. Many men's clinics adapt the decor of waiting rooms to men by hanging posters that suggest a man's world, or more gender-neutral posters, which adds to this make-believe-that-you-are-in-your-own-world game. The separate spaces for men are cited by Profamilia's staff members as crucial in attracting men to the clinic. In the words of Efrain Patrino, a counselor at the clinic in Bogotá: "The first month that we opened the clinic we did 100 vasectomies. We saw that it worked, [and] it worked because men had a separate space. Before that, a man would come into the Profamilia clinic and find 35 women waiting in the waiting area, and they all looked at him. With the clinic for men, we now had a separate entrance for him, and it was easier [for the men to come into the clinic]" (AVSC 1997f: 20).

The fourth tactic used to draw men to the clinic thus consisted of carefully designing the clinic's space. A closer look at the men's clinic in Bogotá reveals how Profamilia went to great lengths to transform the clinic into a man's world. The decor and lighting were designed to give the clinic a high-tech image and to guarantee the client's privacy. The well-marked reception area was designed with brushed-metal countertops where clients could wait to be called for services. On the other side of the reception desk, the designers installed tinted sliding-glass doors "to provide privacy to clients and staff in each of three counseling cubicles" (AVSC 1997f: 12). The first and second floors of the clinic, where the medical examining rooms are located, also have newly designed waiting areas. Profamilia has thought carefully about the design of the clinic, and also about the design of the staff's uniforms. The—mostly male—staff is well dressed in blue-striped shirts and ties. All this adds to the image that the visitor is in a world familiar to him, something that resembles an office more than a family planning clinic.

Another area that is important in understanding the work that goes into configuring men as clients of the men's clinic is the way the staff members treat their new clients once they arrive at the clinic. Initially, Profamilia's men's clinics operated like the women's clinics. Clients had to wait their turn and then visit one of the examining rooms. The staff soon learned that this system, which worked for women, did not work for men. Men often experienced difficulties in identifying and talking about their needs with the receptionist, thus ending up in the wrong examination rooms. Many male clients articulated their needs in terms of health reasons when actually they were seeking help for social problems with their relationships or with other personal issues. Profamilia's counselors have ascribed this attitude to the fact that men are conditioned not to talk about their private worries. The men's clinic in Bogotá therefore had to change its intake procedures for men; they adopted a routine in which every client receives "a brief counseling session before he selects or is sent to a medical service" (AVSC 1997b: 21). Before implementing this system, "men often paid for one service and then realized in the medical examining room that they needed another" (AVSC 1997b: 21). The current counseling system was designed in such a way that men see a counselor both before and after they have seen a doctor. These counseling sessions are considered by the staff as important occasions where men "learn to articulate their needs, resolve their doubts, and reduce their anxiety" (AVSC 1997b: 21).

The counselor has become the key person in adapting the family planning services to the new clients. Counseling can thus be considered as a crucial technology in operating a clinic for men. The practices of the clinic in Bogotá indicate that counseling has a dual function: it is used to make men feel at ease in the clinic, and it functions as a tool to discipline men into acceptable clients of the family planning clinic. Due to the counseling sessions, men do not disrupt the routine and efficiency of the medical services, as is exemplified by the experiences of a urologist at the clinic in Bogotá: "When we have 30 patients to see in a day, we can't offer much information. With counseling, the patient's questions are often answered and many of his doubts already resolved when he arrives in the examining room" (AVSC 1997b: 21).

Finally, the range and type of services offered by the men's clinics in Colombia illustrate that Profamilia has made major changes in its services to make them more attractive to men. The services of the men's clinics in Bogotá include more than the obvious topics one would expect to find in a family planning clinic. In addition to family planning services (vasectomy and condoms); STD and HIV services; laboratory services for sperm counts, hormonal, urine and blood testing; and fertility testing and treatments, the clinic also provides urological services and general medicine (AVSC International 1997b: 15). In 1997 plastic surgery was added to the services of the men's clinic in Bogotá. The aim of this service is "to provide men with a low-cost option" (AVSC 1997b: 15). The clinics in Medellín and Cali offer the same variety of services, except for plastic surgery and HIV testing (AVSC 1997f: 15). The profile of these clinics is thus much broader than that of a traditional family planning clinic: they are actually clinics specialized in male health. This wide range of services was explicitly selected by Profamilia to attract men to visit its clinics. Providing more traditional family planning services such as vasectomies was considered too narrow a base for operating a men's clinic. The inclusion of more general medical services enabled Profamilia to subsidize the costs of the family planning services. The provision of general healthcare services for men thus functions as yet another important tool for enrolling enough male clients to make the clinic cost-efficient. Without these services, the men's clinics would not survive.

A reflection on these practices of the men's clinics in Colombia teaches that these clinics are not incompatible with a traditional machismo culture, as one would be inclined to think. On the contrary, men's clinics like the ones operated by Profamilia can be understood as efficient tools for integrating men into family planning. Establishing separate clinics for men enables family planning organizations to adjust the female, private domain of the traditional family planning clinic to the preferences, attitudes, and norms of male clients. In this way, they succeed in attracting more men to family planning services than the traditional family planning clinics. Nevertheless, these adapted infrastructures do not work for all men. The typical client of the men's clinics in Colombia is approximately thirty years old and from the middle class. More recently, the clinics have also attracted older clients (forty-five years and older) by offering prostate exams and treatment. Younger men of lower income, however, do not frequent the men's clinics in Colombia.[10] Men's clinics thus cannot be considered as a panacea for including men in family planning or improving health services for men.

Sport Physicals as Cover

To analyze the work involved in attracting men to visit men's clinics, it is useful to look at yet another clinic in a different cultural setting. Like the clinic in Bogotá, the Young Men's Clinic (YMC or La Clinica de Jovenes Hombres) in New York City features in the literature as a model program for this new type of clinic.[11] According to a flyer it has published, the clinic serves approximately five hundred young men (1,000 visits) each year and has a staff of six paid workers: two physicians, a physician assistant, a social worker, a laboratory technician, and a director, Dr. Bruce Armstrong, who is also the clinic's founder (AVSC 1997d: 32). Due to his work at the Mailman School of Public Health and the Medical School of Columbia University, Armstrong is able to recruit public health and medical students to work for free at the clinic as part of their training. The students assist the YMC's staff by conducting the intake of clients and providing health education (Armstrong interview 1997). The YMC is New York City's only reproductive health clinic for men and is jointly operated by the Center for Population and Family Health, a division of the Mailman School of Public Health at Columbia University, and by the New York Presbyterian Hospital's Ambulatory Care Network Corporation (AVSC 1997d: 30). The clinic is located in a low-income, inner-city neighborhood in the Washington Heights section of New York City, where a majority of the predominantly Hispanic (mostly from the Dominican Republic) and African-American population are unemployed or not in school (AVSC 1997d: 34) and have very limited access to health care (Armstrong interview 1997). Initially, the clinic was located on the fourth floor of Presbyterian Hospital, but it moved to a building in the middle of the neighborhood as part of the hospital's policy to take some ambulatory services out into the community (Armstrong interview 1997).

The relevant question for this chapter is the extent to which this effort to bring family planning services closer to the people has been effective in bringing men into the clinic. As in Colombia, many American men tend to have ambivalent attitudes about admitting that they need medical help (Bernardes and Cameron 1998; Nahon and Lander 1993). Although men aged seventeen and older, especially those living in the inner city of large cities such as New York, are at high risk of contracting sexually transmitted diseases (STDs), they do not feel comfortable or do not see the need to come forward for medical services (Armstrong interview 1997). Many men will not think of stopping by a clinic, particularly if the clinic is a family planning clinic or an STD clinic, the latter due to the stigma associated with not being sexually healthy (Armstrong interview 1997; AVCS 1997f: 7; Edwards 1994: 78). In a survey of Californian men, a large percentage (70 percent) mentioned that they considered birth control a "female responsibility" (Steinhauer 1995). This implies that the YMC staff has had to put extra effort into trying to recruit male clients. In this case, efforts had to be directed to a specific section of the male population of the neighborhood, due to the YMC's policy of considering young men between the ages of twelve and thirty as their major audience. A closer look at the practices of the YMC shows that the clinic's staff has adopted recruitment techniques very similar to the ones used by their colleagues in Bogotá, although there are interesting differences as well.

First, the YMC uses extensive outreach activities to bring men into the clinic. From the beginning, the YMC staff considered community outreach as a crucial element of providing services for men (AVSC 1997f: 7). In its early years, YMC's staff spent a considerable amount of time, "far beyond normal working hours," talking to people who would be in a position to refer young men to the clinic and attending neighborhood events (AVSC 1997c: D-10; AVSC 1997d: 35). Bruce Armstrong enrolled the help of public health students to visit the pediatrics wards and the emergency room at Presbyterian Hospital to inform physicians about the newly opened clinic and to ask them to refer their adolescent male clients to the clinic. Given the scarcity of healthcare services for this group in the neighborhood, the physicians were very willing to cooperate, as they considered the YMC "another site where they could refer adolescent clients" (AVSC 1997d: 30). Over time, physicians provided an increasing number of referrals to the YMC. The clinic's most important recruiting strategy consisted, however, in outreach activities on the streets and in the playgrounds to build trust and interest in the clinic (AVSC 1997c: D-10). The focus of attention was on the playgrounds frequented by young men to play basketball, to break-dance, or simply to hang out. Public health students went to these playgrounds to videotape the neighborhood youth and told them that they could visit the YMC to see themselves on tape. Students were even specially recruited to play basketball and to chaperone dances (Armstrong interview 1997). This strategy worked: some young people indeed went to the clinic to watch the videotapes. After the videotapes had been played, the public health students organized group discussions on sexuality and contraception and informed the visitors about the services of the clinic. In this way, the public health students and the clinic became very visible in the neighborhood. These frequent meetings worked both ways. Young men from the neighborhood became involved in the work at the clinic. One of them developed a logo for the clinic to put on T-shirts, which were distributed at neighborhood events and at the clinic (AVCS 1997f: 34).

A second strategy used to attract male clients was to adapt the services of the clinic to men. Ever since its inception, the YMC has included sports physicals as one of its services. In this way, they ensured that the clinic would have something to offer that would be of interest to its potential clients, something that went beyond family planning services. Since physicals are required before joining a sports team, a large number of neighborhood youth now have access to a clinic where they can obtain their health certificates. The practices of the YMC indicate that these sports physicals had a dual function. In addition to providing the healthcare services needed by the neighborhood's young male population, they also made it easier for many young men to visit the clinic and request other services (AVSC 1997d: 30). Whereas the clinic in Bogotá used a separate entrance to encourage men to visit the traditionally feminine world of the family planning clinic, the clinic in New York City offered sports physicals as a "cover" for going to the clinic. By visiting a clinic that offers sports physicals, clients do not run the risk of anyone knowing they are asking for medical help in matters other than physical examinations. As Bruce Armstrong says: "And that [including exams for sports] would also make it safer for them, that they could come to the clinic and not have to worry that 'My mother's watching.' They can always say 'I came here for a sports physical' " (Armstrong interview 1997).

To promote these services, the YMC staff also approached local sports coaches, who proved to be an excellent source of referrals (AVSC 1997d: 30). In this manner, the YMC transformed a visit to the clinic into something that fit into the routines of the daily life of the young male population of the neighborhood. To quote Dr. Cohall, a physician at the YMC: "Traditionally, family planning clinics have . . . really spent a lot of time and effort dealing with women's issues. Historically, women have been 'better' consumers than guys; they come in more regularly and ostensibly for reproductive health care. There is more of a feeling that it's a routine thing for them to come in for services . . . We wanted to get guys to come in and, in a sense, see if we could make it routine for them, too" (AVCS 1997f: 34).

In addition to sports physicals, the men's clinic in New York offers a broad array of services, broader than one would expect to find in a clinic specialized in reproductive health. In addition to family planning and reproductive health services (including condom provision, STD diagnosis and treatment, HIV counseling and testing, male reproductive health exams, and sexuality and health education), the YMC offers primary healthcare services (sports, working papers, and school physicals, and comprehensive health exams), social work services, and short-term mental health counseling (AVSC 1997d: 30; Young Men's Clinic flyer). The YMC would even like to expand its services to include "job training; obtaining graduate-equivalence degrees; understanding and treating depression; and management of anger," but they do not have sufficient resources to realize this (AVSC 1997d: 33). The YMC has chosen this wide range of services in order to adapt its clinic to the preferences and needs of its clients. Prior to the clinic's establishment, Bruce Armstrong already had some knowledge of the needs of Hispanic adolescents. In 1984 he had worked on a study about the attitudes of Hispanic men and women toward contraception and family planning services. By conducting focus groups with young men, Armstrong "learned a lot about how they felt, about the services at the clinic [the Young Adult Clinic, a family planning clinic initiated in 1976] and how they perceived the clinic to be inclusive of men in name only" (AVSC 1997d: 30). Armstrong also enlisted the help of some of his students at the School of Public Health to conduct structured interviews with school teachers, sports coaches, and other providers in the neighborhood about the health needs of young men in the community (AVCS 1997f: 33). According to Armstrong:

> We had the family planning clinic since 1976. And it was predominantly women, but there were some men involved, too. I mean, you'd find men in the clinic, sometimes, as you do now. But there were very small numbers, and I think people said, "Why is this the case?" So we did some focus groups and some research, and we found out that there were a lot of men who said they wanted to be involved [in family planning], but that there were certain things about it that they felt uncomfortable with. The main thing on their mind was things like, "It's too embarrassing to go there. Men are supposed to know these things," so men's attitudes about getting help were a bit of a barrier. You know: "Is it a manly thing to do? To go to a family planning clinic?" Those kind of beliefs and attitudes. So, we did that, we did the focus groups, and then we interviewed people from the neighborhood quite a bit, and we found that there were other things, too, that were important, like many of the men that we inter-

viewed said that first, health services were so lacking for young men in this neighborhood that if you really want the men to come forward, if you're really interested in that, then you must do more than just family planning—give them the exams that they need for sports, and school, and so on. (Armstrong interview 1997)

A third strategy used to recruit male clients was to create an attractive space for them. In contrast to the clinic in Bogotá, the YMC has not created a special space for men. Located in the same building as the family planning clinic, the staff at the men's clinic use the same supplies that are used for their female clientele. The men's charts are kept in the same chart room as the women's, only in a different section. The only thing that is different is the staff, although some nurses and physician assistants work with both male and female clients (Armstrong interview 1997: 3). From the outside, the clinic does not even look very much like a clinic. A sign simply says "Medical Center," but there is no sign to make people aware that there is a men's clinic inside the building, which reflects the clinic's policy of attracting men by means other than family planning services. In the case of the YMC it is the cleanliness of the clinic, rather than specific signs or separate entrances, that serves to make the clinic attractive to its new clients. The clinic is located in a renovated, attractive, and clean place. In other contexts, these may not be important features. In the neighborhood where the clinic is located, however, the cleanliness of public places has a significance that goes beyond the mere absence of dirt (AVSC 1997d: 31). Many of the clinic's visitors are not used to clean, attractive facilities. In a neighborhood where little is new or clean, not even healthcare services, people value these—at first sight—obvious facts. As Bruce Armstrong said: "If you're poor and coming from the villages in the Dominican Republic . . . they're not used to this. So when they walk in, even though it's free . . . they say 'Oh, this place is really nice.' And it tells them something about our credentials, and about our seriousness" (Armstrong interview 1997). One male client expressed his experience as follows: "Well, I was going to the public health clinic to get a physical, but they're so dirty. Everybody talks about how horrible they are. But when I heard this place was new and clean, I decided to come" (AVSC 1997d: 34).

A fourth tool the YMC has used to attract clients is the offer of services free of charge for those who cannot afford to pay or do not have any medical insurance, which actually is true of many of the clinic's potential clients. The free services are frequently mentioned as one of the reasons why the young men of the neighborhood come to the YMC and why they choose to return (AVSC 1997d: 33; Armstrong interview 1997).

The YMC's strategies for attracting male clients have been very successful. In the mid-1990s the clinic had to turn away clients during clinic hours. Specific promotional efforts are no longer needed, since the clinic is now very well known in the neighborhood (AVSC 1997c: D-10). In 1997 the YMC therefore expanded its clinic hours for men to two sessions: one on Monday nights and one on Friday afternoons (AVSC 1997f: 42; Edwards 1994: 80; Armstrong interview 1997). However, the YMC's strategies for attracting men also included a risk. Most of the approximately one thousand men who visit the clinic each year come to the clinic for physical examinations (75 percent) or STD testing and treatment (25 percent). To realize its aim as a family planning and sexual health clinic, rather than as a general health clinic, the YMC had to develop additional strategies to transform the needs of their male clients from sports physicals and STD tests to include family planning and extended sexual health needs.

An initial tactic the YMC adopted to transform the needs of their new clients was to organize specific activities in the waiting room. The waiting room is not just a place where the clients wait before they are called by one of the physicians or the social worker. If there are enough men waiting for their turn, the otherwise dull waiting room is transformed into a lively, intensive discussion and information place. Two public health students, in a quite casual way, show slides of the male and female reproductive organs, followed by a story about how a girl and a boy discuss whether to have sex or not, with slides again that show the effects of sexually transmitted diseases (STDs), and ending with a discussion and demonstration of how to use condoms.[12] The aim of these sessions is to provide health education, to teach men specific skills related to sexuality and contraception, and to discuss topics such as male involvement in family planning and the prevention of sexually transmitted diseases (Armstrong interview 1997; Diazgranados and McKracken interview 1997). The students try to involve the waiting men in their activities. Although not everybody participates, even men who sit far away from the discussion tend to listen to what is happening. Usually, one-third of the group actively answers questions or—in the story part—offer their suggestions about how boys and girls discuss sex and contraception. In this manner, clients hear of very different experiences and opinions about sexuality, not only from the public health students but also from the other men in the waiting room. The YMC staff feels that these discussions help to change beliefs, and changing beliefs is considered vital to including men in family planning. To quote two of the public health students who have led the health and sexuality education sessions in the waiting room:

We're not going to change their lives in one group, so what we introduce, just to get them thinking, are ideas, for instance, the fact that you can plan to have sex, that you can talk about it. You can't change attitudes once because attitudes are ingrained. That's an emotional thing. Behaviors, that's really tough. . . . But you can change beliefs. . . . You can change the belief, for example, well, here are two women who say, "We don't feel offended if a guy brings up the issue" [the use of contraceptives]. Maybe get one or two guys to say, "Yeah, my girlfriend, she's never been offended by that. In fact she loves me more because I ask about it." Guys will say, "I would think a girl was smart if she came with a condom." We got that tonight. Or, "that she's clean, because she protects herself." (Diazgranados and McKracken interview 1997)

Usually, the discussions in the waiting room are very intense. The public health students take the time to make the men feel comfortable—"We don't just rap"—and try to get them talking with each other. To help the men feel at ease and willing to talk, the public health students are trained in specific conversation techniques, particularly in making normalizing statements and self-disclosure. To avoid humiliating men who don't have the correct answers to questions, which is very likely to happen if you have learned that, as a man, you should know certain things, the staff has learned to ask questions such as: "How many of you have heard of STDs?" rather than "How many of you know about STDs?"—and to acknowledge that they, and many other people, have also made mistakes and that it is part of being a human being (Armstrong interview 1997). The same techniques are used by the medical students, who record the psychosocial histories of the clients when they first visit the clinic. If a client, for example, tells the provider that he is worried about impotence or if he asks how normal it is to have asymmetrical testicles, the provider is trained to answer, "That's a concern many men have at some point in their lives. We all experience that," and then proceeds to inform the client about impotence or how to examine testicles for testicular cancer (Armstrong interview 1997). These conversation techniques are a central part of the YMC's approach to its clients. According to Armstrong:

We train our staff this way . . . because of our belief that many men, especially living in the inner city like us, feel very disconnected, feel very disempowered, like "I'm twenty and going nowhere," like "I am twenty and I dropped out of school and I can't get a job." That feels terrible. We train our students and our staff not to say things like, "Oh, really, you only went to the ninth grade? So when did you drop out of school?" We don't say that. We teach them to say: "Oh, really, you went through the ninth grade? What happened that you decided to leave?" That's a huge difference, and that's the approach we take. We're not perfect, but we try that. (Armstrong interview 1997)

These group discussions not only serve the purpose of transforming the needs of the male clients, they also shape the emotional climate of the clinic. As Bruce Armstrong put it: "It sets a tone in the waiting room in the clinic, that we really notice you, that we really do care about you . . . My point is that there's an emotional tone to a clinic like this when they [the public health students] are out there doing that. . . . It really relaxes them. . . . And you know what else? It relaxes the staff. It relaxes the people at the desk. . . . It is like a domino effect. . . . I think you can see it filtering into the history-taking that we take individually on these nights. There's a much more cooperative feeling between the patients and the staff " (Armstrong interview 1997).

In addition to the activities in the waiting room, the YMC has developed careful procedures for intake in order to transform the needs of its clients from requests for sports physicals to family planning and sexual health needs. After the check-in at the reception desk and the education sessions in the waiting room, every client who first visits the clinic has a fifteen-to-twenty-minute intake session with a medical student who takes the client's history. The intake form illustrates how the YMC transforms men who visit the clinic for sports physicals into potential family planning and sexual health clients. The clinic visit form includes not only the medical and social history of the client, but also issues such as the use of contraceptives, intimate relations, sexual experience, and sexual health complaints (AVSC 1997d: 32).

If a client mentions social or psychological problems, the medical student informs the YMC's social worker about the client's special concerns, which are consequently discussed during a special counseling session (AVSC 1997d: 32). Then the client gets a lab screening (where he is screened for sickle-cell anemia, syphilis, STDs, and tuberculosis), or is seen by the medical provider (where he gets his physical examination), or goes to the social worker (who does the HIV counseling and testing) (Armstrong interview 1997). These encounters with the service providers are not just used to check the general health or the lab test results of the client. They have an important function in creating and stimulating a need for family planning services. According to Armstrong:

We try to maximize, at every opportunity we can, to go after the guy's beliefs. So when a guy comes to the clinic for a routine testing, let's say for syphilis or sickle cell anemia, we tell them they really need to come back to the clinic in a week or so to go over these results with somebody because you don't want syphilis to be hiding out in your body or anything like that. You don't want to be anemic and tired. So we try to entreat them with finding out the results of their lab work, their body, right? But when they come back to the clinic . . . ideally, we don't do this all the time because the staffing is too short, that could become another what we call "teachable moment." Let's say, you come back, and I look at your arm, and I say, "Oh great, negative for tuberculosis." And then I look at the chart, and I read that the medical student who spent a lot of time with you Monday night said: "This young fellow is very motivated to prevent pregnancy, and he's going to try to talk with his girlfriend this week about getting her to come to the family planning clinic." If it works the way we plan, I'd say to you at this point, "Oh, so this is negative. Tell me, have you used condoms since I saw you last? Have you had a chance to talk to your girlfriend?" (Armstrong interview 1997)

These practices show the precarious nature of the conditions under which a men's clinic is able to exist and survive in the United States. Although family planning and reproductive health have been major aims of the YMC, the clinic owes its success in recruiting clients primarily to the fact that it does not profile itself as a family planning clinic for men.

Like the men's clinic in Bogotá, the clinic in New York has had to adopt carefully designed strategies to configure men as clients of the clinic. In Colombia as well as in the United States men are most likely to visit a men's clinic if the clinic offers services that go beyond family planning and sexual health. In both cultures there exists a wide gap between the rhetoric about the New Man (described in chapter 2) and the identities and lived experiences of men. The survival of men's clinics thus entails hard work and clever detour strategies to overcome these cultural constraints. One such strategy that seems to work is to introduce these clinics as comprehensive healthcare clinics rather than family planning or reproductive health clinics. To quote Bruce Armstrong: "What we have done is we've created other opportunities or reasons for them to come forward. When they come forward, we do the best we can to provide them with comprehensive health care, with family planning and reproductive health still being a main part of that service" (Armstrong interview 1997).

The problem that the YMC faces is not how to get men in the door, but how to continue finding adequate resources to guarantee the quality of its services in the near future. The innovative way in which the YMC's director has recruited medical and public health students to fill staffing gaps is a crucial but fragile basis for running a clinic because it is so tightly connected to the specific personnel who now run the clinic. Even with its present staffing, the clinic has to put great effort into staffing the clinic: "The problem here is if you don't have the clinical services at the other end, you can't create a need that's so great . . . then you can really be creating a monster because now you've created the need, and you've tapped into a need that the guys have, but you don't have the resources to come through with the product. . . . If you take me, for example, and you freed me up from teaching in the medical school, and teaching in the school of public health—all those things—I could turn this neighborhood on fire with male involvement" (Armstrong interview 1997). The resolution, therefore, may be that if the YMC does not continue to get enough resources, it runs the risk of becoming a victim of its own success.

Handle With Care

The practices of the men's clinics in Colombia and the United States thus exemplify the complex material work that is needed to configure men as clients of family planning clinics and to include men in family planning and reproductive health services. Although there are differences between these two clinics, the practices I have described reveal a remarkable similarity: one cannot offer men family planning or reproductive health services in the same way that one offers these services to women. Men's clinics can only come into existence and survive with major adaptations to attune services and spaces to the preferences, attitudes, and norms of men. This includes the organization of extensive community outreach activities; specific adaptations of space, such as providing separate entrances and waiting rooms; and an expansion of services to include more than family planning and reproductive health services alone. Men in Colombia and the United States are not likely to visit a men's clinic that does not offer sports physicals or other general health services.

These practices of adapting services to men have far-reaching consequences involving the creation of a new category of patient. At first glance, one might expect to find a category of patient in which men are classified in terms of type of contraceptive use, or a specific sexually transmitted disease, or maybe a disorder of the reproductive organs. Although these topics feature on clinic forms, they have not led to the classification of patients of men's clinics in terms of organs or diseases. On the contrary, the rhetoric and practices of men's clinics have constructed the patient in terms of a whole person. The Clinica para Hombres in Colombia and the Young Mens' Clinic in New York both reject a reductionist approach in which men are represented in terms of a number of diseases rather than as individuals. In an article in *Family Planning Perspectives*, the director of the YMC summarized this approach as follows: "It's not just a penis; there's a person connected to it. We need a whole-person approach that includes social services and health education" (Edwards 1994: 82). Serving young men "holistically" is a crucial part of the YMC's profile. This can be partly understood in the context of the clinic's location: an impoverished, low-income, inner city neighborhood in New York. Due to this background, providers have developed a strong commitment to do more for clients than simply meeting their medical needs. The fact that many of the YMC's clients face unemployment has made each provider "go the extra mile" in taking care of the whole person when men visit the clinic (AVSC 1997d: 33). Serving these men goes far beyond providing health care; it also entails discussing life in general (AVSC 1997d: 33). Ever since the clinic's inception, the concept of "the whole person" has become part and parcel of the YMC's policy to serve men. The concept originates from adolescent medicine. The fact that the director of the YMC teaches Adolescent Health at Colombia University, and that one of the providers had a fellowship in this specialty, thus functions as an important resource for the clinic's policy to treat men as "whole persons" (AVSC 1997d: 32; Diazgranados and McKracken interview 1997).

The holistic approach is, however, not specific to the YMC. The Men's Clinic in Colombia has also adopted a holistic approach. Like the YMC, the clinics in Colombia offer their clients services that go beyond family planning and reproductive health. One provider at the clinic in Bogotá formulated the clinic's policy to treat men holistically in terms very similar to those used by the YMC director: "We don't see the patient as a prostate gland . . . but as a man with a need. I look for the person behind the need. For the client, this means that the doctor provided a good service but also recognized the patient as a person. This is important . . . because sometimes a man comes for medical attention but really what [he] wanted more was counseling and attention" (AVSC 1997b: 30). Respecting the individuality of each client rather than grouping clients into specific categories of disease is a crucial part of health care for men in the clinics in New York and Colombia.

This holistic approach is new in the world of family planning and quite different from the approach that dominates family planning clinics for women. Family planning clinics for women do not offer their clients such a broad array of services as the men's clinics. Since, historically, the medical profession has focused almost exclusively on the reproductive organs of women rather than men, almost every part of the woman's reproductive body has been institutionalized within a variety of medical specialties, most notably gynecology, obstetrics, and maternal health care. The rise of these medical specialties has disciplined women and healthcare providers to articulate and categorize women's needs in a reductionist way. Given this situation, women now come to clinics asking for specific services (a pregnancy test, a pap smear, etc.) and clinics classify women's needs in narrow service categories. In contrast, men are not (yet?) disciplined to articulate their needs in such a reductionist way, and men's clinics do not have the habit of classifying men's needs in narrow service categories. Consequently, the female patient of a family planning clinic is more likely to be reduced to a specific disease rather than to be seen as an individual.

As new patients of family planning clinics, men are defined not only as "whole persons," but they are also represented and treated as persons who need care. Care is another important ingredient of the services offered to men in both countries. For the YMC, again, this can be understood in the locally specific context of the clinic, whose major clients are poor Dominican men, as is evident in the following quote:

> If you're a poor man, especially a poor man of color, if you're black or Hispanic living in the inner city, especially in the poorest of neighborhoods, of which we have many in this country, it's really not surprising how some of them say: "Who cares about me?" They don't have access to good health care. . . . When you address these issues with men and they really feel like they are being taken care of by somebody who really cares about you, like our clinic . . . We get patients that really like the services. They think we're good at it. Because they know that we care about them. You can tell by their faces—week after week after week—that they know we care. We're too slow; they don't like the waiting time, but they know we care about them. . . . People know we care so they come back to us. (Armstrong interview 1997)

Although situated in a completely different cultural context, the clinic in Bogotá shows a similar construction of men as patients who need care, as exemplified by Efrain Patrino's account of his experiences as a counselor in this clinic: "I am trying to bring more caring to the situation. Men often come in with aggression. We need to show caring. In addition, if we want to provide a quality service, we can't do it in a rushed way" (AVSC 1997b: 29). As I described earlier, the clinic in Bogotá uses specific counseling sessions to reduce the doubts and anxieties of male clients (AVSC 1997b: 21).

Finally, men are defined not only in terms of needing care, they are also represented as patients who have to be taken care of in their own right. In the context of the men's clinics, the new clients are represented as autonomous individuals who have the right to reproductive health care. As we saw in the previous chapter, this type of categorization is remarkably different from traditional family planning clinic discourse, where the need to include men in family planning is defined in terms of men's responsibilities to their female partners. The clinics in Colombia and New York City adopt a critical attitude to the men-as-partners approach developed in international population policy arenas such as the U.N. Conferences of Population and Development and in international family planning organizations such as the AVSC. Bruce Armstrong described the dilemmas that this policy has created in practice as follows: "So on the one hand you want to talk to him about responsibility, but I think I would want to question, Where's your responsibility to him? Where is society's responsibility to men? I don't think that for many men there is access to the kind of care that they need. . . . You can't keep saying that men should be more responsible, that men should be this and men should be that, if you're not willing to provide them with access to the means that they need" (Armstrong interview 1997). At the YMC, men are therefore not considered as patients who need health care because of their responsibilities for their partners, as is shown in the account of Al Cohall, a medical provider at YMC: "Men deserve to be seen and taken care of in their own right, and not just as partners of women. In family planning circles, the reason why you get men in is so they don't give infections back to women, rather than dealing with the man's health issues [which we attempt to do]" (AVCS 1997f: 33).

In the context of the men's clinics in Colombia and New York the new patient in the family planning clinic thus comes to be defined as a person who should be handled with care, in a double meaning of the word. On the one hand, the practices of the men's clinics reveal how providers put great effort into adapting their services to their clients in order to avoid making men feel uncomfortable, embarrassed, insecure, or stupid. On the other hand, the clinics try to maximize the quality of the care they offer their new clients.

Conclusions

We can conclude that family planning clinics have indeed made room for men. Over the last two decades, family planning organizations have tried to reorganize the infrastructure of family planning clinics to accommodate men. Most countries in which services for men have been established have integrated these services into already existing family planning clinics or primary healthcare clinics. Since financial resources for programs and services for men are scarce, most clinics give limited space to men and have made only minor, low-cost adaptations in the existing infrastructure. To demarcate the spaces for male clients, clinics have established separate waiting areas or separate entrances for men, or changed their decor to look less women-centered. As we have seen, this demarcation of spaces for men has not always been unproblematic. Allocating space to men in the predominantly female world of family planning clinics is not simply a matter of logistics; it requires renegotiating gender relations, both among and between staff and patients. The introduction of male clients has challenged gender routines and norms in provider–client relations and disrupted the gendered pattern in work relations that characterized the world of family planning prior to the emergence of the new client.

In addition to this integrated approach, a small number of family planning clinics, most notably in Brazil, Colombia, and the United States, have chosen to establish a separate new infrastructure for men: the men's clinic. The world of family planning thus provides an exceptional cultural practice compared to other public domains. Whereas the 1970s saw the emergence of women's houses, women's pubs, women's motor clubs, women's adult education programs, and so on, the 1980s witnessed the birth of the male clinic. In this case, men rather than women were set apart. Establishing men's clinics required a lot of work, including building separate facilities, hiring staff with specializations other than those found in traditional family planning clinics, and, on several occasions, hiring male staff. Moreover, the operation of men's clinics required the initiation of special activities to encourage men to visit the clinic. To configure men as clients of family planning clinics, service providers had to go to great lengths. Getting men in the door not only required the organization of extensive outreach programs, but also involved the development of carefully designed detour strategies to overcome the hesitation and reluctance of men to visit such unfamiliar places. To encourage men to visit these traditionally female spaces, the men's clinic in Bogotá transformed the clinic into a man's world: the clinic was designed with high-tech features to look like an office rather than a family planning clinic. Separate entrances and waiting rooms in integrated clinics had a similar symbolic and material function: men remain separated from the female domain, which facilitates a situation in which they become less painfully aware of where they actually are. Another strategy used to attract male clients consisted of expanding the services of the clinic to provide sports physicals and other general health services.

Configuring men as clients of family planning clinics thus involved a careful balancing between hegemonic masculinity, which considers family planning clinics as a female world, and non-hegemonic masculinities, which represent men as taking responsibility for family planning. The conventionalized performance of gender roles, which delegates family planning to women, puts a severe constraint on the existence of family planning programs and services for men: men's clinics can only succeed in attracting male clients if they do not profile themselves as family planning clinics. In Colombia and the United States, men are only likely to visit a men's clinic that offers services that go beyond family planning and sexual health. Non-hegemonic masculinities can obviously be performed only away from public scrutiny.

Most importantly, the introduction of men into the world of family planning implies the construction of a new category of client. The rhetoric and practices of the men's clinics in Bogotá and New York show how the new clients of family planning clinics have come to be represented as "whole persons" who deserve to be handled with care, both socially and physically. The fact that men are hesitant to visit a family planning clinic and often have problems in articulating their needs has led to the paradoxical situation where men receive more comprehensive health care in family planning clinics than women. In the short history of his existence, the men's clinic patient has thus received a special status as compared to women. In this respect, my account of the men's clinics mirrors studies about the entrance of men into other female domains. The enrollment of men in the traditionally female profession of nursing has given male nurses positions that women in the profession usually don't have, or, if they have them, women have worked harder to get there.[13] In the case of men's clinics, something similar seems to happen. This time, it is not the healthcare provider but the patient who receives special treatment because of his male gender. The introduction of this new type of clinic and patient into the world of family planning may therefore have important consequences for the quality of care in this domain. On the one hand, the introduction of men's clinics may lead to a reorientation and improvement of services for the family planning clinic's traditional clients: women. This seems to be happening in the family planning clinics in Colombia, as exemplified in the evaluations of Profamilia's family planning programs for women and men:

> In the male-only clinic, the staff there is always prepared, they are superactive to whatever question they [the men] have. They grumble that men are impolite, but it is that they [men] are more demanding. It is a gender issue . . . having separate spaces showed us how things are different. Our

male experience taught us how important the privacy issue was. If we asked them in public when they last had sexual experience, they would refuse to answer. Women would often answer in a low voice. The men's clinic taught us the importance of privacy because they [men] complained from the beginning. They started changing how we look at the issue of privacy for women as well. (AVSC 1997b: 32)

To solve the problem of privacy, Profamilia decided to offer special counseling sessions to all male clients. Although they would prefer to offer counseling to women as well, they don't have these facilities yet, due to the great number of women visiting their clinics (AVSC 1997b: 32). The introduction of men's clinics may thus eventually result in an improvement of services for women, if there are enough resources. On the other hand, the emergence of men's clinics may also lead to a further differentiation in quality between services for women and men. Whatever happens, configuring men as clients of family planning clinics has created a special status for men.

In recent decades men were not only newcomers in the world of family planning, they also first became enrolled as test subjects in medical clinics involved in the clinical trials of new male contraceptives. The next chapter explores how men became disciplined as participants of male contraceptive trials.

8

"The First Man on the Pill": Disciplining Men
as Reliable Test Subjects

· · · ·

None of us have ever seen a male method introduced. There is no track record for male methods since the condom, going from basic studies to market place. It's not like an antibiotic where there are fifty antibiotics introduced and the next one is small change really. So this is a truly revolutionary event, introducing a new male method. I mean that is just unheard of really in anybody's experience.—William Bremner, University of Washington, 1994

Clinical trials are a peculiar type of testing. They not only require material resources such as the availability of drugs, instruments to measure the effects of the drugs, and forms and statistical procedures to register and produce data, they also depend on the collaboration of human beings, known more formally as the trial participants. Clinical trials thus represent a very specific practice of configuring the user. Whereas most other configuring processes take place in the absence of users, clinical trials, as with other user tests, require the presence and cooperation of potential users.[1] As Stephen Epstein has suggested, "Clinical trials are a form of experimentation that requires the consistent and persistent cooperation of tens, hundreds, or thousands of human beings—subjects—in both senses of the word—who must ingest substances on schedule, present their bodies on a regular basis for invasive laboratory procedures, and otherwise play by the rules" (Epstein 1997: 691). One of the major aspects of clinical testing thus consists of ensuring the cooperation of trial participants. For researchers, this is a complicated endeavor because test subjects talk back: they may decide to discontinue with the experiment, or fail to comply with the procedures of the trial (Epstein 1997: 33).[2]

In male contraceptive trials, ensuring the cooperation of test subjects proved to be even more complicated than usual. First, the researchers and clinicians involved in male contraceptive trials faced a new situation because, for decades, contraceptive testing had been focused on women. Contraceptive researchers, predominantly men, were therefore not used to experimenting on men, as is illustrated in the quote above. Second, men were not used to being subjected to contraceptive trials or any other form of medical experimentation or examination relating to their reproductive organs. Whereas women have been, and still are, subjected to widespread experimentation and testing practices, such as screening programs for breast and cervical cancer, procedures for assisted fertility, physical examinations related to pregnancy and the use of contraceptives, and clinical testing of new contraceptives, such routine practice has been virtually absent for men. Consequently, noncompliance was a serious problem in the early male contraceptive clinical trials. In the 1970s many researchers reported problems in ensuring compliance and reported high dropout rates, sometimes even amounting to half of the test population (Foegh 1983: 25; Guille et al. 1989: 123). In a trial published in *Contraception* in 1979, researchers described how few men followed the instructions recommending the use of alternative contraceptive methods to prevent their female partners from becoming pregnant if the method on trial happened to fail (Barfield et al. 1979: 123). In the late 1970s a French research group decided to leave the field of male contraceptive research because trial participants failed to comply with treatment (Guille et al. 1989: 123).

This chapter examines the work that is involved in disciplining men to be reliable test subjects in clinical trials. I will show how this endeavor was dependent on the creation of specific procedures and, most importantly, on a renegotiation of masculine identities. As we saw in chapter 1, the predominance of modern contraceptive drugs for women has disciplined both men and women to delegate the responsibility for contraception largely to women. In the latter half of the twentieth century, contraceptive use thus came to be excluded from hegemonic masculinity. The development of new contraceptives for men required the destabilization of these conventionalized performances of gender identities concerning contraception. As we saw in chapter 6, family planning discourse has been a major domain for articulating new identities of men as users of contraceptives.

This chapter shows how the clinical testing phase of a new technology should be considered as another site where the articulation of identities of men takes place. Clinical trials have functioned as a cultural niche in which participants perform non-hegemonic masculinities. Adopting the concepts of projected and subjective identities, I will describe the renegotiation of male identities as a dual process involving both the projection of masculine identities, as articulated by others, to the trial participants, and the articulation and performance of identities as created and experienced by men.[3] I will describe how male contraceptive researchers have configured trial participants by articulating specific representations of masculine identities. For their part, men participating in contraceptive trials have articulated and performed masculine identities that largely matched the researchers' projected identities.

Selection Procedures as Tools to Ensure Compliance

Since men are not accustomed to being subjected to contraceptive testing, and reproductive scientists are not in the habit of having men as test subjects, the clinical testing of hormonal contraceptives for men can be considered a novelty. Given the newness of the situation, one important question concerns the extent to which male contraceptive testing required specific procedures to discipline men as trial participants. Let us first take a look at the selection procedures. As in other forms of clinical testing, male contraceptive researchers used specific procedures to select participants for the trials. Some of these so-called "inclusion criteria" were explicitly articulated and formulated beforehand, and others emerged as a result of the contingencies of locally specific institutional practices. The explicit criteria articulated in recruitment advertisements, protocols, and WHO guidelines for selecting volunteers included age (most researchers recruited men between 21 and 45, whereas the WHO guidelines recommended a range of 18 to 50 years[4]) and health condition (men were to be in good general health, including normal semen production) (University of Manchester 1993; WHO/HRP 1992b: 13). The implicit criteria used for the selection of trial participants included socioeconomic status and, in some cases, ethnic background and having a stable relationship. Although most researchers do not impose restrictions on ethno-cultural background, religion, or education (WHO/HRP 1976: 6), the test population for the male contraceptive trials nevertheless showed a specific selection of men. In the United States and Europe the trial participants were predominantly white, relatively young men with an above-average educational background, and usually included a high percentage of students, due to the location of recruitment (university settings). In some cases, the preference for higher socioeconomic status and education was explicitly chosen by the researchers. In Los Angeles, for example, male contraceptive researchers preferred to work with men from well-educated, advanced economic groups because they expected that this would facilitate a better compliance (Swerdloff interview 1993). In Seattle, however, male contraceptive researchers decided to exclude busy executives because of previous negative experiences with men who did not comply with the demands of the test because of work obligations (Paulsen interview 1994). One issue related to socioeconomic status concerned the payment of volunteers. In most trials, the participants were not paid because unpaid volunteers were believed to be more reliable than paid individuals: the latter might be motivated by the pay rather than by interest in the trial (Foegh 1983: 13, 36). This choice may imply an exclusion of the poor. In most trials, participants were, however, reimbursed for travel expenses and for the time they spent in the trials (Thau interview 1993).

Thus far, the selection criteria are not specific for male contraceptive testing but reflect practices in other drug testing situations where test populations are predominantly white, well-educated, younger men.[5] In this respect, the multicenter WHO clinical trials were an exception because they included a much wider variety of men of ethnic backgrounds. One of the criteria used to select trial participants was, however, specific for male contraceptive trials. Although not specified in the protocols or advertisements of most clinical trials, researchers selected men with "stable relationships." This implicit selection criteria reflected one of the major worries of the male contraceptive community—that trial participants and future users would be unreliable in using contraceptive methods. In "Birth Control after 1984," published in *Science* in 1970, Carl Djerassi, one of the developers of the Pill for women, was among the first to articulate the problem of the unreliability of men in matters of contraception: "This leads to the third difficulty—namely, the male's generally lesser interest in, and greater reservations about, procedures that are aimed at decreasing his fertility. If the agent were to be administered orally, men would probably be even less reliable about taking a tablet regularly than women have proven to be, and efficacy could probably be determined on a large scale only through long-term studies of married couples" (Djerassi 1970: 948).

Although most clinical trials in the last three decades have consisted of testing contraceptive injections rather than pills, most researchers have preferred to work with couples. To solve anticipated problems with noncompliance, researchers have put their faith in the female partners of the trial participants. Procedures for clinical testing, both in the United States and Great Britain, illustrate the crucial role of women in transforming their husbands and partners into reliable test subjects. First, female partners functioned as key actors in motivating men to participate in the trial. To quote from the experiences of the researchers involved in clinical trials in the mid-1990s:

"Quite often you get, particularly the patients recruited from Family Services, it's the women who saw the leaflet or poster and who initiated the contact and she's phoned us for more information" (Kinniburgh interview 1998). Men who participated in the two WHO multicenter clinical trials reported that one major reason for participation was that they had been encouraged to do so by their female partners (Ringheim 1995: 76). Researchers actively exploited the positive attitude of women toward male contraceptive trials. They usually asked women to come along for the first visit to the clinic, as is exemplified by the intake procedures used in clinical trials in Manchester: "We always ask whoever is interested to get in touch with us and then we always ask them to come together as a couple. . . . I think it's essential because one of the driving forces of the husband volunteering comes from the female partner. It certainly was our recent experience that it is the wife or the female who has seen the advertisement or whatever and that encouraged the husband to come along. So the female partner is a very key person during recruitment and throughout the studies" (Wu interview 1994).

As the last part of the quote indicates, female partners also fulfill other roles in clinical trials. This is also illustrated by the procedures used in clinical trials in Seattle: "First of all the wife, the live-in, whoever, we always invite them to come at the same time. We want both of them to come to the informational meeting where we tell them what we are doing . . . and then we ask them to think about it and we give them a document, a consent form and they both have to sign it . . . the way we operate is that we try to include the women" (Paulsen interview 1994).

During the trials, women are not only included in informed consent procedures, they also act as agents to monitor changes in their partners. In the trials in the U.K., female partners were asked to keep records of any changes in the sexual activity or behavior of the trial participants (Wu interview 1994), a fact also illustrated by the procedures used in Edinburgh: "We have a questionnaire that the partners answer every twelve weeks, so four times in the study. And it basically asks questions about their partner's behavior and sex drive and sex life and are you having sex more often, is your partner wanting sex more often, is he more irritable, less irritable, that sort of thing. Then there is a gap there for any comments. We normally get quite good feedback from the partners as well. Normally it's not just a matter of ticking of the boxes and that's it, they normally write a comment at the end as well" (Kinniburgh interview 1998).

In Manchester, female partners fulfilled a similar monitoring role, which revealed yet another crucial aspect of women's role in ensuring the com-

pliance of trial participants: "We see them [the female partners] intermit-
tently. They also keep a menstrual record. We have to keep in touch with them
as a couple, because if there is any failure the female partner will be the first to
tell us, or to tell the participant. So we also have in the past asked them to keep
a confidential diary of sexual intercourse just to make sure that people are not
preventing pregnancy by abstaining" (Wu interview 1994).

In trials in which the contraceptive activity of hormonal compounds is
measured by the number of pregnancies rather than sperm count as an indicator of the suppression of sperm production, female partners thus played yet
another role, namely as subjects to determine the efficacy of the contraceptive
on trial. In these trials, the selection criteria specified that only couples would
be allowed to participate, as described in the publication of the first formal
efficacy trial organized by WHO and published in The Lancet in 1990: "Healthy
men between 21 and 45 years of age were eligible if they were in a stable
relationship in which both partners wanted contraception" (WHO 1990b: 956).

Advertisements to recruit trial participants for the WHO trial also asked
explicitly for "couples," as shown by the press release issued in July 1993 by
the University of Manchester, one of the participating centers in this trial: "Dr.
Wu is now urgently looking for about 30 male volunteers to take part, with
their partners, in an 18-month trial. So the race is on to find suitable couples
in the North West. The man should be between 21 and 45 years of age and the
female partner under 35. They do not have to have had children previously, but
they should be people in stable relationships" (University of Manchester
1993). For this efficacy trial, the selection criteria also included specific requirements for the female partners, for example, an age limit. The choice to
select couples rather than individual men is exceptional compared to the
clinical testing of other drugs. Some researchers even consider the couple
rather than the man as the test subject[6]: "We are treating the couple. It just
happens that we're giving the male the injection" (Paulsen interview 1994).

To discipline men as reliable test subjects, researchers not only enrolled
their female partners but also relied on other tools to ensure compliance.[7] In
Edinburgh, researchers asked men who were interested in the trials to come
and see the researcher in charge of the trials at least twice before they started
taking any medication. Men who failed to turn up for these meetings were
excluded from the trial:

> People who failed to turn up for the first two meetings, we sort of weed
> them out. I mean there are some people who come along once and I
> never see them again. I phone them up and say, "You've missed your

appointment, do you want another one?" But quite often they tell you, "Oh, I have changed my mind." And the first meeting is quite intensive. I go through all about the study, answer questions, there are question-naires about. . . . And they're with me for probably an hour. And they have a blood test and a full physical examination including examination of the prostate gland which is a rectal so if anyone's not certain they usually don't turn up for that or they say before that. I think most of the men, if they've gone through that, either you'll never see them again or they'll sign up and come back. And there's quite a lot of dropout at that point. I'd say between three and four out of ten men who do come to that first meeting don't go on to the study. So that's wasted and they change their minds or they just don't come back. So I suppose that's mainly where the selection process goes on. (Kinniburgh interview 1998)

In the two large-scale WHO clinical trials, researchers adopted similar pro-cedures. Men who turned up two days late for any injection (the mode of administration of the contraceptive on trial) were excluded from the study for "protocol violation" (WHO 1990b: 956). Due to these experiences with non-compliance WHO has included a specific requirement in the selection crite-rion for future trials. In *Guidelines for the Use of Androgens in Men* WHO has added the criteria that men "should be able and willing to keep all appointments for the entire study period" (WHO/HRP 1992b: 13–14). In Germany, researchers have used a standardized personality questionnaire to test the reliability of men interested in contraceptive trials (Akhtar et al. 1985: 664).

Medical Care, Camaraderie, and Humor as Tools to Ensure Compliance

Men who passed the selection procedures were subsequently subjected to a whole range of medical examinations and laboratory tests. The protocols of most trials include physical examinations (including measurement of body weight, liver and prostate size, and testes volume, as well as blood pressure, heart rate, and the occurrence of acne), measurement of hormone values, semen analysis, routine clinical chemistry, liver function tests, blood and urine analyses, and monitoring for sexual function.[8] The laboratory tests are usually performed at least twice within a two-to-four-week period. In addi-tion, trial participants have to visit the clinic for the administration of the contraceptive on trial (once a week, in the case of hormonal injections) and to produce a semen sample (usually every four weeks) and a blood sample (usu-ally every three months) (Wu interview 1994). Practices during the trial show

how the procedures used to discipline men into reliable test subjects are not restricted to the selection phase of clinical testing. To ensure compliance during the entire period of the trial, researchers offer trial participants special services and treatments. Sessions to take blood and semen samples and other laboratory tests are usually organized in the evening to accommodate the men's work schedules (Matsumoto interview 1994). Moreover, researchers spend quite some time in sharing the results of the medical examinations and laboratory tests with trial participants:

> Each time they arrive we need to go through what's happened the pre-vious four weeks. I think that's quite unusual. . . . Men aren't really used to seeing a doctor on a regular basis. It's quite unusual for them. So you get told a lot of small things, but we encourage that. "Oh, well, I had a bit of cough last week," or "I stubbed my toe," or something very small. But strictly because we don't know exactly what effects we might be having, we want to encourage them to tell us everything. They want to know if the tests are okay and they're quite pleased to be involved and to have this attention. They're not used to the attention from doctors. I think it's quite good, they think to themselves maybe it's good for their health to have all this attention, all these blood tests. (Kinniburgh interview 1998)

Practices of clinical trials thus show how these tests have a dual function. For researchers clinical tests function as tools to investigate contraceptive efficacy and the side-effects of contraceptive compounds. For the participants, clinical trials function as a health check that keeps them motivated to visit the clinic on a regular basis.[9] Medical examinations during the trials provide men with attention and health care they do not request or receive in other places, which reflects the growing awareness among men of the importance of health issues that emerged in the 1980s (Nahon and Lander 1993). Researchers in Seattle also emphasized the importance of free medical care in ensuring compliance:

> We are very successful with keeping volunteers going. That has a lot to do with recruitment but it also has to do with the fact that we have a monthly clinic and we set it up so that it is an evening clinic, after hours and so they come, get their exam, their blood drawn, drop off their sperm counts and get to know the investigators pretty well. They get examined very carefully, so they get medical care, if they have a cold, we take care of that, if they have a little acne, we . . . Yes, that might motivate people to stay and there is some camaraderie in a sense that is built up over the years. They get some feedback about what is happening to the sperm

counts, they get laboratory evaluations, so they see what the cholesterol is doing, what the blood count is doing. A lot of the volunteers like to see that feedback. (Matsumoto interview 1994)

The practices of testing in Seattle thus indicate yet another important component of ensuring compliance. Researchers not only pay a lot of attention to the health of the trial participants, they also try to create a friendly, non-hierarchical atmosphere. Asked about their experiences, men who participated in the first large-scale WHO trial mentioned that they appreciated the camaraderie they had found at the clinic (Ringheim 1993b: 8). Humor plays an important role in this,[10] particularly when dealing with semen samples. As I described above, prior to the 1990s the efficacy of hormonal contraceptives was measured by counting the number of sperm in the male volunteer's semen. To gain access to semen, reproductive researchers had to rely on the cooperation of trial participants to provide semen samples by masturbation, which was not a routine practice in laboratories involved in clinical testing. Published articles from the 1970s and 1980s illustrate that there was an uneasiness about reporting on this part of the trials. Although most "method" sections of the articles included a detailed description of all other measurements, the fact that semen samples were obtained by masturbation was mentioned in only half of the articles (Soufir et al. 1983: 627; Barfield et al. 1979: 122). Many articles stated only that "semen was collected" without specifying how. The experiences of men participating in the WHO trials reflect a similar uneasiness with this part of the trial among trial participants: "I don't think the needles [the trial consisted of testing a hormonal injection] were as bad as the idea of hanging outside collection rooms waiting for one to become vacant. People know why you are standing there with your white paper bag" (Ringheim 1995: 78).

Camaraderie and humor have been very useful not only as ways to cope with the uneasiness related to masturbation, but also to reduce the tensions men experienced related to the effects of the hormonal compounds on their sperm production (Paulsen interview 1994). As David Kinniburgh, one of the researchers involved in the clinical trials in Edinburgh in the mid-1990s, described it: "A lot of men on the trial were worried that their ability to make sperm would be damaged for life or that it would make them unable to perform. Most men also feared that it would affect their sex drive" (quoted in Marlin 1998). One of the trial participants in Edinburgh expressed his worries: "You shouldn't tell a guy that without counseling. It's a big part of your masculinity" (Men as partners 1997: 36).

The practices of clinical testing of contraceptives for men thus show how researchers had to put great effort into disciplining men to be reliable test subjects, which required a variety of social skills.[11] As in the testing of other drugs, the reliability of trial participants is a crucial requirement in establishing stable relationships between researchers and trial participants. For male contraceptive trials, however, reliability is a concern that goes beyond the relationship between researchers and test subjects within the secluded and relatively malleable domain of the laboratory. In contrast to the testing of female contraceptives, where any pregnancy can be directly identified as a failure of the contraceptive method (or in the case of contraceptive pills, as indicating noncompliance of the trial participant), contraceptive failures in male contraceptive trials can never be excluded, because the untreated partner can become pregnant by having sex with someone else (WHO 1990b: 958). The assessment of contraceptive efficacy of hormonal compounds thus required specific procedures to ensure the compliance of the female partners of the trial participants, a highly peculiar practice compared to other drug testing. In this context, the selection of "couples" or "men in stable relationships," as described above, can be considered an adequate, although not 100 percent effective, tool to avoid skewing the data due to the extramarital sex of the female partner of a trial participant.

In this process, researchers not only configured the trial participants, but they also configured the future users of male hormonal contraceptives, as noted by British researchers involved in clinical trials in the early and mid-1990s in Manchester and Edinburgh:

> The men we think this will appeal to are those in stable relationships and those prepared to share the burden and benefits of partnership. (Fred Wu, investigator in Manchester, quoted in Shankland 1993)
> The Pill will appeal to couples where trust has built up and men want to take responsibility for what happens between the sheets. (David Kinniburgh, at the Medical Research Councils' Reproductive Unit in Edinburgh, quoted in Marlin 1998)

The selection of couples in stable relationships was not just introduced as a tool to make men into reliable test subjects. Equally important, it was constructed to create a distinctive niche for male hormonal contraceptives. In reaction to skepticism about the acceptability of the new contraceptive, which was voiced by groups of feminists, healthcare providers involved in AIDS prevention, and journalists who suggested that men are unreliable in matters of contraception or that hormonal contraceptives (as non-barrier methods) do not help to prevent AIDS, researchers configured the potential user of reversible, non-barrier contraceptive methods as men in monogamous, stable relationships where the partners trusted each other.[12] By configuring the users as couples in stable relationships, researchers simultaneously constructed the non-user: men in casual relationships, as was noted, again, by researchers in Edinburgh and Manchester:

> It won't work for the 17-year-old at the nightclub looking for a contraceptive but will for men in relationships. (David Kinniburgh, quoted in Smith 1997)
>
> A woman would be mad to believe a chap she met in a night club who said: you're all right love, I'm on the Pill. (Dr. A. Bellis from Manchester, quoted in Sweetenham 1994)

Disciplining men as reliable test subjects and future users thus entailed the construction of users as men with stable, monogamous relationships and the construction of promiscuous men (and women!) as non-users.

The procedures introduced to discipline men as reliable test subjects have been quite successful. As against the complaints about noncompliance articulated in reports of clinical trials in the 1970s and mid-1980s, reports in the 1990s were much more optimistic about compliance. Dropout rates after the initial screening procedure have been estimated at approximately 10 percent, which is much lower than the dropout rate in female contraceptive trials, which can be as high as 30 percent (Paulsen interview 1994; Wu interview 1994; WHO 1990b: 958).

Clinical Trials as Sites to Negotiate Masculine Identities: The Responsible, Caring Man

Disciplining men as reliable test subjects not only required specific procedures. Intriguingly, it also involved a renegotiation of male identities. As I have described in the introduction, this renegotiation can be understood as a dual process in which clinicians and others articulate the gender identities of men participating in the trials. Documents used to communicate with the media and the trial participants, such as posters and press bulletins to recruit trial participants and leaflets to inform trial participants about the procedures of the trial, are important sources through which to study these projected identities. These documents provide trial participants with identities to reconcile their new role as contraceptive trial participants with their subjective identities. The rhetoric of these texts shows how male contraceptive researchers and public relations officials constructed a specific image of the potential trial participant. In Seattle, men who applied to be trial participants received a leaflet entitled "Questions and Answers," first introduced in 1994, which opens with the question, "Why is a male contraceptive needed?" (Paulsen, Bremner, and Matsumoto 1994: 6). After a short description of the contribution male contraceptives can make to reduce the "exponential population growth," the document continues to highlight the importance of male contraceptives for enhancing "equality between men and women": "However, the primary value of a male contraceptive may be that it will allow couples to share not only the benefits but the responsibilities and risks of contraception. While the development of contraceptive agents has allowed women to control their fertility and thus has been an important factor in freeing them from most traditional roles, the responsibility for contraception has remained almost exclusively a female role" (Paulsen, Bremner, and Matsumoto 1994: 6).

Documents used to recruit men in the U.K. contain a similar emphasis on sharing responsibility between the sexes as a major reason why it is worthwhile for men to participate in the trials. A press release from the University of Manchester's Communications Office dated 9 July 1993, issued for the purpose of recruiting male trial participants for the second large-scale WHO clinical trial, articulated the need for new male contraceptives: "The move towards providing more options for male contraception is really reflecting social trends that equality between the sexes should extend to Family Planning. Of course, it also has important implications for the Third World, where the population explosion is uncontrolled" (University of Manchester 1993: 2).

As happened with policy documents, researchers thus actively reframed the need for contraceptives for men as a tool to enhance equality between women and men in the expectation that men would be attracted by this appeal to their altruism. In both the documents quoted above, the potential trial participant is configured as a man who wants to contribute to helping his partner as well as people in Third World countries.[13] The poster used in Edinburgh to recruit men for clinical trials in the mid-1990s exemplifies this altruistic image, although it also adds a third interesting motive. The poster begins with the following three questions:

Interested in helping develop a new contraceptive pill for men?
Fed up by the lack of choice for men?
Want to help your partner get off the female pill?

In contrast to most of the documents used to recruit and inform male volunteers, this poster explicitly addresses men in terms of their individualistic interests. Taking part in clinical trials is portrayed as relevant for men because it may increase their choice of contraceptives. Most researchers configure male contraceptive trial participants, however, as men who are willing to share the responsibilities and risks of contraceptives with their partners, as we have also seen in the previous section, thus constructing the image of men as responsible, caring partners.

The ways in which men who participated in the contraceptive clinical trials organized by WHO between 1987 and 1994 articulated their motives to participate in these trials provide interesting insights into how these men performed and articulated masculine identities.[14] Focus group discussions and questionnaires completed by men in five clinical centers, in Bangkok (Thailand), Edinburgh and Manchester (U.K.), Singapore, and Sydney (Australia), show how the image of the responsible, caring man has become part of the identity of these men. Many men participating in this acceptability study portrayed themselves as men willing to take the responsibility for contraception (Ringheim 1996a: 6):

> It's about time fellas start taking responsibility for this kind of thing. I hadn't been wandering around with the burning desire to take part in male contraceptive trials.(Ringheim 1996a: 7)
>
> I think men have been allowed to be lazy about this. I don't know who decided it, but it always seemed to be pushed on the woman to be responsible. (Ringheim 1996a: 7)
>
> A man should have 50 percent of the responsibility. This attitude is becoming more common. Women are not objects. They're the same as us. We're equals. To some older guys, women are second-class citizens. In this country [U.K.], they go to the pubs and leave the women at home. I think it will probably take 20 years before this dies away, but a male contraceptive would appeal to my circle of friends. They are like me and think men should be responsible. (Ringheim 1996a: 87)

Demonstrating prior awareness of the potential for problems, the majority of men who participated in the acceptability studies (61 percent), particularly men from the clinical centers in Edinburgh, Singapore, and Sydney, articulated their motivation in terms of helping their partners who experienced problems with the female Pill (Ringheim 1996a: 6):

> It's got to do with the fact that my wife gets depressed when she takes the Pill, and I saw this on the telly and I just rang up. That's the main reason I came on the trial. (Ringheim 1996a: 6)

If she goes on the Pill again there is always the risk, isn't it? And my way of thinking is, once she's taken the risk for a few years, I'll take the risk. Then you halve it. (Ringheim 1996a: 8)

My wife taking estrogens was like the shrew that couldn't be tamed. She would wake up depressed . . . and after a period of time I said, "Honey, it's the Pill, stop taking it, I don't care, I'll use condoms, or other forms of birth control, I'll go on the program that my friend is on, but you stop taking the Pill right now." (Ringheim 1995: 76)

Participants in the WHO trial in Bangkok also explained their motivation by referring to problems with the female Pill, although they articulated concerns about their partners' forgetting to take the Pill (Ringheim 1995: 77). Incentives to participate in the trials were expressed not only in terms of problems with the female Pill, but also of dissatisfaction with the use of condoms or vasectomy as means of contraception in stable relationships (Ringheim 1995: 77; Ringheim 1996a: 81). The motives to participate in the trials thus also contained non-altruistic components: the trials could help men to avoid the use of condoms or vasectomy. Another motive which shows the self-interest of men participating in the trials is the argument that the trial enabled them to be in control of their own fertility (Ringheim 1996b: 86; Ringheim 1995: 77). The dominant image articulated by male trial participants, however, was their interest in sharing responsibility for contraception with their partners.

The language used by these trial participants reflects how they considered taking responsibility for contraception as a largely unfamiliar and exceptional activity for men in long-lasting relationships or marriage. By taking part in contraceptive trials, men thus actively performed nonhegemonic masculine identities, which unmistakably reflected the researchers' projected identities of responsible, caring men. Participants in the trials in Sydney constructed self-images in which they saw themselves as different from other men:

We all know that at this stage of time, it's not socially acceptable for men to use male contraception. We are doing this because we are different. (Ringheim 1993a: 22)

I figure that the people who are doing this program are a different kind of guy anyway, we're not SNAGS [sensitive new age guys]. I hate SNAGS. . . . I don't think we are typical of white Australian middle-class society.[15] (Ringheim 1993a: 22)

Some of the Australian trial participants also explicitly articulated their new role in terms of masculine identities: "I think that men have always had soft

sides, gentle sides, nurturing sides, but for a long time they have been re-
pressed. To a certain extent all these norms, morals, and values are raised into
prominence because we are precisely in that period of change so people are
forced to think about 'Do men have to do things a certain way?' and 'What's a
typical male?' " (Ringheim 1993a: 11).

In assuming nonhegemonic identities, male trial participants did not receive much support. Most male colleagues and friends considered their decision to participate in a contraceptive trial as rather peculiar, as shown by the
experiences of trial participants in Sydney:

> You still get people who would say "What are you doing that for, can't
> your wife take the Pill or something?" It seems like the abnormal rather
> than the normal, the idea that the bloke, apart from condoms, would
> actually take any part of sexual responsibility for contraception, par-
> ticularly not one which involved needles. (Ringheim 1993a: 23)
> I told a lot of males about it because . . . I felt quite proud about the fact
> that I was on it. I thought it was a great thing to do. Probably out of the
> maybe fifty guys I told, X [another man participating in the trial] was the
> only one who considered it. . . . I thought a lot more people would have
> said that sounds great. (Ringheim 1993a: 23)
> [They] weren't particularly interested in the contraceptive side effects,
> they were more interested in the anabolic effects. (Ringheim 1993a: 23)
> They worry for us most of the time. My boss does. (Ringheim 1993a: 23)

Trial participants thus had to defend and negotiate their new identities. Interestingly, these men received much more encouraging reactions from women,
particularly their female partners (Ringheim 1993a: 25). As I have described
above, women played a crucial role in encouraging their partners to participate in the trials (Ringheim 1995: 76; Ringheim 1993a: 13). A significant
proportion of the participants in the acceptability studies (23 percent) mentioned the encouraging role of their partners as a main reason for participation (Ringheim 1996b: 76). As one of the British men expressed: "Quite
honestly, I never would have volunteered if my wife hadn't complained. My
motto is: 'If it isn't broken, don't fix it.' I think most men are only too happy to
have women use contraception. We know they have problems sometimes.
Why would we want to share that? But when the wife says: 'I've had it. Use a
condom or get the snip [vasectomy],' then we begin to look around and
realize, there isn't much else for men, is there?" (Ringheim 1996b: 86).

The reasons why women adopt this role is quite obvious: the participation
of their male partners in the trial frees them, although only temporarily, from

the use of contraceptives, at least if they are monogamous. In many studies investigating the experiences of women with the Pill, a substantial number of women have expressed their dissatisfaction with oral hormonal contraceptives or other current methods, as is reflected in the previously quoted remarks of men participating in the male contraceptive trials.[16] To quote two female partners of the British trial participants:

> I thought it was absolutely brilliant. I loved it. The break from the Pill really gave me a chance to get my head straight. I've always suffered from depression. I didn't always know it was the Pill until I went off of it. (Ringheim 1996b: 84)
>
> The trial was an interesting experience for him. We'd do it again. I found it great. I didn't have to do anything. Nice not to have to think about it. I wasn't worried about pregnancy. I was relaxed. We definitely had more sex, but I was also more receptive. I felt happy that he was taking responsibility. (Ringheim 1996b: 84)

Women thus used the clinical trials as a site to renegotiate the responsibility for contraception with their male partners. By doing this, they actively engaged in the construction of nonhegemonic masculine identities: caring, responsible masculinities of various types.

"Astronauts in the Sperm World"

To negotiate this nonhegemonic male identity, contraceptive researchers and male trial participants also relied on hegemonic representations of masculinity. The illustration and caption on the poster used in Edinburgh—First Man on the Pill—exemplifies this imagery in a nutshell (figure 2).[17] The upper half of the poster shows a picture of an astronaut standing on the moon with a flag in his hand, with the word "Exclusive" in a balloon-text near his head. The left side of the picture says, in capital letters, "FIRST MAN ON THE PILL." In a funny and clever way, the poster suggests that men who decide to become volunteers are performing a heroic act, like the man who first set foot on the moon. Participation in a male contraceptive trial is thus portrayed as an exciting new endeavor.[18] Potential trial participants are portrayed as adventurous men who want to explore a territory where no one has gone before.

Space metaphors were also adopted by trial participants. One participant in the second large-scale WHO clinical trial at Sydney described himself and his colleagues as "astronauts of the sperm world" (Ringheim 1993a: 10). Other male volunteers constructed images with similar connotations. They

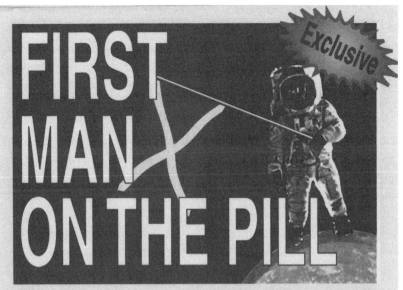

FIRST MAN ON THE PILL

Exclusive

Interested in helping develop a new contraceptive pill for men?

Fed up by the lack of choice for men?

Want to help your partner get off the female pill?

We are looking for volunteers to take part in a study for 6 to 12 months. You will take a daily hormone pill to stop sperm production and have a small pellet inserted under your skin to reduce side effects. You will need to use some other contraceptive for the first 6 months.

You need to be between 18 and 42, and be generally fit and well. We will see you every 4 weeks for a blood test and sperm count.

We do not expect many side effects.

Other men in Edinburgh have taken these pills with no problems, but we need more help.

For more extensive information call or write to
Dr David Kinniburgh
0131 229 2575 ext. 2105
Centre for Reproductive Biology,
37 Chalmers Street,
Edinburgh,
EH3 9EW

Please take a card >

Figure 2. Poster used to recruit men for clinical trials in Edinburgh.

identified themselves as pioneers in the development of a new male contraceptive method for men, which they felt was important to them (Ringheim 1993a: 7). Others described "the excitement of trying something new and possibly risky" as the most important feeling of being a trial participant. Researchers and trial participants thus transformed participation in a clinical trial into a brave, pioneering act.

The way in which male contraceptive researchers and the female partners of trial participants described men participating in contraceptive trials also adds to this image of the brave man. In reports of the trials, male volunteers were praised for their commitment to the trial and for their perseverance in enduring the demands of testing. In the report of a French clinical trial published in 1983, trial participants were given credit for their compliance: "The authors wish to thank the 6 men for their strict adherence to the protocol's requirement in spite of the constraint of their professional lives" (Glander 1987: 631). Including trial participants in the acknowledgments section of a clinical trial report is rather exceptional; usually only funding agencies, pharmaceutical firms providing drugs, technical assistants and secretaries, or laboratories that have performed specific tests are included in such acknowledgments. Other reports of male contraceptive trials also credited their male trial participants: "The volunteers . . . took a keen interest in the research and felt very responsible for fulfilling their part of the studies, although they were not paid" (Foegh 1983: 7).

In the report of the second large-scale WHO trial and in WHO's April 1996 press release reporting the results of the trial, the trial participants were portrayed similarly. In the press release, Dr. Giuseppe Benagiano, the director of the WHO's Human Reproduction Program, praised all the men who had ever volunteered to participate in a WHO trial: "The willingness of men to volunteer for the recently completed study, and other similar WHO-supported studies in the past, as well as their motivation and commitment to continue with the protocol of weekly injections, demonstrates the interest in—and demand for—a reversible male contraceptive of this type" (WHO 1996–1999). Benagiano not only praised the volunteers for their commitment, he also used them as examples to articulate the need for the new method. Male volunteers thus have a dual role in these reports: they figure as trial participants and as "prototypes" of future users. The rhetoric that appears in scientific journal articles exemplifies this transformation of trial participants into future users. In abstracts and method sections, these male trial participants are portrayed as active agents rather than passive test subjects. Instead of the usual phrases, such as "the subjects were given an intramuscular injection" (Belkien et al.

1984: 417), or "experiments performed on 10 normal volunteers" (Skoglund and Paulsen 1973: 358), or "a male contraceptive trial was undertaken in 23 men" (Bain et al. 1980: 365), trial participants are described as "men requesting contraceptives" (Guerin 1998: 187; Foegh 1983: 7; WHO/HRP 1996: 625, 821; Guille et al. 1989: 118). This subtle shift in discourse, in which agency is attributed to the trial participants, suggesting that they have taken the initiative or asked for the trial, transforms trial participants into initiators of the new technology.

Finally, the female partners and friends of the British men participating in the contraceptive trials also contributed to highlighting the special role these men played:

> It's absolutely noble. The man's so brave. (Ringheim 1996b: 82)
> I thought it was very noble of him to have injections. I go hysterical with needles. I wouldn't have been able to do that. (Ringheim 1996b: 82)

Researchers, trial participants, and their female partners and friends thus all actively constructed the image of the brave, pioneering man.

Conclusions

We can conclude that the organization of clinical trials for the testing of hormonal contraceptives for men required a lot of extra work compared to the testing of other drugs. Researchers had to create specific tools to ensure the cooperation of the test subjects. Since men were not accustomed to being subjected to contraceptive testing, and researchers were not used to having men as test subjects in contraceptive trials, the testing required specific procedures. To configure men as reliable test subjects, clinicians selected men in stable relationships. Test subjects and future users of the new technology came to be represented as monogamous men. Women also played a crucial role in configuring men as reliable test subjects. Female partners were important actors in encouraging men to take part in the trials and to ensure their cooperation during the clinical testing. Last, but not least, these women were creative agents in articulating masculine identities. Women used the clinical trials as a site to renegotiate responsibility for contraception with their male partners. By doing this, they actively engaged in articulating the image of the caring, responsible man.

Most importantly, men taking part in the clinical trials of male hormonal contraceptives in turn performed this projected identity. By participating in the clinical tests, men consciously or unconsciously performed an aspect of masculine identity that conflicted with hegemonic representations of mascu-linity—that men are not inclined to take responsibility for contraception. As we have seen, a majority of the men participating in contraceptive clinical trials portrayed themselves as altruistic men who wanted to relieve their female partners from problems experienced with the female Pill. We can thus con-clude that the clinical trials have functioned as sites for the co-construction of a new technology and a new male identity: the caring, responsible man. This image has dominated male contraceptive discourse in the scientific commu-nity and in policy circles since the late 1960s and was also adopted by clinical trial participants. This does not imply that hegemonic masculinities were completely absent from these narratives. To negotiate this new male identity, clinicians and trial participants relied on dominant cultural representations of masculinity that portray men as brave and pioneering subjects. Remarkably, being in control of reproduction is not a central aspect of these narratives. This is in sharp contrast to other technologies recently introduced for male re-productive bodies, most notably Viagra. The discourse surrounding Viagra is dominated by a modernist rhetoric which foregrounds the capacity to be in control of one's body as "the proper and appropriate order of masculine things" (Mamo and Fishman 2001: 16). Taken together, the debates on Viagra and the male Pill thus show a reification of hegemonic masculinity which emphasizes men's mastery and control of sexuality rather than reproduction as essential aspects of masculinity (Mamo and Fishman 2001: 17; Connell 1995). The virtual absence of representations of men being in control of contraception can be understood in the context of the contested nature of male contraceptives. An articulation of the users of the new technology in terms of men being in control of conception would run the risk of providing critics and opponents of new male contraceptives with arguments to reject the new tech-nology. An image in which male contraceptives are portrayed as drugs that serve the interests of men, particularly if it emphasizes men's control over contraception, conflicts with feminists' advocacy of women's autonomy in reproductive matters.

This chapter has shown that researchers were quite successful in renegoti-ating masculine identities. This renegotiation, however, met with resistance among other relevant actors in constructing the cultural feasibility of new male contraceptives, most notably the news media, which is the subject of the next chapter.

9

On Masculinities, Technologies, and Pain:
The Testing of Male Contraceptives
in the Clinic and the Media

· · · ·

In the last fifteen years testing has attracted a lot of attention in science and technology studies. Both historians and sociologists of technology have emphasized the crucial role of testing to understand the dynamics of technological development (Constant 1983; MacKenzie 1989; Pinch, Ashmore, and Mulkay 1992; Pinch 1993). These studies have focused almost exclusively on testing in the laboratory or in specifically designed test locations, and, for medical technologies, in the clinic. Due to this focus, what counts as testing has largely been described in terms of the activities of scientists, engineers, manufacturers, and clinicians. Testing, defined as "the processes in which the workability of a technology is established" (Pinch 1993: 26), thus seems to be restricted to the domain of scientific experts. In these studies, nonscientific experts figure only as witnesses or audiences to a test, or as "guinea pigs" or users of a technology.[1] In this way, science and technology studies have reproduced the still dominant hierarchy of institutional discourses by prioritizing the right of scientists to speak. Moreover, this approach has tended to favor one specific type of text as a unit of analysis: the academic journal article.

   This is not to say that science and technology studies have completely neglected other institutional discourses. Journalistic texts have been a favorite research site for STS scholars, particularly for those trying to understand the dynamics of public controversies in science and technology.[2] Although most constructivist studies of science and media relations have treated journalistic texts as secondary to scientific texts,[3] other scholars have dismissed the hierarchy of scientific and journalistic texts. They refuse to prioritize scientific reports as primary texts and acknowledge the contribution of journalistic texts in the construction of scientific claims. Following this argument, I regard scientific texts and journalistic texts as equally important sites for analyzing the testing of technologies.[4] As Madeliene Akrich has suggested, the construction of representations of users is an important part of technological innovation and the testing of a technology (Akrich 1995).[5] Akrich's work reflects, however, the same prioritization of scientific texts by restricting the analysis of representations of users to those articulated by innovators. In this chapter, I will show how scientific experts are not the only actors who construct specific representations of the prospective user. In the case of male contraceptive technologies, journalists have played an active role in articulating and demarcating the identities of the potential users of this technology-in-the-making. For my analysis, I will systematically compare three different types of texts:

1. The scientific report of a multicenter clinical trial, organized by the World Health Organization (WHO) and published in *Fertility and Sterility* in April 1996, of a testosterone injection;
2. The press bulletin of this trial released by WHO on 2 April 1996;
3. The media coverage of this trial in Dutch and British newspapers.

My central questions are: What is on trial, and where? To what extent is the testing in the media, as represented in journalistic texts, similar to or different from the testing in the clinic, as represented in scientific texts? I analyze these texts in a symmetrical way, by focusing on their basic storylines.[6] What type of account is given about what is going on in the testing of male contraceptives?[7] I will show how scientific and journalistic texts construct completely different accounts of the technical and cultural feasibility of the technology-in-the-making, including contrasting sets of images of future users.

Testing in the Scientific Article

Prior to the 1970s women were the main focus of reversible birth control technologies in the twentieth century. The introduction of men as targets for the development of contraceptive technologies in the late 1960s thus meant a revolutionary shift in focus in the contraceptive world. It required an organizational infrastructure that was not yet in place. As we saw in chapter 2, the main actors who took up the challenge to create the conditions required for the development of new male contraceptives were not private-sector agencies, but public-sector organizations such as WHO. WHO has been, and still is, one of the main actors in promoting and coordinating research in the area of new male contraceptives. One of its first efforts was to establish a worldwide laboratory network for the synthesis of suitable contraceptive compounds. The second effort consisted of the organization of two large-scale clinical trials. The scientific report of the second trial, in which four hundred men in nine countries in Europe, Asia, and the United States participated, was published by the WHO Task Force on Methods for the Regulation of Male Fertility in the April 1996 issue of *Fertility and Sterility* (WHO/HRP 1996). The publication is written in a style characteristic of the scientific genre. The article adopts the passive voice and the researchers are absent in the text (they figure only in a footnote, which mentions the principal investigators at the fifteen centers in the nine countries that participated in the trial). The realistic effects of the text are created by the inclusion of descriptions of methods, subjects, and instruments and the inclusion of tables and references to previous trials. The opening paragraphs are quite intriguing. The article, entitled "Contraceptive Efficacy of Testosterone-induced Azoospermia and Oligospermia in Normal Men," opens with an abstract, followed by a paragraph with a legitimization of the development of new male contraceptives and a paragraph describing the previous WHO multicenter trial and the hormonal prototype that was selected for the trial. I quote: "Reversible male contraceptive methods, comparable in efficacy to female methods, would allow more men to participate in regulating the couple's fertility. Despite their limited effectiveness or reversibility, up to one third of contraceptive couples rely on currently available methods that involve men. The new male methods closest to practical implementation are hormonal contraceptives" (WHO/HRP 1996: 821–22). The fact that the authors chose to begin this article with an articulation of the need to develop new male contraceptives suggests that the authors may believe that the usefulness of this technology, even after more than twenty-five years of extensive literature, still needs to be argued. Remarkably, WHO does not specify the contexts in which new male methods are needed. Instead of specifying the need for new male methods, WHO anticipates possible criticism of the need for new male contraceptives, which suggests that men will never use them. They claim that up to one-third of "contraceptive couples" already use male methods, despite their "limited effectiveness."[8] According to WHO, there already exists a huge audience that is waiting for a new method.

The opening text of the WHO article includes another intriguing message for the reader. The authors emphasize that the prototype of the technology that is on trial (a weekly intramuscular injection of 200 mg of testosterone enanthate) should not be considered as a practical contraceptive method. The prototype used in this trial was selected because of "its safety, reversibility, and efficacy in suppressing spermatogenesis" and not because it was expected to be effective in a practical way. Again, the authors of the text anticipate possible criticism concerning the acceptability of the new male contraceptive method. The introductory text thus reveals WHO's apparent perception of the contested nature of the technology. The technology is contested in two ways: in terms of the need for a new male contraceptive method and in terms of the acceptability of the specific method on trial (a weekly hormonal injection).

Let us take a closer look at the body of the text. What are the most important topics in this report? Since the authors put so much emphasis on the need and acceptability in the introductory text, the naive reader would expect to find a more detailed analysis of the need for new male methods and the acceptability of the method. A further discussion of the need for new male methods is, however, absent from the text. The acceptability of the method is indeed discussed in the text, but only as a minor part of the article. The authors describe how the acceptability of the method was assessed in three different ways: by monitoring the possible side-effects of the injection; by monitoring psychological reactions to the injection; and by organizing group discussions to assess the experiences of the participants and their partners.

A central concern in the assessment of the acceptability of the hormone injection, however, was the monitoring of side-effects. The effects of the injections on variables such as weight, testis size, blood pressure, liver function, and cholesterol and hormone levels are described in two paragraphs and one table on the last two pages of the article. The assessment of the psychological reactions to the injection, and the assessment of the opinions of the participants, are even less central in the text. The psychological reactions are mentioned in two sentences in the section on results (p. 825) and six sentences in the discussion section (p. 828) with the following conclusion: "The low incidence of psychological reactions is consistent with the lack of behavioral changes in a placebo-controlled study of healthy normal men given T enanthate and contrasts with reports of psychological disturbances among anabolic steroid abusers" (WHO/HRP 1996: 828). The results of the group discussions are deemed worthy of only four sentences, which conclude that "the study underlined the acceptability of an injectable method, particularly if based on longer injection intervals" (p. 820). A more extended report of the assessment of the experiences of the participants and their partners was published in a separate article written by a single author (Karin Ringheim), and not in the name of WHO (Ringheim 1995).[9] More information on the acceptability of the injections can be gleaned from the section on "Discontinuations," where the authors note that fourteen men (3.8 percent) stopped the injections due to psychological changes (changes in mood or aggression), twenty-one men (5.1 percent) stopped the injections out of dislike for the injection schedule; and dislike of the frequency of injections or pain was mentioned by nine men (2.4 percent). The high compliance of the participants is presented as evidence to show "their commitment to share responsibility for family planning" (p. 828). Acceptability and side-effects are thus not important topics in the text, neither in terms of space nor content. In the abstract of the article, the authors announce that they monitored only minimal short-term side-effects. In the discussion session, they conclude that long-term effects (on prostate or cardiovascular disease) "can be determined only by appropriate long-term surveillance when such methods are widely used in the community, as for female hormonal methods" (pp. 828–29).

The section on "Discontinuations" also contains a specific representation of the potential user as a member of the group of men who are willing to share responsibility for contraception with their partners. WHO thus constructs an image of the responsible, caring man. By adopting this image, which clearly conflicts with hegemonic cultural representations of men, WHO embraced a project that is potentially much broader than the development of a new technology. The endeavor to make new male contraceptives includes the articulation and defense of new representations of masculinity. Reproductive scientists working on male contraception have to uphold the image of the "caring man." In their text, they reject the idea that men are not willing to use a new contraceptive by arguing that men have always played a large role in family planning. The opening paragraph of the article in Fertility and Sterility, in which the authors emphasize that many people are already relying on the use of male contraceptives, exemplifies this advocacy role of scientists.

The most important topic in this article, however, is neither the user nor the acceptability, nor even the efficacy, of the new male contraceptive method. The authors of the Fertility and Sterility article describe how the contraceptive efficacy of weekly testosterone enanthate injections had already been tested in a previous trial organized by WHO in the late 1980s and published in The Lancet in 1990. The most important topic in Fertility and Sterility is a redefinition of the criteria for assessing the contraceptive efficacy of contraceptives for men. The authors report how, in the first trial, WHO had faced the problem that weekly injections could not completely suppress sperm production. In 30 percent of the men the sperm concentration did not go to zero, but went to very low levels. This observation presented a major stumbling block in the development of hormonal male contraceptives. If testosterone could not always switch off sperm production completely, and if azoospermia (the condition in which sperm concentrations in the semen are reduced to undetectable levels) is the sole criterion for concluding that a man is no longer able to fertilize his partner, then hormonal methods can never be made into effective and safe contraceptives.

The question crucial to the further development of male hormonal contraceptives was thus: can men with low sperm concentration also be infertile? The second large-scale WHO trial was of crucial importance for the continuation of the entire endeavor to develop male hormonal contraceptives. The major conclusion drawn in *Fertility and Sterility* was that the clinical trial indicated that men in whom sperm concentrations were reduced to three million or less per milliliter of semen were no longer fertile. Or, as the authors concluded in the discussion section:

> The level to which sperm output must be reduced by a hormonal method to ensure adequate contraceptive efficacy has remained uncertain, and an expert consultation in 1977 was divided whether azoospermia or severe oligospermia was necessary. A previous multicenter study demonstrated that hormonally induced azoospermia provided reliable and reversible contraception up to 12 months, but it was considered appropriate to examine the contraceptive efficacy in the 30% of men who remained oligospermic. The present study, using the same hormonal regimen, has demonstrated that 98% of men can be suppressed to azoospermia or oligospermia and such suppression provides effective contraception. . . . Although the study was not testing a method, these findings enhance the prospects for hormonal contraceptive methods for men since many potential regimens readily can achieve such levels of spermatogenetic suppression. (WHO/HRP 1996: 827)

The testing of a hormonal contraceptive method thus led to a redefinition of (artificially induced) infertility. Before the trial, only men in whom sperm production had been reduced to zero (or undetectable levels) were considered infertile. After the trial, men with low sperm concentrations also came to be considered infertile.

The strategy to redefine the boundaries of fertility enabled WHO to adjust the criteria for assessing the contraceptive efficacy of a method. Based on this trial, WHO could now claim that hormonal methods that suppress sperm production to three million or less per milliliter are highly effective, safe contraceptives. So, the most important news from this trial was the rescue of the trajectory of the development of hormonal contraceptives for men.

Testing in the Press Bulletin

On 2 April 1996 WHO sent a press release to over two thousand addresses, by fax, e-mail, and regular mail. The press release was also made available to news agencies and wire services attached to the United Nations in Geneva (Khanna 1996), and not without success: the WHO press bulletin resulted in worldwide media coverage. But why should scientists actually bother to communicate with the media? Why is the press so important? As scholars in science and technology studies have noted, the introduction of new technologies requires cultural interventions to create a demand for and acceptance of the new technology (Knorr-Cetina 1993). There is a lot of cultural work to be done for scientists who want to introduce a new technology, especially if the technology is a cultural novelty. The development of new male contraceptives is definitely a cultural novelty. As we saw in chapter 1, innovation in the field of male contraceptive technology has been absent from the R&D agenda of scientists and industry for a very long time. Since the 1950s, scientists have successfully introduced thirteen new contraceptive methods for women, whereas the contraceptives available to men are by and large the same as they were four hundred years ago (Davidson et al. 1985). The media provide, in principle, a very appropriate tool for cultural intervention: they reach the public, the professional community, and industry. Scientists in the field of male contraceptive research are fully aware of the importance of the media in creating cultural acceptability for their technology. Two quotations illustrate this, one from Geoffrey Waites, the former manager of WHO's Male Task Force, and another from William Bremner, one of the pioneers in male contraceptive research at the University of Washington in Seattle:

> Well, you have to be an advocate all the time. In the way that I think is not necessary if you are working with females. It is well accepted that the responsibility and the consequence of failure are there on the female, so it's obvious that the work there is relevant. But there are areas of prejudice and areas of vested interest in science, which are serious constraints for the development of this technology. (Waites interview 1994)
> It takes a lot of salesmanship, it takes a lot of giving talks and talking loudly. And to some extent getting information out to the public. So I'm glad to see that you are writing something about it. We try to be fairly

available when we get called up by the newspaper, or the magazines, or the radio. We have to talk about it because it's a very poorly understood area, of course by the public and even by professional people. (Bremner interview 1994)

It is in this context that we understand why WHO decided to release a press bulletin to communicate the results of their large-scale clinical trial to the media. Press bulletins are an interesting though often neglected type of document in the study of science–media relations (Hagendijk and Meeus 1993)— interesting because they represent what the scientific community (scientists or, in many cases, university press offices) considers the most relevant news they want to communicate to the public. What news did WHO want to bring to the public? To what extent was this message different from the message they communicated to the scientific community? The press bulletin, issued under the headline "WHO Completes International Trial of a Hormonal Contraceptive for Men," begins as follows: "A major breakthrough in the development of a new contraceptive for men is reported today in the results of a four-continent, two-year clinical trial published by the World Health Organization (WHO) in the journal *Fertility and Sterility*" (WHO 1996b). Compared to the presentation of the results of the trial to the scientific community, the press bulletin adopts a completely different strategy and tone. Now, the results of the trial are presented as "a major breakthrough in the development of a new contraceptive for men." In the *Fertility and Sterility* article, the results were presented as merely the testing of a prototype that was still far from a new male contraceptive method. The opening paragraph of the press release, however, emphasizes the effectiveness of the new contraceptive (98.6 percent), "which is comparable to the effectiveness of hormonal methods for women such as the oral contraceptive pill." The trustworthiness and importance of the news is created by an emphasis on the extensive testing of the technology (two years in four different continents), the involvement of WHO and its respectful and powerful allies (the World Bank and the United Nations, who are named in the concluding paragraphs of the bulletin as co-sponsors of the Human Reproduction Program of WHO), and reference to the scientific journal in which the results were published. The credibility and importance of the news is further enhanced in the second paragraph of the bulletin with the inclusion of a quotation from the Director of the WHO Human Reproduction Program, Dr. Giuseppe Benagiano: "The findings in the WHO study have brought us a step closer to developing a hormonal contraceptive for men." The message for the public is not the testing of a prototype (as it was presented to the scientific community) but the testing of a very promising, highly effective new male contraceptive, one that can bear comparison with the gold standard in contraceptive methods: the oral contraceptive Pill for women.

Another important topic in the press bulletin is the need for new male contraceptives. In the third paragraph, the authors articulate the need for the new technology. Here, WHO tells a story similar to the one addressed to the scientific community. It legitimates the development of new male methods in terms of the need to "expand the options available to couples who wish to plan their families." The remaining text of the two-page press bulletin is devoted to a description of the centers in which the trial took place, the characteristics of the participants, the treatments with hormones, the criteria to assess the efficacy of the treatment, the results of the trial ("only four pregnancies occurred"), and an homage to the participants.[10] The participants are presented as the heroes of the story, and this serves to legitimate the need and demand for new male contraceptives in the eyes of readers: "The willingness of men to volunteer for the recently completed study, and other similar WHO-supported studies in the past, as well as their motivation and commitment to continue with the protocol of weekly injections, demonstrates the interest in—and demand for—a reversible male contraceptive of this type" (WHO 1996b). The press bulletin thus represents the prospective user in a manner similar to that presented in the Fertility and Sterility article. Both texts represent users as men who are willing to share responsibility for contraception with their partners.

Compared with the trial participants and the users, the specifications of the artifact are less central in the press release text. Only in the section which describes the details of the trial is the reader told that the new contraceptive for men is delivered in the form of a weekly injection. The headline and the first three paragraphs do not mention the delivery system of the contraceptive. In the concluding paragraph WHO further reflects on the fact that the contraceptive is an injection and the reader is informed that "the need for weekly injections by the use of testosterone enanthate, is considered a drawback." However, this constraint is presented as a technical problem that can easily be solved. The reader of the press bulletin is told that WHO is studying longer-acting contraceptives with a three- to four-month interval between injections.

The press bulletin thus tells an optimistic story about a major breakthrough in the development of new male contraceptives. Topics that featured in the Fertility and Sterility article, such as possible health risks, psychological effects, or the cultural acceptability of the new method, are not included in the press bulletin. There are thus important differences in the ways in which WHO communicated its findings to the scientific community and to the media. These differences can be understood in terms of the differences in audiences of the two texts. Whereas *Fertility and Sterility* is aimed at the scientific community, the press bulletin is addressed to the public at large. Press bulletins can function as important tools for convincing audiences other than the scientific community of the feasibility of new technology. In the case of male contraceptive technologies, it is not only the public that has to be convinced of the importance of this new technology, but also another important actor: the pharmaceutical industry. As described in chapter 1, industry is still very reluctant to invest in the development of male contraceptive methods. It is therefore not surprising that WHO should adopt a more optimistic and glamorous style for the press bulletin. The press bulletin can thus be read as an attempt to use the media as a tool to articulate the technical and cultural feasibility of the new male contraceptive by emphasizing the effectiveness of the technology and the motivation and commitment of the participants in the trial.

Testing in the Mass Media

To what extent have the media played a role in enhancing the technical and cultural feasibility of the new technology? At first glance we may be tempted to conclude that the media have indeed contributed to the demonstration of the effectiveness of the technology. The WHO press bulletin resulted in worldwide media coverage, including local and national radio, television, and newspaper reports in Europe, the United States, and China.[11] However, the content of the news articles reflects a gloomier picture. The media, at least in The Netherlands and the U.K., did not unquestioningly reproduce the optimistic story of the press bulletin.[12] To the contrary, the storyline of the Dutch and British newspaper articles was completely different from the storyline of the WHO press bulletin.

Whereas the WHO press bulletin tells the story of a very promising, highly effective new male contraceptive in which men are the heroes, the news media tell stories in which side-effects and pain are the most important topics and in which men are portrayed as victims. What is happening here is that journalists put the trial results to another test. This time it was not the artifact that was on trial, but the potential user. In this testing, journalists enrolled a new type of expert. In contrast to the *Fertility and Sterility* article, the news media cited members of the public as experts, including a number of well-known personalities, and scientists figured merely as commentators on public opinion. Two examples from Dutch national newspapers will illustrate this difference. On

10 April 1996, De Telegraaf, one of the major Dutch daily newspapers, published an article by two (female) journalists in the section "Woman" which opened with a lead text in which a man tells the reader that he cannot appreciate a male contraceptive injection: "I already have a fat belly. Who can guarantee that those hormones won't give me breasts?" The article includes the opinions of three other men and one woman, along with their pictures with captions showing their negative attitudes toward the new male contraceptive (Ketting and Wieringa 1996). Another leading Dutch newspaper, De Volkskrant, used its special column, in which well-known Dutchmen are asked to give opinions on a topic of the day, to discuss the pros and cons of a male contraceptive pill. This article presented a curious grouping of people (eight men and two women) who were considered to have valuable opinions on this issue: three writers, one actor, a television programmer, a football player, a politician, and three medical professionals, who were presidents of medical professional societies (Vries 1996).

A comparison of this testing in the media with the testing in the clinic reveals a remarkable difference in the criteria used for the testing of the new male contraceptive. Whereas the redefinition of the criterion to assess the efficacy of contraceptive methods was the major aim of testing in the clinic, the testing in the media focused almost exclusively on the acceptability of the new technology. Dutch newspapers emphasized that it was very likely that both men and women would reject this new technology. Women were portrayed as opponents of male contraceptives because they do not trust men in matters of contraception. In De Volkskrant one female writer concluded: "It is a great invention that will please feminists in theory and ideology. But the injection will hardly be used in practice, I think. Women don't trust men with this, they want to keep it in their own hands. Imagine that you have to control your partner: 'Darling, did you take your injection?' . . . I'm afraid that this is again a feminist victory that is good for nobody" (Vries 1996). Under the headline, "Where are the Cheers for the Buttock-Injection?" a journalist in the Haagse Post/De Tijd told his readers that the male injection might be as reliable as the female Pill, but he simultaneously raised the question: "How reliable are men?" The journalist cited the results of a nine-year survey of female visitors to a Dutch family-planning clinic to try to convince readers that women would never accept this technology: 80 percent of the women said "no" to the idea of a new male contraceptive because they did not trust their partners with contraceptives (Leclair 1996).[13]

The theme of trust and reliability also featured prominently in British press coverage. In the U.K., coverage was undertaken almost exclusively by female journalists, who raised the question of whether men could be trusted to take responsibility for contraception (King 1999: 15):

> The Pill for men might be around the corner—but there's just one little problem. How can women trust guys who say: It's all right, I'm on the Pill? (Nicoll 1998)
>
> Work on the "male pill" has been all but killed off by the reality that women do not trust men to take it. (Sunday Times, 22 September 1996)

Dutch and British journalists were equally convinced that the majority of men would never use male contraceptive injections. Here, the criterion was not trust, but pain. In contrast to the WHO press bulletin (where pain is not mentioned at all; it was only described in Fertility and Sterility, as one of the reasons why some volunteers stopped with the injections), journalists emphasized the painful nature of injections in the buttocks. Three leading national Dutch newspapers (De Telegraaf, Trouw, and De Volkskrant) constructed the image of a painful technology and oversensitive men, using headlines like: "The Injection-Pill for Men is Reliable but No Fun" (Trouw), or "No INJECTION in My Buttock" (De Telegraaf). The article in De Telegraaf also included a photo of a man trying to inject himself. Journalists constructed this image by quoting the opinions of "the men/women in the street" (Telegraaf) or of well-known Dutchmen (De Volkskrant):

> They need a weekly injection in the buttock? Oh, you can forget it. There is no man who will do that. Men are very oversensitive to injections. (a female writer, quoted in Vries 1996)
>
> Terrible. A hypodermic injection. I don't like to do that any more. . . . Imagine me sitting there in a waiting room with all these men who can already feel the pain in their buttocks. (a male actor, quoted in Vries 1996)
>
> An injection is painful and men are ten times more sensitive to pain than women, I have been told. So, I don't see a breakthrough for a male contraceptive. (a male physician, quoted in Vries 1996)

In the HP/De Tijd, one journalist chose the role of participant-observer of the discussions among his colleagues and fellow journalists. I quote again: "Although the male participants in the trial were enthusiastic about the buttock-injection, Dutch men don't seem to like the idea at all. Giggling, they discussed the side-effects that the guinea pigs (those poor guys) had to endure in the trial" (Leclair 1996). The editors of the Algemeen Dagblad even tried to convince their female colleagues that the new male contraceptive would have a negative impact on the national economy, because men would have to stop working for one hour a week to get their injections (Leclair 1996).[14]

As in Holland, many British journals characterized the weekly injections as inconvenient and painful (King 1999: 18). According to one journalist in *The Guardian*: "I wouldn't mind taking a contraceptive pill but I'm not having any injections in my bum, because that would put me right off sex. A pill is easy to swallow . . . but an injection sounds horrible. I had one in my buttocks once and could not sit down for a week, it was like having a good caning at school." The journalist went on to comment on the interviewed men's views by concluding that his opinion "reflected the painful views of many men" (Johnson 1996). The British news media also raised concerns about the side-effects of the contraceptive on trial. Although adverse effects were not mentioned in the WHO press release, many British articles provided information on the side-effects of the contraceptive injection, including acne, increases in weight and aggression, physical and psychological effects on libido and virility, and long-term implications for health and fertility.[15] Journalists also criticized the use of hormones. A journalist for the *Independent on Sunday*, for example, wondered whether "pumping hormones into men too really [is] the best alternative" (14 April 1996). *The Times* voiced a similar concern and quoted the head of the Association of the British Pharmaceutical Industry: "Giving millions of men a high dose of a potent steroid strikes me as unacceptable" (WHO 1996a: 30). In contrast to the Dutch press coverage, the British press also revealed a great anxiety about the effects of the contraceptive injection on fertility, virility, and masculinity (King 1999: 21).[16] As one journalist in the *Guardian* put it: "Another downside is that men are very delicate creatures who don't like anything which might interfere with their manliness or capacity to make love" (Johnson 1996). A journalist in the *Scotsman* expressed similar concerns, which he referred to as the "deep-seated male worries relating to chemically-induced emasculinisation" (Jourdan 1997). As Cathy King has noted, macho images of men featured prominently in the British press reports on the testing of the new male contraceptive (King 1999).

These journalistic texts contain specific representations of the prospective user. In their texts, Dutch and British journalists represented users as unreliable and oversensitive men. By constructing these images, journalists simultaneously reproduced and contested hegemonic cultural representations of masculinity. The portrayal of men as unreliable corresponds to hegemonic views of masculinity that emphasize the unreliability and disinterest of men toward contraception.[17] These texts thus confirm and legitimate the hegemonic view of gender roles in which the responsibilities and risks of contraception are delegated to women. The image of oversensitive men, however, does not resemble any hegemonic view of masculinity; to the contrary, dominant cultural representations of masculinity portray men as brave and strong (Connell 1995). By representing men as oversensitive to pain, journalists embraced the incorporation of hegemonic feminine representations in which women rather than men are portrayed as the sensitive, weaker sex.

Two journals also added other images of men that went beyond hegemonic representations of masculinity. *De Volkskrant* presented two advocates of new male contraceptives, a football player on the Dutch national team and a physician. They suggested that weekly injections would be no problem at all, and that there were men who would want to have control in matters of contraception (Vries 1996). In these two cases, the journalists explicitly articulated new male identities.

De Volkskrant chose to illustrate its article on the opinions of well-known Dutch men and women with a photo of a shaving-apparatus next to a strip with pills (Vries 1996). And the journalist in the *HP/De Tijd* predicted (although with an ironic undertone): "Within a couple of years there will be contraception pills and plasters for sale at each drugstore. There is no doubt that the advertisement boys will find a nice marketing strategy: black plasters taped on sexy muscular upper arms or carelessly stuck on a shaggy stubbled chin" (Righart 1996).

These texts thus show another set of representations of the envisioned user and of masculinity: users are represented as men who want to have control over reproduction. The visible use of contraceptives (the black plaster) is presented in such a way as to fortify a sexy, masculine image.

The news media coverage of the WHO press bulletin in the Netherlands and the U.K. thus shows a conflicting set of representations of masculinity rather than an articulation of the need and acceptability of new male contraceptives.[18] We thus may conclude that the media did not play a role in enhancing the cultural feasibility of new male contraceptives.[19]

Conclusions

In this chapter I have argued that the testing of the feasibility of a technology is not solely in the hands of scientific experts. The news media must also be considered as important actors in the construction of this feasibility. The development of a new male contraceptive shows that there are important differences between the scientific and the popular press as sites of testing. First, there are differences in testing in terms of the subjects, the aims, the criteria, and the experts. What was on trial in the scientific text and the press bulletin was the artifact and the trial participants. What was on trial in the news media was the potential user and, very remarkably, the partner of the potential user. The aim of testing in the scientific press was the technical feasibility of the technology, that is, the redefinition of the criteria used to assess the efficacy of male contraceptive methods. The testing in the media focused almost exclusively on the cultural feasibility of the new technology, that is, the need and acceptability of injectable contraceptives for men. Although acceptability was also a major topic in the scientific report and the press bulletin, the newspapers applied different criteria to assess the acceptability of the contraceptive on trial. In the scientific article and the press bulletin, the criteria for acceptability centered on the incidence of side-effects and the psychological reactions to the injection. In the media, the main criteria used to assess acceptability were the reliability of men in the use of contraceptives and the pain caused by the injection. Finally, there was a major difference in who should be considered the experts in the testing. The experts in the scientific text and the press bulletin were reproductive scientists, clinicians, and WHO. The experts in the media were "lay people," both men and women.

Second, scientific and journalistic texts presented completely different accounts of the technical and cultural feasibility of the technology:

1. In the context of a scientific report in an international journal specialized in reproductive research, the technology was represented as

—a prototype that is still far away from a new male contraceptive method, and
—a technology that has not yet acquired an acceptable form, although this problem can be solved in a technical way (by synthesis of a testosterone compound that permits longer intervals between injections);

2. In the context of the WHO press bulletin, the technology gained in status. It was represented as

—a major breakthrough in the development of a new contraceptive for men,
—a highly effective new contraceptive comparable to the contraceptive pill for women, and

—an important contribution to equal sharing of contraception between the sexes.

As in the scientific report, technical improvements of the hormonal compound were presented as solutions for problems with the acceptability of the specific form of the technology:

3. In the context of the Dutch and British media, the technology was portrayed as

—a painful technology, and
—a technology that would face problems in becoming acceptable to many men and women.

Finally, scientific and journalistic texts reveal completely different representations of the prospective user. In the scientific report and the press bulletin, users were represented in terms of men who were willing to share responsibily for contraception. In the media, users were primarily represented as oversensitive, unreliable men who would never use a contraceptive injection. These representations of users are not innocent. On the contrary, they can function as tools in enhancing the cultural feasibility of a technology, as exemplified in the texts of WHO, or they can be used to denounce the viability of a new technology, as happened in the journalistic texts. Journalists have used representations of masculinity to argue that new male contraceptives will never be accepted by men and women.

These different accounts of male contraceptive technology show that what counts as a successful test is not solely in the hands of scientists or defined exclusively in scientific journals. News media can play an important role in shaping the fate of test results (Hagendijk and Meeus 1993; Ashmore, Mulkay, and Pinch 1989).[20] Whereas scientists rely on the "replication" of experiments to accept or refute scientific claims, journalists have the powerful tool of literary replication, as James Secord has called it (Secord 1989; Gieryn 1992; Collins 1987). The news media can shape scientific claims by replicating or contesting the results of experiments in newspapers. In the case of the testing of male contraceptive technology, the media refused to replicate the test results. Although the WHO press bulletin resulted in widespread media coverage, Dutch and British newspapers contested the scientific authority of WHO by providing an alternative testing of the new technology. This is a rather exceptional practice because newspapers more often adopt the role of uncritically reproducing what scientists tell them.[21] "Breakthroughs" in the biomedical sciences frequently receive considerable media coverage, which often gives a simplified and overly optimistic picture of what has been claimed (Fox and Swazey 1992).

The question that needs to be answered, therefore, is why journalists in this case departed from this routine. How did Dutch journalists come to compete with WHO in the construction of claims about the feasibility of a technology? Is it the low status of the science in question that facilitates a deconstructive attitude among journalists, as Collins and Pinch have suggested (Collins and Pinch 1979; Collins 1987)?[22] Although the reproductive sciences are not among the top-ten high-status sciences, the alliances with established and respectable organizations such as the WHO indicate that this field is definitely not positioned in the lower ranks of the spectrum of respectability.[23] Moreover, not all the scientific claims of the WHO trial were subjected to a critical deconstruction in the media. Journalists contested only the claims about the cultural feasibility of the male contraceptive injection. The technical feasibility of the contraceptive method was not questioned. So, if the low status of the field does not explain the contesting attitude of the media, what can account for it? I would suggest that the news coverage of the testing of this male contraceptive technology can be ascribed to previous criticism of contraceptive technologies that has created a climate in which the media has already been educated about questioning the promises of contraceptive technologies. Ever since the introduction of the first oral contraceptive for women in the early 1960s, the women's health movement has informed the media and the public of the health risks and the abuse of female contraceptives (Seaman and Seaman 1978; Gelijns and Pannenborg 1993). The skeptical attitude toward male contraceptives is, however, different from concern about female contraceptives, both in terms of the origin and the content of the criticism. In the case of male contraceptives, criticisms are voiced by the media rather than by (women's) health advocates. Moreover, criticism of female contraceptives has focused particularly on health issues and fertility control as symbolic of institutional power over women, whereas male contraceptives have been criticized as incompatible with gender roles and identities. We thus can conclude that those scientific claims that clash with hegemonic representations of gender are likely to become subject to deconstruction by the media. As Lyotard has suggested, "the discourses of stories, histories, myths, biographies, legends, and tales of the future" are important resources in defining "what has the right to be said and done in the culture" (cited in Gieryn 1992: 221). Following Lyotard, Gieryn's study of the role of the media in the cold-fusion controversy showed that narratives are important resources in assigning credibility to scientific claims (Gieryn 1992). Gieryn points to the important role of the media, which function as gatekeepers for what stories can be told or not told in our culture today. By contesting the results of the WHO clinical trial, journalists refused to reproduce the scientific discourse on new gender roles and identities for men. The story of the "caring man" obviously did not fit into the journalists' favorite tales of the future.

10

Articulating Acceptability

· · · ·

Through the years, the most hotly debated topic in the field of male contraceptive research has been the future user. Ever since the demand for new male contraceptives was first articulated, people have questioned whether men would be willing to use a contraceptive pill or injection if it became available. The previous chapter illustrated how the acceptability of the new technology remained a contested issue until the late 1990s. Articulating acceptability is therefore a crucial aspect of the cultural work involved in establishing the feasibility of this technology. In the last three decades, the male contraceptive community and family planning organizations have used several strategies to articulate the acceptability of hormonal contraceptives for men. One of the strategies consists of configuring the user as a man with a specific male identity and demographic background. In chapter 6 we saw how family planning organizations and women's health organizations configured the user in terms of "men as partners" to counter the criticism and distrust of women's health organizations, feminists, and critics within family planning organizations, who were concerned that men would prove to be unreliable in matters of contraception. Reproductive scientists and clinicians represented future users of the new technology as men in stable relationships. In chapter 8 we saw how the couple became the major target for male contraceptive development. The distinction between users and non-users, that is, men with casual sexual relationships, thus anticipated problems with acceptability.

This chapter focuses on yet another strategy used by reproductive scientists and clinicians to articulate the acceptability of the new technology. In the last three decades, the male contraceptive community has enrolled the expertise of social scientists to conduct so-called acceptability studies to investigate the extent to which men (and women!) would favor new contraceptives for men. Although the aim of acceptability studies seems to be rather straightforward, that is, the assessment of the acceptability of the new technology for the potential user, I will show how these studies actually perform a variety of functions: as tools to provide feedback on product development, as instruments to counter skepticism, and, last but not least, as tools to convince pharmaceutical companies of the viability of a market for the new technology. The second part of this chapter focuses on the pharmaceutical industry. The fact that this actor only figures in the first chapters and the last empirical chapter of this book is no coincidence. As I have described in chapter 2, pharmaceutical firms have been very reluctant to become involved in male contraceptive development. Over the last three decades, the absence of the pharmaceutical industry has been a major factor in shaping the developments in this field. Since the late 1990s, this situation has changed. For the first time in the history of male contraceptive research, pharmaceutical firms, particularly the Dutch company Organon, are now showing an active interest in the new technology. I will describe how acceptability studies were one, but by no means the only, factor bringing about this shift. Changes in the hormone market for men and changes in the management of Organon have also played a crucial role.

Acceptability Studies as Tools to Create Cultural Feasibility

Social science research on male contraceptives has a history of almost thirty years. The introduction of this new type of expertise into the world of contraceptive research coincided with the widespread introduction of vasectomy in the early 1970s (Ringheim 1993a: 87). The concept of "acceptability" was defined by John Marshall in 1977 as "a quality which makes an object, person, event, or idea pleasing or welcome" (Marshall 1977: 65). Marshall, a social scientist affiliated with the WHO Special Program for Research in Human Reproduction, played an important role in designing, supervising, and encouraging acceptability studies of contraceptives for men in the 1970s (Davidson et al. 1985: 27; WHO 1979b: 121). The first studies of new contraceptives for men took place in the early 1970s. University-based social scientists conducted several field surveys in which they compared the acceptability of existing male contraceptives with a hypothetical contraceptive pill for men.[1] In the same period, the need for social science research on the acceptability and prevalence of the use of male contraceptives became a priority within the

Human Reproduction Program (HRP) of WHO (Ringheim 1993a: 87). The organization of clinical trials on new contraceptives for men enabled WHO to initiate another type of acceptability study. Instead of studying hypothetical methods, social scientists now focused on the experiences of men actually using a method, although one in an experimental setting.[2] In the last three decades, WHO has conducted several of these so-called experiential acceptability studies (Ringheim 1993a: 89).[3] In the 1990s the Contraceptive Development Network, consisting of four university centers for reproductive biology, in Edinburgh, Hong Kong, Cape Town, and Shanghai, has initiated field surveys focusing particularly on cross-cultural differences in the acceptability of male hormonal contraceptives among men and women (Martin et al. 1997).

Over the years, acceptability studies have served different functions in the field of male contraceptive research. In the 1970s the major objective of these studies was to provide feedback to product development. In "Acceptability of Fertility Regulating Methods: Designing Technology to Fit People" (Marshall 1977), which outlined the basic methodology for acceptability studies, John Marshall described the general goal of acceptability studies as "providing program administrators and biomedical scientists with information that will enable them to modify technology and programs to fit people, rather than modifying people to fit technology and programs" (Marshall, cited in Keller 1979: 230). WHO/HRP's early interest in acceptability studies was largely inspired by the expectation that social science research would provide biomedical scientists and HRP managers with guidelines for developing culturally acceptable contraceptives (Keller 1979: 230). The protocol of the first acceptability study of 1976 clearly reflected this objective:

> In summary, the proposed research on the acceptability of new male fertility regulating methods is intended to help provide biomedical scientists with information at each collaborating site regarding the perceived advantages and disadvantages of the methods. Data will suggest possible modifications which could be made to improve the user acceptability of the male contraceptives, differential preferences for monthly injectables or daily oral pills, perceived positive and negative side effects (including changes in sexuality), and reasons for discontinuation of the method. (WHO/HRP 1976: 3)[4]

In the 1980s acceptability studies came to be used for yet another reason, that is, to counter skepticism about the cultural feasibility of the new technology. In one of the first acceptability studies conducted in the mid-1980s, scientists criticized opponents of male contraceptive research for relying on stereotypical images of the potential user that had never been subjected to empirical investigation:

> One cause of the relative disinterest in male fertility regulating method development among scientific investigators and public and private supporters of contraceptive research has been the widely held belief that a demand does not exist for new male contraceptives. Prevalent stereotypes include the notion that men view family planning as a woman's problem and are neither concerned nor interested. . . . Given that contraceptive research and development priorities should be guided in part by information on the need and demand for new products, it is somewhat surprising that the question "Would men be willing to use a new male contraceptive?" has been the topic of considerably more conjecture and debate than empirical investigation. (Davidson et al. 1985: 1–2)

In the conclusions of the report the authors emphasized that the results of their survey were "clearly inconsistent with prevalent stereotypes" and that men were willing to assume an active role in fertility regulation (Davidson et al. 1985: 21). This use of acceptability studies is not restricted to social science publications. From the 1970s until the present, publications reviewing the state of the art of male contraceptive research routinely include references to acceptability studies to counter skepticism about the motivation of men to use contraceptives:

> The attitudes of men regarding birth control and the family were frequently mentioned by investigators and family planners as having a deterrent effect on research interest in male contraception. . . . The assumed prevailing notions were that (1) family planning was a woman's problem and responsibility because men were neither concerned nor interested; and (2) the male was perceived as sexually capricious, at least prior to marriage. . . . These stereotypic notions have had serious impact on the potential role of the male in family planning in the United States, so much so that scientific investigators questioned the demand for a male contraceptive even if one were available. Family planners ignored men as consumers; drug companies were reluctant to invest in projects that appeared to have little profit; and researchers were discouraged from entering the field because of lack of interest and funding. Recent analysis of male attitudes and perceptions has shown the earlier stereotypes to be false. (Diller and Hembree 1979: 1273)

In this publication, the authors thus used studies of male attitudes as a tool to convince their critics that they had a more accurate picture of the acceptability of the new technology.

A third, and related, use of the results of acceptability studies has been to articulate the need for the development of new male contraceptives. Two reports of acceptability studies organized by WHO in the early 1980s and early 1990s exemplify this function of acceptability studies (WHO/HRP 1982; Ringheim 1995). In "Hormonal Contraceptives for Men: Acceptability and Effects on Sexuality," a WHO report published in 1982, the authors concluded: "In conclusion, this study provides important confirming evidence to strengthen conclusions from other recent studies that because there is considerable user acceptability for male hormonal contraceptives, efforts should therefore continue toward developing and perfecting these methods" (WHO/HRP 1982: 340). Finally, acceptability studies perform yet another crucial function in male contraceptive research, namely, to convince industry of the viability of the new technology. The protocol of the acceptability studies organized by WHO in the late 1980s and mid-1990s as part of the two large-scale clinical trials illustrates this use:

> The Human Reproduction Program (HRP) of WHO and other institutions engaged in contraceptive development have been investigating hormonal methods of fertility regulation for men for more than 20 years. WHO/HRP has played a leading role in this research. Because the introduction of an hormonal contraceptive method for men now appears to be a possibility within 10 years, the Task Force on Methods for the Regulation of Male Fertility wishes to initiate research on the acceptability of its most promising product to date, testosterone enanthate. . . . An underlying question of this research and one that will be of importance to potential pharmaceutical backers is, will it be worth the effort to develop this product? (WHO/HRP 1994: 1)

This expansion in the audience for acceptability studies, from biomedical scientists and critics of male contraceptive research to pharmaceutical companies, implied a redefinition of the concept of acceptability. Whereas acceptability studies in the 1970s and 1980s were based on Marshall's definition of acceptability, which framed acceptability in terms of what makes a product attractive to the user, acceptability now became conceptualized in terms of economic categories such as supply and demand. To quote the WHO/HRP 1994 protocol again:

Acceptability has been defined by Marshall (1977), as a quality (or qualities) that makes an idea (or product) attractive, satisfactory, pleasing or welcome. Broader than the qualities of acceptability are the factors that determine prevalence of use—To what extent will there be a demand or "market" for a new product? To what segment of the market will such a product appeal? (WHO/HRP 1982: 1)

The aim of acceptability studies was thus expanded from assessing the preferences and attitudes of individual men to investigating the potential market for the new technology.

A major part of the WHO/HRP acceptability studies now focused on understanding the extent to which the men participating in the clinical trials were representative of the "general public" or "atypical and thus unlikely to be numerous in the general population" (Ringheim 1995: 79).

Assessing Acceptability

Although acceptability studies have performed different functions in the field of male contraceptive research, all studies organized as part of clinical trials have used more or less similar methods to assess acceptability. The basic methodology consists of investigating the experiences of clinical trial participants with the experimental method and evaluating the discontinuations of men participating in the clinical trials (WHO/HRP 1976: 1). The early clinical trial acceptability studies utilized a comparative approach in which men were asked to compare their experiences with the method-on-trial to existing contraceptives and to rank their preferences for the new method. Ranking preferences was also used in field studies where men were asked to compare hypothetical contraceptive methods with existing methods (WHO/HRP 1976; Martin et al. 1997). Although the number of indicators to assess acceptability has expanded over the years, the types of indicators have remained rather stable, including topics such as overall acceptability compared with existing methods, cultural differences in acceptability, experiences of side-effects, perceived benefits, changes in sexual functioning, preferences for the route of administration, and willingness to use the new method if it were available (WHO/HRP 1976: 6; WHO/HRP 1982: 330; WHO/HRP 1994: 2–3).

Through the years, most of the attention in acceptability studies has been focused, however, on sexuality and the route of administration. The attention to sexuality is clearly reflected in the protocol and reports of the first WHO/HRP acceptability study in the late 1970s. The protocol described the major objective of the study as assessing "users' acceptability and effects on sexuality of recently developed male fertility regulating methods" (WHO/HRP 1976: 1). The authors articulated the need to pay attention to sexuality in acceptability studies as follows: "In view of the important implications changes in sexuality are likely to have for acceptability, it is clearly of high priority to investigate whether, and to what extent if any, the treatment affects the sexual desire and performance of the volunteers" (WHO/HRP 1976: 2). The reports of this acceptability study reiterated this primacy of sexuality over other indicators of acceptability. In the publication of the preliminary results of the study in 1979, the authors mentioned assessing interference of the contraceptive method with sexual function as the first aim of the acceptability study, and went on to report that "the research is also assessing . . . acceptability in different socio-cultural settings" (WHO/HRP 1979b: 121). The publication reporting the final results of the study showed that thirty of the fifty variables studied addressed sexuality (WHO/HRP 1982: 330). The WHO/HRP acceptability studies in the late 1980s and mid-1990s show a similar focus on sexuality; these studies included a separate questionnaire for sexuality with an extensive list of items (WHO/HRP 1994; Ringheim 1995). As happened in the clinical trials, the interference of hormonal contraceptive methods with sexuality thus became foregrounded as a crucial aspect of assessing acceptability.

The other recurring theme in the acceptability studies for new male contraceptives is the route of administration (WHO/HRP 1976; WHO/HRP 1979b). The question of whether injections would be acceptable to men, or whether they would prefer a pill, has been debated ever since research on male contraceptives was initiated. In the population control discourse, which, as we saw in chapter 2, dominated male contraceptive research in the 1960s and 1970s, the ideal male contraceptive would consist of a long-acting injectable method. This specific requirement was formulated in the 1960s in reaction to the appeals of family planning organizations and several governments in developing countries, who stressed the need for alternative contraceptives with an effective duration of up to six months (Crabbé et al. 1983: 243–53). This specification, initially developed for female contraceptive methods, also became an important requirement for male methods. As I have described in chapter 2, in 1975 WHO initiated a large-scale R&D program for the development of long-acting contraceptives, both for women and men.[5] Long-acting contraceptives were, and still are, considered important tools for increasing the efficiency of birth control programs because they aim at minimizing "user failure." This type of contraceptive technology is a good example of "technical delegates": artifacts that are designed to compensate for the perceived "deficiencies" of their users, that is, their unreliability with respect to continuity of use.[6] Although the major emphasis in this early period was on the development of long-acting injectable contraceptives, the field was by no means uniform. Other approaches had been developed as well, such as patches, implants, and pills (Kretser 1974; Schoysman 1976; Arlidge 1997). An explicit debate about the requirements of the ideal male contraceptive emerged only when feminists actively intervened in the field. Feminist health advocates clearly set the terms of this debate: they requested not just a male contraceptive, but demanded a "male twin" of the oral contraceptive that was already available for women (Seaman and Seaman 1978: 29). The emergence of this ideal type is reflected in the scientific literature: in the mid-1970s papers were published with titles like "Oral Contraception for Men" (1974), and "Progress Towards a Male Oral Contraceptive" (1975), and "Towards a Pill For Men" (1976) (Jackson 1975; Kretser 1976).

The development of oral contraceptives for men requires extra work for male contraceptive researchers, however. Oral administration of the available androgens turned out to be ineffective because they are broken down too quickly. To be effective, high doses are required, which may cause liver damage (Bennink interview 1999). The development of the Pill for women initially faced similar problems. When it was decided to develop a pill rather than an injection, Pincus could rely, however, on a large supply of different types of progestins to solve the problem. But this was not the case for male contraceptive researchers, who had at their disposal only a very limited number of androgens.[7] The combined hormonal contraceptive methods used in most trials therefore consist of an injection, an implant, or a patch as the mode of delivery for androgens, and pills as the mode of administration for progestins. The two WHO/HRP trials used a testosterone injection as the mode of administration. Injections of the currently available androgens require, however, weekly administration. As we saw in the previous chapter, the use of weekly injections has met with some resistance, particularly in the news media. Problems with the acceptability of injections are by no means restricted to male contraceptives. The history of medicine shows how the injection has become an icon for the fear of medicine, at least in Western cultures. As historians of medicine have suggested, people fear injections not only because they involve some pain and a small injury. The reluctant attitude toward injections is related to the perception of injections as "bodily intrusion and internal violation" (Arnold et al. 1998). Negative attitudes toward injections seem to be most prominent among Dutch and other citizens of Western Europe (Geest and Hardon 1994:

144). In most non-Western cultures, however, injections have positive connotations. People prefer injections because they are perceived as representing the technological expertise of the Western world, which is considered something good ("far is beautiful") (Geest and Hardon 1994). Other explanations given by medical anthropologists for the popularity of injections among non-Western cultures is that injections correspond to "traditional" views of the central role of blood in disease and health. From this perspective, injections are considered powerful therapy because they bring drugs directly into the bloodstream (Geest and Hardon 1994: 142). The results of the acceptability studies on male contraceptives reflect these cultural differences in attitudes toward injections. The first WHO acceptability study concluded that important cultural differences were involved in the acceptability of injections. Whereas Asian men were prepared to accept injections because they associated them with good health, clinical trial participants from the U.K. and the United States had less positive views of injections (Ringheim 1995: 80). Men participating in the two large-scale WHO clinical trials, which tested weekly injections, did not object to injections as such, but considered the frequency of the injections problematic (WHO/HRP 1996: 828). The field survey conducted by the Contraceptive Development Network among men in Edinburgh, Hong Kong, Cape Town, and Shanghai reiterated the conclusions of the WHO studies on cultural differences in the acceptability of the various methods on trial. The Pill was reported as "the most common first choice" in Edinburgh, whereas men in Cape Town were described as having a preference for a three–monthly series of injections. Chinese men were said to have a marked preference for condoms. The differences between the acceptability of a daily pill and a monthly injection were reported to be small (Martin et al. 1997).

As a whole, the results of the acceptability studies of the last two decades have articulated a positive view of the attitudes of men toward the new technology. The 1982 publication of the first WHO acceptability study reported that the contraceptive-on-trial was rated as more acceptable than either vasectomy or condoms, except for trial participants in Bangkok and Toronto, who preferred vasectomy over the new method (WHO/HRP 1982: 332). The acceptability studies conducted as part of the two large-scale WHO clinical trials reported "participants enthusiasm for a 3-monthly injectable method" (Ringheim 1995: 79). The field study conducted by the Contraceptive Development Network in the mid-1990s concluded that "our results demonstrate that hormonal methods of contraception are acceptable to men in all centers" (Martin et al. 1997).

To articulate the cultural feasibility of new contraceptives for men, scientists have also sought out the opinions of women—an important strategy because the view that women would never accept a male contraceptive pill or injection has been an important argument in the debate over the cultural feasibility of the new technology. A field survey among 450 women in Edinburgh, conducted by the Contraceptive Development Network in the mid-1990s, reported favorable results similar to those for their survey among men. A great majority of the women (94 percent) thought that "a male hormonal contraceptive would be a good idea." (Martin et al. 1997).

Until the late 1990s, the results of acceptability studies were used mainly by male contraceptive researchers and policy agencies. At the turn of the twenty-first century, we have seen an interesting change, in that acceptability studies are now coming to be used by pharmaceutical companies as resources to articulate the cultural feasibility of the new technology.

Pharmaceutical Firms as Agents of Change

In the late 1990s pharmaceutical firms, most notably the German company Schering and the Dutch company Organon, began to show an active interest in the development of male contraceptive technologies (Johansson interview 1997; Bennink interview 1999). This increased attention can partly be understood as a result of the successful articulation of the cultural feasibility of new male contraceptive methods by the male contraceptive community. In this respect, the acceptability studies, particularly those of the Contraceptive Development Network, were timely. When the results of the field surveys among men and women were reported at the Thirteenth Annual Meeting of the European Society of Human Reproduction and Embryology (ESHRE), in Edinburgh in 1997, the representatives of Organon present at this conference were involved in reassessing the priorities for their R&D program for contraceptive technologies. The results of the acceptability studies provided them with resources to counter reluctance within the firm to male hormonal contraceptive development. According to Herjan Coelingh Bennink, who was the newly appointed director of Organon's Reproductive Medicine Program in 1997:

> Nobody actually liked the idea. There was always the same story: the acceptability was non-existent or minor. These opinions, however, lacked any empirical foundation. . . . When I took over this program and tried to lobby to establish a male contraceptive research program at Organon, I attended the ESHRE meeting in Edinburgh where they reported the first

results of the surveys among 450 men and women. . . . For me that was a gift from heaven. Although the decision to start male contraceptive development had already been prepared within the firm, this finally settled the matter. (Bennink interview 1999)

Gender norms have played an important role in Organon's reluctant attitude toward male hormonal contraceptives as a viable product line. Most men working at the firm opposed the development of new male contraceptives because they simply didn't like the idea of contraceptive injections or pills from a personal point of view (Bennink interview 1999). For decades, the firm had relied on what Madeleine Akrich has described as the I-methodology: a practice of technological development in which experts take themselves as referents to assess the needs of future users (Akrich 1992). The results of the acceptability studies provided the new director with resources to challenge the view of "the middle-aged male management" that contraceptives were a matter for women (Bennink interview 1999). Following the meeting in Edinburgh, Organon, which was already involved in several small-scale studies initiated by male contraceptive researchers in Edinburgh, Manchester, and Seattle, for which the company had provided the hormonal products, publicly announced that the firm expected to begin commercial production of a hormonal contraceptive for men in the year 2000 (Arlidge 1997).

In addition to the acceptability studies, the results of clinical trials have also played a role in Organon's decision: "In the early 1990s I participated in a discussion to launch the first feasibility study. . . . But WHO had not yet published its results, and David Baird [the director of the Contraceptive Development Network] had not yet conducted his surveys. There were clearly fewer arguments then" (Bennink interview 1999).

Currently, Organon runs a male contraceptive R&D program, including a long-term basic research program for the development of nonhormonal contraceptive agents using molecular biology techniques to intervene in spermatogenesis; a middle-term program involving twenty chemists and pharmacologists to synthesize new androgens; and a clinical trial program, including phase II and phase III testing for the commercial production of a hormonal contraceptive, that is, for a combination method of progestagen and androgen, that is expected to be on the market within approximately five years.[8] Moreover, Organon is involved in negotiations with WHO on the production of the androgen (testosterone bucyclate) tested by that organization.

By deciding to begin the commercial production of a hormonal contraceptive for men, Organon has chosen to market a product that is not yet considered "the ideal hormonal contraceptive" (Bennink interview 1999). The method will consist of a pill or an implant and an injection: "We think we can make an acceptable method with the existing products, although the combination of a pill and an injection will be acceptable only for people who are extremely motivated to use such a method. Maybe the frequency of the injection is not ideal. Anyway, we can get going and get away from the endless theorizing over these matters" (Bennink interview 1999).

The choice of this specific formulation of the product was made in close collaboration with leading experts in the male contraceptive community. In December 1999 Organon convened a meeting of experts so as to discuss ideas for product development with reproductive scientists from the United States and Europe. In the late 1990s, such contacts between pharmaceutical firms and male contraceptive researchers were formalized in the so-called Summit Meeting Male Contraceptives, an annual meeting of investigators, public-sector agencies such as WHO and the Population Council, and pharmaceutical companies (Bennink interview 1999). These developments show that the pharmaceutical companies have finally become part of the existing networks on male contraceptive development, which had been restricted to public-sector agencies and university-based researchers for more than three decades.

The decision to begin the production of a contraceptive considered "not yet ideal" can partly be understood in the context of the increased commercial interest in drugs for male reproduction that I described in the introduction to this book. In the last decade, androgens have come to be of increasing interest to pharmaceutical firms, not as contraceptives but for hormonal replacement therapy (HRT). In the United States, twelve companies have become active in HRT research. In Europe, Schering's sales of androgen have increased compared to previous decades. The market value of hormonal methods for men has increased by 20 to 30 percent every year since 1993 (Johansson interview 1997). For the first time in the history of androgen development, pharmaceutical firms have actively approached public-sector agencies such as the Population Council to discuss HRT product development for men. According to Elof Johansson, the director of the Population Council's Center for Biomedical Research in New York:

> I think it's the same thing that happened in women when steroids came on, that there has to be a sort of critical mass. Enough people have to be interested, and there have to be openings, and they [industry] have to see the profit possibility. And the profit possibility has been in the hormone

replacement therapy. And at the same time, when Schering, for instance, who is now the number one company in steroid hormones, asks: "Where are the next big areas?" Well, certainly males are the next big area because decline in hormone production starts at about the same time in men and women, about when you turn forty. . . . I think the reason that the escalated interest came in this country was the development of the testosterone patch. . . . Then companies saw that there was a market, and more companies developed patches for men. And they sold well, so it became a snowball effect. And now there is development all over, and companies are beating a path to our door to talk with us about product development. (Johansson interview 1997)

The introduction of hormone replacement therapy for men thus had an important function in clearing the way for the use of hormones as contraceptives. Interestingly, the dynamics of the hormone market for men show the opposite of what happened to the hormonal drug market for women, where the hormonal contraceptive paved the way for a widespread acceptance of hormonal replacement therapy for women (Johansson interview 1997). Due to developments in HRT products for men, pharmaceutical firms have come under more pressure to get their share in the hormonal market for men. For Organon, a decision to postpone the commercial production of a hormonal contraceptive for men until more "user-friendly" methods of administration could be developed implied running the risk of losing the relative lead the firm has enjoyed in the area of male contraceptive development. In contrast to other companies, Organon was in the position to exploit technological opportunities within the firm: the company could rely on hormonal products they had developed for other purposes. For the progestagen component of the new contraceptive, the firm uses a hormonal implant developed as a hormonal contraceptive for women, whereas the androgen component consists of a modified testosterone product developed as a therapy for hypogonadal men (Bennink interview 1999). The development of hormonal products more acceptable to future users, such as less frequent injections or pills, would require a much longer development trajectory and delay the marketing of a male hormonal contraceptive by at least ten years.

The major constraining factor is the paucity of available androgens, a problem I described earlier, in chapter 2. In contrast to progestagens, which have been one of the major drugs on the hormone market for women, resulting in the availability of a broad variety of different products, attempts to optimize existing androgens have largely been absent from the agenda for many years.

Consequently, the actual choice of a specific androgen is limited to a handful of products. The decision to work with existing products enabled Organon to shorten the development trajectory considerably because these products have already been subjected to previous testing and do not require animal studies or phase I clinical testing (Kersemaekers interview 1999). The choice to begin the commercial production of a "not yet ideal" product can thus be understood as a strategy to establish a leading position in the contraceptive hormonal market for men.

Yet another development contributed to Organon's initiative to become actively involved in male contraceptive development, namely, the appointment of a new director for Organon's Reproductive Medicine Program. In 1997 Herjan Coelingh Bennink, a gynecologist who, as head of Organon's Clinical Development Department, had lobbied in vain for the company's involvement in male contraceptive R&D, was promoted to director of the Reproductive Medicine Program and thus took charge of the policy and strategy of Organon in this area. This position enabled him to introduce drastic changes to Organon's R&D activities on contraceptives: he prioritized contraceptives for men over the development of immunological contraceptive approaches for women, a line of development that had been part of Organon's R&D program for ten years and was excluded from further development. Instead, he initiated the three programs focused on male contraceptive development I described above. Coelingh Bennink's advocacy of Organon's involvement in male contraceptive R&D was inspired by both economic and normative incentives: "We cannot permit ourselves to focus only on women and ignore men. That is wrong, commercially as well as strategically. It is half of the market. . . . Moreover, I think it's almost unethical not to include men" (Bennink interview 1999).

The change in attitude toward male contraceptive development within the pharmaceutical industry can thus be understood also as a result of the advocacy of a dedicated program director.

Most importantly, the decision to start the commercial production of a hormonal contraceptive for men can be considered as the ultimate strategy to enhance the cultural feasibility of the new technology: "We could have decided as well to work on the ideal compound: you make a nice oral androgen and a better progestagen. But then it takes ten years before we actually can begin. . . . I think it's more important to show in practice that there is a niche for male contraceptives" (Bennink interview 1999). The actual production of a new contraceptive for men thus became a tool for inducing cultural change.

Conclusions

Reflecting on developments in the field of male contraceptive research in the last decade, we can conclude that acceptability studies have played an important role in articulating the cultural feasibility of hormonal contraceptives for men. Most importantly, acceptability studies conducted in the mid-1990s have been instrumental in challenging the status quo in the field of male contraceptive research. After three decades of research inactivity, pharmaceutical companies finally have become actively involved in R&D in this area. In the end, the efforts of the male contraceptive community to attract the interest of industry have payed off. We have seen how the results of acceptability studies and the two large-scale WHO clinical trials provided advocates of male contraceptive innovation within Organon with the resources needed to overcome the reluctant attitude toward this technology that for decades had prevented the pharmaceutical company from becoming involved in this field. We can thus conclude that acceptability studies and clinical trials have been instrumental in convincing companies of the cultural and technical feasibility of male hormonal contraceptives.

We are in a crucial phase in the development of the new technology. In the last three decades, the proponents of new contraceptives for men have been successful in creating a sociotechnical network to overcome the material, cultural, and social barriers to male contraceptive innovation. As I described in chapter 2, the network of university-based reproductive scientists, clinicians, family planning organizations, and public-sector agencies provided a protected space to develop knowledge, expertise, techniques, and chemical compounds, and to articulate the cultural feasibility of the new technology. The key step for successful technological innovation, however, is to ensure that the technology-in-the-making will be able to survive outside this protected space (Schot and Rip 1997). For male contraceptive innovation, this implies that the technology should be able to survive outside the niche of nonprofit-sector agencies and university laboratories and clinics. The current involvement of pharmaceutical companies indicates that male contraceptive technological innovation is going through this phase of transition. Pharmaceutical firms are key actors for successful technological development because they have the resources necessary for the widescale production and marketing of drugs. We can thus conclude that the alternative sociotechnical network established in the last three decades has been successful as a "demonstration network." As I described in chapter 3, demonstration networks are aimed at "demonstrating the feasibility of a new technological option for a collective good" (Laredo 1994). This chapter has shown how demonstrating the feasibility of a new technology not only includes material work, such as synthesizing hormonal compounds, but also cultural work, that is, articulating the acceptability of the new technology.

Finally, this chapter has demonstrated the importance of actors who take the trouble to counter disbelief in the cultural feasibility of a new technology. Organon's decision to enter the field was made only after years of active lobbying by a dedicated manager. By linking such heterogeneous elements as economic market strategies, ethical incentives, and a belief in the cultural need of the new technology, Coelingh Bennink succeeded in convincing his colleagues of the viability of male hormonal contraceptives. In the late 1990s pharmaceutical companies thus finally became involved in male contraceptive innovation.

11

Technologies of Trust

· · · ·

My argument throughout this book has been that the constraints on the development of new contraceptives for men cannot be ascribed to intrinsic properties of bodies or technologies. My concern has been to provide a corrective to perspectives that create the impression of gender asymmetry in contraceptive technologies as an inevitable process of technical logics. The previous chapters have illustrated how technologies are the materialized result of negotiations, selection processes, contingencies, and technological choices, embodying socially and culturally constituted norms and practices. In this biography of the male Pill, I have tried to trace all the social and cultural work involved in developing a technology that challenges dominant cultural narratives on masculinity. Including men in the contraceptive research agenda required changing established sociotechnical networks and the related vested interests of experts, clinics, industry, and social movements that have focused for a long time almost exclusively on women. Most importantly, the development of new contraceptives for men involved a mutual adjustment of technologies and gender identities. This story of a technological innovation thus becomes ultimately a story of the design of masculinities in the last decades of the twentieth century. It is time to return to the central questions I posed in the introductory chapter. Who acted as the agents of sociotechnical and cultural change? What were the major constraints faced by the proponents of new male contraceptive technologies? And, last but not least, how and to what extent did the advocates of the new technology succeed in overcoming these constraints?

Agents of Sociotechnical and Cultural Change

Women have been the main focus of reversible, physiological contraceptive technologies in the twentieth century. The introduction of men into the world of contraceptive development may therefore be considered as revolutionary. In contrast to many historical accounts of revolutions and technological innovations, my analysis of technological innovation in contraceptives for men shows how technological change cannot be ascribed to a single political or scientific hero. For this technology, the impetus to change the status quo was a much less centralized endeavor, spread over many actors from different social worlds, each with a different agenda. Most importantly, the demand for the development of new contraceptives for men was first articulated by actors outside the scientific community rather than by reproductive scientists or clinicians. It was only following social pressures from political leaders in China and India and feminists in the Western industrialized world that contraceptive technologies for men were added to the research agenda. Both groups can be considered as "gender-benders" because they aimed to break away from gendered patterns in contraceptive development and use, although for very different reasons. Whereas political leaders articulated the need for new male contraceptives in terms of the technology's potential for limiting population growth, feminists framed the need for technological innovation in terms of sharing the risks and responsibilities of contraceptives between the sexes. For the second time in history, feminists thus played a crucial role in technological innovation in contraceptive development. In the 1950s, it was Margaret Sanger, a representative of the first feminist wave of the twentieth century, who succeeded in getting scientists to work on the development of a contraceptive drug for women.[1] In the 1970s, the second wave of feminism initiated a debate on the risks of contraceptives for women and first demanded a male equivalent of the female Pill. Technological innovation in contraceptives thus reveals a pattern in which social movements, most notably the feminist movement, have been major actors in initiating technological change.[2] My account of the history of contraceptive development for men thus provides a corrective to the history of technology and innovation literature which highlights the role of economic change and government policies in technological innovation. In addition to political leaders and feminists, family planning organizations also played an important role as gender-benders.[3] Because of their creative agency, men, "the forgotten 50 percent of family planning," came to be included in family planning discourse, thus breaking with a past in which family planning services had been almost exclusively focused on women.

Although the feminist movement played an important role as an agent of sociotechnical and cultural change in the world of contraceptives, feminist voices were by no means unanimous. The past three decades show a picture in which feminists have acted both as advocates and opponents of new contraceptives for men. This peculiar pattern can be understood in terms of differences in the politics of feminists. As with other topics in the feminist movement, feminist debates on contraceptives show contrasting ideological views of the role of women and men in matters of contraception. For radical feminists, women's control over their own fertility has been, and still is, the main frame of reference for evaluating the advantages and disadvantages of contraceptives. From this perspective, they opposed the advocacy for new contraceptives for men because they considered the new technology a threat to women's autonomy. In contrast to this view, liberal feminists argued that the new technology would enable men to take responsibility for contraception, thus sharing the burden of contraception with women. The differences in feminist politics concerning contraceptive technologies for men can also be understood in terms of differences in generations in the feminist movement. Feminist advocacy for new male contraceptives was particularly strong in the early 1970s, when women's health advocates protested against the health risks of female contraceptives. This protest was initiated by feminists who were among the first generation of women using the contraceptive Pill, and experiencing serious side-effects from the high dosages of hormones in the early pills. Although criticism of the side-effects of the Pill continued to be voiced in the 1980s and 1990s, the younger generation of feminists did not campaign for new male contraceptives but lobbied extensively for the development of new safe contraceptives for women.

Ambivalence toward the new technology was not restricted to feminists. The pharmaceutical industry shows an even more profound dual face. As I have described, at the turn of the twenty-first century, pharmaceutical companies changed from being reluctant actors opposing the cultural feasibility of the new technology to proponents of new contraceptives for men. My account of the impetus of technological change in contraceptive technologies thus shows how the position of collective actors on a new technology is not stable. Whereas the feminist movement simultaneously acted as advocate and opponent of the new technology, the pharmaceutical industry changed its position through the years from a reluctant actor to an advocate of the new technology.

One group of potential agents of change remained remarkably silent. In contrast to the development of female contraceptives, where the feminist movement as spokesperson of women has been one of the crucial actors in initiating contraceptive innovation, men as the future users of the new technology have been completely absent as agents of change. Neither the articulation of the need for new male contraceptives nor the advocacy of technological innovation has been part of the political agenda of the men's movement.[4] This silence magnifies the persistence of those cultural narratives in which contraception is considered a woman's job.

Overcoming Resistance: Constructing Alternative Sociotechnical Networks

The advocacy of new contraceptives for men severely challenged the status quo in contraceptive development in the 1970s. Alliances between reproductive scientists, medical professionals, family planning organizations, pharmaceutical firms, and social movements had developed into extensive and stable sociotechnical networks oriented toward the development, diffusion, and use of female rather than male contraceptives. The conditions for radical technological change were thus very poor. Path dependence in the field of contraceptive technologies and reproductive biology had resulted in a situation in which basic and clinical knowledge of male reproductive biology, expertise and techniques to synthesize male contraceptive drugs, and infrastructures for the clinical testing of new male contraceptives had remained largely unexplored, underdeveloped, and marginal. In addition to these sociotechnical barriers, the advocates of new male contraceptives were also confronted with resistance. Ever since the idea of a male contraceptive pill or injection had been first articulated, heterogeneous groups of actors, including scientists, clinicians, journalists, feminists, and pharmaceutical entrepreneurs, had questioned whether men or women would accept a new male contraceptive if it were available. As I have described, the history of the development of new male contraceptives shows many traces of resistance, including refusal to take part in R&D (the pharmaceutical industry) and refusal to collaborate in the recruitment of clinical trial participants (gynecologists), disinterest in the organization of clinical trials (urologists and andrologists), a reluctant attitude toward conducting male contraceptive research (reproductive scientists), and the active production of counternarratives representing men and women as anti-users of the new technology (journalists and feminists).

The Male Pill shows how advocates of the new technology have used multiple strategies to overcome the constraints and resistance confronting male contraceptive innovation. The most important strategy has been the creation of alternative sociotechnical networks. In the case of male contraceptive technologies, path creation depended largely on the building of new sociotechnical networks in which public-sector agencies, most notable WHO, played an important role. My analysis shows the importance of intermediary organizations for technological innovation in cases where crucial actors for drug development, that is, pharmaceutical firms, do not participate in drug development. As I have shown, WHO has played a major role in coordinating the scarce and scattered expertise in male reproductive biology and contraceptive research and in stimulating new activities in the emerging field of male contraceptive research. In addition to its role in coordinating and stimulating male contraceptive basic research, WHO also played an important role in trying to overcome the constraints of the lack of available research materials by organizing a worldwide laboratory for the synthesis of new hormonal compounds. Finally, WHO and other public-sector and university-based organizations played a major role in overcoming barriers to male contraceptive research by creating networks of academic centers with the expertise, skills, and facilities to conduct clinical trials. This strategy was used to solve the problems of inadequate test locations and the recruitment of a sufficient number of men for the phase II clinical trials.

The created networks provided a protected space in which scientists and clinicians could break away from the routines, practices, and interests that had directed the development of contraceptive drugs exclusively toward women. Most importantly, the creation of alternative sociotechnical networks set in motion transformative processes within and between heterogeneous groups of actors that were beyond the capacities of each individual member. The sociotechnical networks of governments, scientists, clinicians, feminists, and public-sector agencies gave access to skills and resources necessary for realizing changes in research agendas, in the programs of family planning organizations, and in the cultural norms and practices concerning male responsibility in matters of contraception. The groups of actors who had previously not been involved in contraceptive development, that is, WHO, governments, and feminists, enabled the network to mobilize resources to overcome major barriers to male contraceptive development. WHO gave credibility and respectability to the quest for new male contraceptives, a crucial contribution because reproductive research in general, and male contraceptive research in particular, were marginal, not highly respectable fields in the academic world. Governments, particularly China and India, were successful in granting political relevancy to the technological innovation and played an important role in the establishment and survival of the WHO's Male Task Force. Feminists, finally, were important actors in transforming contraceptive technologies from tools to reduce population growth to methods to distribute equally the responsibilities and health risks of contraceptives among women and men, thus extending the market for the new technology to the Western industrialized world. As I have described, women's health groups were able to mobilize family planning organizations and the United Nations to include male responsibility for family planning on their agendas. These are crucial transformations because the quest for new male contraceptives will ultimately fail if men are not willing to use them, or family planning organizations are not inclined to include them in their programs.

The major question is the extent to which the advocates of new contraceptives for men have succeeded in overcoming the barriers to technological innovation. Since the technology in question has not yet concluded its trajectory, it is impossible to give a definite answer. This is one of the difficulties and challenges of writing a biography of a technology-in-the-making. A reflection on the developments of the last three decades, however, indicates that most strategies used to overcome resistance have been rather successful, particularly the strategy to create a protected space for the synthesis and clinical testing of hormonal contraceptive compounds. Whereas in the early 1970s male contraceptive research was restricted to a handful of researchers scattered all over the United States and Europe, the late 1990s show a picture of a small but stable research community consisting of various international networks capable of organizing phase II and phase III clinical testing. Most importantly, the technology-in-the-making has left the virtual walls of the protected space. As I indicated in chapter 10, a key step for successful technological innovation is to ensure that the technology will be able to survive outside the protected space. Although it is still too early to draw any definite conclusions, the current involvement of pharmaceutical companies indicates that male contraceptive technological innovation is going through this phase of transition. Pharmaceutical firms are key actors for successful technological development because they have the resources necessary for the widescale production and marketing of drugs. We can thus conclude that the creation of an alternative sociotechnical network has been successful as a strategy to overcome the barriers in male contraceptive technological innovation. The creation of networks has enabled scientists and clinicians to transform male hormonal contraceptives from "hopeful monstrosities" (Mokyr 1990), a promising technology that does not perform very well, into a technology that meets the standards of industry.

Although the strategies to overcome barriers to male contraceptive innovation have been successful, there is one important drawback: male contraceptive innovation shows a very slow pace of development. Whereas contraceptive drug development usually covers a period of approximately fifteen years, the development of male hormonal contraceptives has already taken more than three decades. As I have described, the development trajectory of hormonal contraceptives for men encountered several delays. Both of the approaches to hormonal contraceptives for men currently on trial (WHO's single hormonal compound consisting of testosterone enanthate, and the combination hormonal compounds consisting of a testosterone and a progestin used by the Contraceptive Development Network and Organon) have been available already for two decades. Although the technical feasibility of male hormonal contraceptives was demonstrated as early as the late 1970s, it took ten years for large-scale clinical testing to begin, and another five years before pharmaceutical companies considered the results convincing enough to include male hormonal contraceptives on their R&D agendas.

I suggest that there are two different, but equally important, explanations for this delay. First, the slow pace of development can be understood in the context of the specific infrastructures in which this technological innovation takes place. Although the created alternative sociotechnical networks were successful in mobilizing resources to overcome major barriers to male contraceptive development, the networks could not rely on any previous experience or routines in such a heterogeneous, collaborative endeavor. It is therefore not surprising to note that most activities, including collaborative efforts to synthesize and test hormonal compounds, were very time-consuming. The case of male contraceptive technological development thus shows the limitations of technological innovation that emerges in a protected space.

Second, the delay in male contraceptive development can be ascribed to cultural constraints. My biography of the male Pill shows that technologies in conflict with hegemonic masculinity have a hard time coming into existence. All of the actors involved in male contraceptive development, including the advocates, have had serious doubts about the cultural feasibility of the technology. As I described in chapter 10, cultural views of gender among the employees of Organon were a major disincentive for the pharmaceutical company to becoming involved in this technological innovation. It was only after a large-scale acceptability study that Organon decided to include male hormonal contraceptive R&D on its agenda. Cultural notions of masculinity have also delayed the clinical testing of hormonal contraceptive compounds. As I described in chapter 5, the low acceptance of health risks of contraceptives in the male contraceptive community and culture at large, particularly where men are concerned, has had a major impact on the assessment of safety of the compounds on trial. Most strikingly, the assessment of health risks of male contraceptives reveals the structuring role of gender norms in constructing standards of safety. During the three decades of testing, the risks of interference of hormonal contraceptive compounds with sexual function has been the most debated side-effect. This concern reflects a cultural preoccupation with norms of masculinity than can best be summarized as "no tinkering with male sexuality." This preoccupation with male sexuality in contraceptive research shows a definite gender bias. As I have described, a similar concern for female sexuality only emerged in the contraceptive scientific community three decades after the introduction of the hormonal contraceptive Pill for women. Finally, another constraining factor for the clinical testing of hormonal contraceptives for men has been the ethical and political concerns related to the risk of abortion to terminate unwanted pregnancies of women whose partners had participated in the clinical trials in case of contraceptive failure.

The major conclusion to be drawn from this history is that successful technological innovation depends not only on sociotechnical networks. Cultural transformations are an essential, but often overlooked, part of technological innovation.

Configuring the User: Articulating and Performing Masculinities

The second part of *The Male Pill* therefore consists of an analysis of the cultural work involved in technological innovation. To understand how actors have tried to accomplish the cultural feasibility of male hormonal contraceptives, I have looked particularly at the ways in which they configure the user. As I have argued, the articulation of gender identities of future users is an important but as yet unexplored aspect of the work involved in configuring the user. I have described how the creation of the cultural feasibility of new contraceptive technology for men required a destabilization of conventionalized performances of gender identities. The predominance of modern contraceptive drugs for women has disciplined men and women to delegate the responsibilities of contraception largely to women. In the latter half of the twentieth century contraceptive use became excluded from hegemonic masculinity. The advocacy of new contraceptives for men severely challenged these stabilized conventions. Technological innovation in contraceptives technology thus became a quest to renegotiate masculine identities. I have therefore suggested that the development phase of a new technology should be viewed as a cultural niche in which actors articulate and perform nonhegemonic masculine identities to create the cultural feasibility of a technology.

My analysis shows how this cultural work was performed by a hetero-geneous group of actors, including reproductive scientists, clinicians, femi-nists, men who participated in the clinical testing, the female partners of trial participants, family planning organizations, and journalists.[5]

Reproductive scientists configured users as men who were willing to share responsibility for contraception with their partners. This articulation of the user can be understood as the result of alliances between the worlds of femi-nists and scientists. Due to interactions between feminists and scientists, the discourse on hormonal contraceptives for men became increasingly framed in terms of sharing health risks and responsibilities between the sexes. The practices of the clinical testing of male hormonal contraceptives show a fur-ther refinement of this image of the caring, responsible man.[6] To configure men as reliable test subjects, clinicians selected men in stable relationships. Test subjects and future users of the new technology came to be represented as monogamous men. This articulation of the user also implied a construction of the non-user. The configuration strategy excluded a large proportion of the male population. Men in casual relationships, less committed couples, single men who wanted to protect themselves from paternity claims, and bisexual men came to be represented as non-users. Clinicians thus reiterated and sustained conventionalized performances of gender that emphasize hetero-normativity as an important aspect of masculine identities.

The practices of clinical testing show intriguing new actors in technological innovation: the female partners of the men who participated in the clinical testing. As I have described, these women played a crucial role in configuring men as reliable test subjects. Female partners were important actors in en-couraging men to take part in the trials and in ensuring their cooperation during the clinical testing. Last but not least, these women were active agents in articulating masculine identities. Women used the clinical trials as a site to renegotiate responsibilities for contraception with their male partners. By doing this, they actively engaged in articulating the image of the caring, responsible man.

Most importantly, men taking part in the clinical trials of male hormonal contraceptives reiterated this projected identity. By participating in the clinical tests, men consciously or unconsciously performed an aspect of masculine identity that conflicted with hegemonic representations of masculinity, that is, that men are not inclined to take responsibility for contraception. As we have seen, a majority of the men participating in contraceptive clinical trials por-trayed themselves as altruistic men who wanted to help their female partners who had experienced problems with the female Pill. This does not imply that hegemonic masculinities were completely absent from these narratives. To negotiate this new male identity, clinicians and trial participants relied on dominant cultural representations of masculinity that represent men as brave and pioneering subjects.

Remarkably, being in control of reproduction is not a central aspect of these narratives. This stands in sharp contrast to other technologies recently introduced for male reproductive bodies, most notably Viagra, a drug for the treatment of male impotence. The discourses of Viagra are dominated by modernist rhetoric which portrays the capacity to be in control of one's body as "the proper and appropriate order of masculine things" (Mamo and Fishman 2001: 16). The fact that the notion of being in control of reproduction is largely absent from male contraceptive discourse can be understood as a strategy to reconcile conflicts in interests between the advocates of new contraceptives for men and radical feminists who considered male contraceptives as a threat to women's autonomy in matters of reproduction. A representation of male contraceptives as a technology to enhance men's autonomy and control of reproduction would have encouraged radical feminists to reject the new technology altogether. It was only in the local practices of the men's clinics in the United States and Colombia that the subject identities of men were articulated in terms of autonomous individuals who have the right to reproductive health. The debates on Viagra and the male Pill thus show a reification of hegemonic masculinity that emphasizes men's mastery and control of sexuality as an essential aspect of masculinity rather than reproduction (Mamo and Fishman 2001: 17; Connell 1987; Connell 1995). Again, being in control of or taking responsibility for reproduction is excluded from hegemonic masculinity. Male contraceptive discourse thus involved deferring to hegemonic masculinity as much as designing it.

The renegotiation of masculinities to accomplish the cultural feasibility of new contraceptives for men was not restricted to laboratories and clinics. I have argued that the world of family planning is an equally important location to understand the processes involved in configuring men as users of contraceptive technologies. Prior to the late 1960s, family planning discourse had been focused almost exclusively on women, thus reiterating and reinforcing dominant cultural narratives on gender and contraception. I have described how feminists and family planning organizations have been important actors in articulating new identities of men as users of contraceptives to counterbalance dominant cultural narratives on masculinity, male sexuality, and birth control embedded in family planning research traditions, policies of national and international family planning agencies, and women's health organizations.

Feminists have been important agents of change by transforming family planning discourse towards reproductive health concerns rather than demographic incentives. As a result, national and international family planning organizations strengthened their efforts to include men in their programs. However, the problem was not just that men were absent from family planning discourse, which could have been solved simply by adding men as a target group in family planning policies and services. I have described how, prior to the 1970s, family planning discourse was dominated by cultural narratives that portrayed men as opponents of family planning. In family planning policy documents, research publications, and family planning services, men, particularly in developing countries, were represented as having a preference for large families, as having no incentive to control their fertility, as being more promiscuous than women, and as being against family planning. A major part of the cultural work therefore consisted of attempts to counterbalance these dominant cultural narratives on masculinity and family planning. I have described how family planning researchers and organizations articulated a contrasting set of representations of men that emphasized that men have a very positive attitude toward family planning. Most importantly, the advocates constructed a new male identity reflecting nonhegemonic masculinities. "Men as partners" became the new term to capture this identity. Another major strategy in the advocacy of male involvement in family planning consisted of redefining what should be considered as the major barrier to increasing the participation of men in family planning. Instead of blaming men, the problem of men and contraception was redefined as a problem of failing family planning services and male contraceptive technologies.

As in the scientific community, the endeavor to include men in family planning shows traces of resistance. I have described how the advocacy to include men in family planning met with resistance from feminists. Again, we see how feminists acted both as advocates and opponents of cultural change. Whereas liberal feminists had been important in articulating the need to include men in family planning, radical feminists considered these attempts as a serious threat to the achievements of the women's health movement to make family planning policies congruent with policies to increase women's autonomy. Moreover, feminists suggested that policies to include men in family planning ran the risk of increasing gender inequalities if they didn't acknowledge the power relations between women and men. I have described how family planning organizations put much effort into consolidating these conflicting interests between male-oriented family planning initiatives and women's health advocates. By introducing a vocabulary defined from the perspective of women, which redefined family planning as a relational rather than an individual issue, family planning organizations tried to reconcile their activities to include men in family planning with feminists' concern of women's autonomy.

Configuring men as users of family planning services was not restricted to articulating the identities of users. I have shown how changing family planning discourse to include men also required a lot of material work. The incorporation of men as clients in the world of family planning literally meant making room for men. Prior to the 1970s, family planning clinics were almost exclusively women's spaces. A large part of the cultural work therefore consisted of creating infrastructures to configure men as clients of family planning services. I have described how men and family planning advocates established special clinics and services for men. The 1980s witnessed the birth of the men's clinic. A major conclusion of my analysis is that men's clinics can only come into existence and survive if professionals make major efforts to adapt their services and spaces to the preferences, attitudes, and norms of men. Configuring men as clients of family planning clinics included the organization of extensive outreach activities and specific adaptations of spaces, such as making separate entrances and waiting rooms, and expanding the services to include other than family planning and reproductive health services, such as sports physicals and other general health services.

In these processes of configuring the user, men came to be represented as "whole persons" who should be handled with care—care in a double meaning of the word. On the one hand, the practices of the men's clinics revealed how providers put much effort into attuning their services to their clients in order to avoid making men feel uncomfortable, embarrassed, insecure, or stupid. On the other hand, the clinics tried to maximize the quality of the care given their new clients. The fact that men are hesitant to visit a family planning clinic and are considered as having problems articulating their needs has led to the paradoxical situation where men receive more comprehensive health care in family planning clinics than women. In the short history of his existence, the male client of family planning clinics has thus received a special status compared to that of women.

Finally, there is yet another location that has been important in renegotiating masculinities to create the cultural feasibility of hormonal contraceptives for men: the news media. Although skepticism about cultural feasibility was also registered by other actors, resistance toward the new technology has been particularly strong among journalists. As we have seen, journalists represented men and women as anti-users. Dutch and English newspaper reports emphasized that it was very likely that both men and women would reject this new technology. Women were portrayed as opponents of male contraceptives because they do not trust men in matters of contraception. Men were represented as unreliable and oversensitive to the pain caused by contraceptive injections. A similar skepticism has been articulated by radical feminists, who argue that men cannot be trusted in matters of contraception. I have described how feminist discourse on new male contraceptives presented two conflicting images of masculine identities: the "caring man" and the "unreliable man." Whereas the advocates of male contraception constructed an image of men who would be willing to share health risks and responsibilities for contraception with their partners, the opponents of the new male contraceptives represented the users as men who could not be trusted. Feminists and journalists became locked together in perpetuating hegemonic representations of masculinities that emphasize the unreliability and disinterest of men in matters of birth control. Like feminist discourse, journalistic discourse was not univocal. We have seen how journalistic discourse also articulated identities of men that go beyond hegemonic representations of masculinity. In one Dutch newspaper, future users of male hormonal contraceptives were represented as men who would not have objections to contraceptive injections and who would want to have control in matters of contraception. These representations are, however, rather marginal. Most journalistic texts articulated gender identities incompatible with male contraceptives, thus denouncing the cultural feasibility of the new technology.

In summary, we can conclude that male contraceptive technological innovation included the articulation and performance of multiple and contrasting masculinities, which functioned to enhance as well as to denounce the cultural feasibility of the new technology. Configuring men as users of contraceptives thus shows both successes and failures. A consideration of the practices of family planning shows that cultural work in this domain has definitely been successful. Whereas prior to the 1970s men were almost completely absent from family planning discourse, the 1980s and 1990s witnessed the increasing incorporation of men as users of family planning services. The separate clinics for men established in this period succeeded in attracting more men to family planning services than had been the case in the traditional, women-oriented family planning clinics. The practices of clinical testing of the new technology show a similar picture. Through the years the clinicians' strategies to recruit men and to ensure their compliance has largely succeeded in configuring men as reliable test subjects. Most importantly, the clinical trials functioned as an important site in which to articulate and perform masculinities that incorporated contraceptive use as an action compatible with masculine identities.

Failures to configure men as users of hormonal contraceptives were particularly manifest in journalistic discourse. The news media articulated masculinities and femininities that portrayed contraceptive use by men as incompatible with hegemonic masculinity. In the end, journalistic discourse does not seem to have had much impact on the actors involved in the development of hormonal contraceptives for men. We have seen how pharmaceutical companies have given more credence to social scientists' surveys and clinical reports than to journalistic sources. Acceptability studies among both men and women, articulating positive attitudes toward the new technology, have played an important role in convincing industry of the cultural feasibility of the new technology. Finally, pharmaceutical companies adopted the ultimate strategy of making male hormonal contraceptives into an acceptable technology through the establishment of an R&D program to produce hormonal contraceptives, and thus to end the theoretical debates on the cultural feasibility of the technology.

Conclusions

Although the long and winding road to the development of hormonal contraceptives for men has not yet come to an end, the quest for new male contraceptives has had a definite impact. Activities in laboratories and clinics and the ongoing debates in the news media have transformed male reproductive bodies from invisible bodies into public bodies, thus breaking with the practices and traditions that have long dominated medical and bodily discourses. Most importantly, technological innovation in male contraceptive technologies has also exposed gendered routines and conventions concerning contraception to reconsideration. The Male Pill shows how technologies have the capacity to make visible and to destabilize dominant cultural narratives of gender. Trust is one of the major themes in these narratives, articulated particularly by the opponents of male contraceptive drugs. In feminist and journalistic discourse, "men cannot be trusted" has become a familiar phrase through the years. This argument reflects and reinforces positivist views that consider masculinity as something singular and immutable. My analysis suggests another picture, in which masculinity emerges as multiple, complex, and fluid.[7] Discourses on male contraceptive technological innovation have revealed a mixture of hegemonic and subordinate masculinities that are not stable but the result of ongoing transformations. At the beginning of the twenty-first century, women and men are renegotiating gender identities and relations, as is exemplified in discussions on the Internet in January 2000 following the report of a male contraceptive clinical trial in England.[8]

> Woman X: Women must maintain control as much as possible of the contraceptive process. The fact is if the man is non compliant in taking his medications the woman, not he, will be the one that has an unwanted pregnancy.
>
> Woman Y: While I certainly see your point as a practical matter, I do think such a position has a deleterious effect on the way we value our relationships and the level of trust we expect to cultivate. I have had some relationships wherein I felt that level of trust, and others wherein I didn't. I would like to at least leave open the possibility for creating relationships with a high degree of trust and mutual responsibility.
>
> Woman Z: In reply to X, who thinks male contraception will deprive women of control and that men will be irresponsible: Sure, some men will forget their pill, as some women do. It might STILL be to a woman's advantage to take that risk in return for her partner bearing the side effects of medication. . . . If you think a guy is responsible enough to rent an apartment with him, or have a joint checking account, or to move to another city with him, or have kids with him, letting him be the birth-control user seems like a funny place to draw the line.

Technological innovation in male contraceptives thus facilitates a situation in which hegemonic masculinities are destabilized and nonhegemonic masculine identities are articulated and gain momentum. In these processes, femininity is interrogated as well. As Bob Connell has suggested, masculinity is always constructed in relation to femininity (Connell 1987: 183). As the discussion on the Internet illustrates, the advocates of male contraceptive drugs are articulating femininities that challenge the view that women do not trust men in matters of contraception. These examples also illustrate the trade-offs women have to make when it comes to contraception.

Male contraceptive innovators anticipated the discussions on trust by configuring the user as couples with stable, monogamous relationships where trust is well established. In my biography of the male Pill, this technology emerges as a relational drug. As with other reproductive technologies for men, such as Viagra and IVF techniques for the treatment of male infertility, male contraceptive innovation reveals a peculiar pattern in which couples rather than individual men figure as the patient (Ploeg 1998; Mamo and Fishman 2001: 26). Although these technologies have given visibility to male reproductive bodies, they still tend to hide them by representing men in relational terms rather than as individuals. This representation strategy is often legitimized by referring to the fact that only women can become pregnant, thus again making men's contribution to contraception invisible.

Another way in which male contraceptive innovators could have anticipated the problem of trust would have been to modify the technology to ensure compliance. Remarkably, this has not happened. By configuring the user as a couple with a trusting relationship, reproductive scientists and clinicians delegated the responsibility of compliance to people rather than to the artifact. This is in sharp contrast to the development of contraceptives for women, where reproductive scientists have developed long-lasting contraceptive injections and implants to ensure compliance. One perceived disadvantage of the contraceptive Pill was that it delegated all responsibility to women, who could intentionally or unintentionally neglect to exercise it. By developing long-lasting injections, the responsibility became delegated to the artifact. The major incentive for this innovation was not that men would not trust women to take contraceptives but to configure women as reliable contributors to reduce the population growth. An explicit discussion of the need to modify the mode of administration of male contraceptives to make men into reliable contraceptive users is, however, absent from male contraceptive discourse. The fact that the current modes of administration include injections and implants cannot be ascribed to an explicit choice to ensure compliance, but is rather the result of a lack of hormonal compounds that can be taken orally. Moreover, no consideration of how the new technology differs from condoms, the first being an invisible, and the latter a visible technology, and how this might shape the trust of women in men as contraceptive users, is taken into account in the technological design. A reflection on the inspectability of contraception as it relates to users and co-users is largely absent from male contraceptive discourse.[9] In summary, male contraceptive drugs can thus best be portrayed as technologies of trust. The efficacy and the acceptability of the technology presupposes and depends on trusting relationships between women and men.

Male contraceptive discourse also shows a variety of identities attributed to the new technology. Whereas the advocates portray the new technology as a tool for enhancing gender equality, feminist opponents represent the technology as a threat to women's autonomy. These different representations show the interpretative flexibility of technologies (Pinch and Bijker 1987). As constructivist theories of technology suggest, technologies do not have intrinsic properties, but are inscripted with different meanings by different groups of actors. Male contraceptive technologies are not inherently emancipatory, nor intrinsically oppressive. This is not to deny that technologies have gender politics.[10] Whether technologies will be emancipatory or not depends, however, on their contexts of use. How technologies perform socially and culturally is not an intrinsic property of the technologies, nor something that can be determined during the development phase. A specific technological design can only prestructure but never determine a specific use.[11] Even after specific representations of use and users are incorporated into the design, the technology's meanings and uses are not fixed. Users, and many other actors, can adopt, modify, or reject the technology's intended meanings or use (Akrich 1992; Akrich 1995; Bijker 1987; Cowan 1987; Clarke and Montini 1993; Oudshoorn 1996; Kline and Pinch 1996). What technologies eventually will become should thus be considered as the result of a co-creation of the many actors involved in the development, production, diffusion, and use of the technology (Lie and Sørenson 1996; Saetnan, Oudshoorn, and Kirejczyk 2000; Oudshoorn and Pinch 2003).

My story thus shows that there are no easy answers. Men are not inherently unreliable, and technologies are not intrinsically emancipatory. Gender and technology are neither fixed nor univocal, but mutually constitutive. New male contraceptives may enable men to perform masculinities that include responsibility and care. As happened to women with the female Pill, the male Pill may discipline men as reliable contraceptive users. Whether this will happen or not lies ultimately in the hands of its users. Whatever happens, one thing is certain: male contraceptives have become an inevitable factor in the dynamics of change in the gendered social order.

Notes

· · · ·

1. Designing Technology and Masculinity:
Challenging the Invisibility of Male Reproductive Bodies
in Scientific Medicine

1 Viagra has been described as having had the fastest takeoff of any other new drug, outpacing such quick starters as the anti-depressant Prozac, one of the best-selling drugs in the United States (Handy 1998: 39).

2 This does not imply that impotence was completely absent from public discourse prior to the late twentieth century. For instance, studies of divorce show that impotence, often called by other names, was articulated as a reason for divorce by women in New England as early as the seventeenth century (D'Emilio and Freedman 1997: 25). I thank an anonymous reviewer for making me aware of this history.

3 The history of medicine shows that there were two previous attempts to include the "aging male" in the agenda of modern reproductive medicine. In the 1890s, medical scientists such as Brown-Séquard and Voronoff advocated the use of extracts of testicles or gonadal transplantation as a medical therapy for aging men. The scientific community, for the most part, reacted with hostility to Brown-Séquard's claims. In their eyes, the clock was being set back to the dark ages of quackery. From the earliest times, the testis has been linked with male sexuality, longevity, and bravery. The Greeks and Romans used preparations made from goat or wolf testes as sexual stimulants. The therapeutic claims of Brown-Séquard about the effects of testis extracts on the sexual activity of men caused a controversy among clinicians and laboratory scientists. There was such a strong resistance that Brown-Séquard's reputation as a distinguished neurophysiologist was eventually ruined and he was marginalized in the scientific community (Corner 1965: iv).

A second attempt to introduce testicular therapy for aging men took place in the early decades of the twentieth century. Practitioners in France and the United States transplanted monkey (and other) testes into men and animals, a practice that became known as "the monkey gland affair." Like the early testes extracts therapy, this gland transplantation became the subject of public debate and controversy in the 1920s. This controversy was even greater and more long-lasting than that surrounding Brown-Séquard. The practice of testicular transplantation lasted through the 1930s and 1940s, after which the surgery gradually began to lose credibility. For a more detailed description of these attempts to include male aging bodies in the medical agenda, see Oudshoorn 1997.

4 To be sure, I don't mean to suggest that there have been no changes in the perception of the female body in different times and cultures. Nevertheless, western medical discourses on reproduction reveal a rather universal focus on the female body.

5 Although there had been two previous attempts to establish a medical specialty devoted to the study of the male reproductive functions, it was not until the late 1970s that andrology became a definite branch of medical science (Niemi 1987; Moscucci 1990: 32, 33).

6 Condoms made of animal materials have been in use as a means of contraception since the 1600s (Clarke 1998).

7 See Clarke 1998; Lissner 1992; Setchell 1984; and Tone 2001 for a more extended analysis of the history of the development of male contraceptives.

8 The need to develop a contraceptive pill for women was first articulated by Margaret Sanger, a women's rights activist and pioneer of birth control in the United States throughout the first half of the twentieth century. Sanger, arrested and jailed for opening the first birth control clinic in New York in 1916, believed that the most important threat to women's independence came from unwanted and unanticipated pregnancies. She advocated birth control as a basic precondition for the liberation of women (Christian Johnson 1977: 1). In 1951, at the age of 72, Sanger approached Gregory Pincus, an American reproductive biologist who specialized in the study of hormones, and persuaded him to start research on contraceptives; he eventually became one of the "fathers" of the first oral contraceptive for women.

9 For an extensive analysis of the role of promises and expectations in technological development, see Lente 1993.

10 Morton Hair, a researcher at St. Mary's Hospital, University of Manchester, as cited in an interview with the BBC News, 25 October 1998, reporting the results of a clinical trial with hormonal contraceptive implants for men.

11 The production of eggs as well as sperm depends on the secretion of two pituitary hormones (LF and FSH), which can be suppressed by many steroidal hormones, including testosterone, estrogen, and progesterone. Many oral contraceptives for women, which consist of various combinations of steroidal hormones, are effective because they inhibit the secretion of pituitary hormones. Many of the hormonal contraceptives for men that have been tested since the 1970s are based on the same mechanism (Bremner and de Kretser 1975: 390).

12 See, e.g., Latour and Woolgar 1979; Gilbert and Mulkay 1984; Bijker, Hughes, and Pinch 1987; Latour 1987; and Bijker and Law 1992.

13 Other exemplary studies of the focus on practice and work are Knorr-Cetina 1993; Latour and Woolgar 1979; Lynch 1985; and Star 1989.

14 The concept of networks is used in two different theoretical approaches in the social studies of science and technology: the social construction of technology approach (SCOT) and actor-network theory (ANT). Both traditions emphasize, however, different elements in the networks. The SCOT approach restricts sociotechnical networks to human actors. In this theoretical perspective, the development of technology and technological change is understood

in terms of the activities and interests of various social groups who may give different meanings to technological artifacts and who favor different technological options (Pinch and Bijker 1987; Bijker 1995). In ANT, sociotechnical networks include both human and non-human actors (Callon 1987). In this approach, agency is not restricted to human actors: technological artifacts and other material entities are also represented and analyzed as actors. The concept of sociotechnical networks has been introduced by Elzen, Enserink, and Smit (1996) to describe interactions between human entities as well as interactions between human entities and technological artifacts. They use the term *sociotechnical* to emphasize that social and technical developments always go together. In contrast to traditional social-network approaches, the sociotechnical network approach thus includes the role of technology in the analysis of social change. Similar to SCOT, and in contrast to ANT, agency is restricted to human actors. This is not to say that technological artifacts cannot act. The adherence to an analytical difference between humans and non-humans is considered relevant, however, for questions concerning the accountability of human actors in socio-technical change (Oudshoorn, Brouns, and Oost forthcoming), and for the development of tools to guide technological development (Elzen, Enserink, and Smit 1996: 102).

15 Some scholars actually refer to cultural interventions involved in the development of science and technology, but the emphasis in this literature is very much on the social rather than the cultural construction of technology. See, for example, Knorr 1993, who mentions cultural interventions as an important aspect of the creation of facts and artifacts but who does not further explore the cultural work that goes into technological innovation.

16 To be sure, I don't mean to suggest that gender is restricted to the cultural dimensions of technology. Many feminist scholars have shown how technological development is shaped by and shapes gendered social relations, including gender divisions of labor. Exemplary studies include Cockburn and Ormrod 1993 and Wajcman 1991. I, therefore, suggest that a gender analysis of technology should include both the social and the cultural dimensions of technology.

17 For nice exceptions to the neglect of identities in technological development, see Cockburn and Ormrod 1993; Kammen 2000; Ploeg 1998; Klinge 1998; Rommes, Oost, and Oudshoorn 1999.

18 A similar criticism has been voiced by Roger Silverstone and Leslie Haddon, who argue that scholars in media studies and technology studies should go beyond a conceptualization of user-technology relations in terms of "isolated individuals" whose relationship to technology is restricted to technical interactions with the artifacts (Silverstone and Haddon 1996: 52). See Oudshoorn and Pinch 2003 for a more detailed overview and discussion of the literature of user-technology relations.

19 Although my argument is very likely to be valid for the relationship between technology and identities in general, I will restrict my analysis to gender identities.

20 Actually, gender theorists adopting ethnomethodological and interactionist approaches have been the first to describe the ongoing processes of gender presentation and gender attribution involved in categorizing people as belonging to a specific gender as "doing gender" (Garfinkel 1967; Goffman 1976; West and Zimmerman 1987). An early example of this sociological work on gender-as-process is Kessler and McKenna's *Gender: An ethnomethodological approach* (1978); it it, the authors describe how we come to impute sex-identity

to people based on how they perform gender. Butler's theory of performativity has enriched the view of gender-as-doing by incorporating theories of the speech act, psychoanalysis, and poststructural philosophy.

21 Butler's work represents a multidisciplinary approach that combines theoretical perspectives developed in Austin's theory of the speech act, the poststructuralist philosophy of Derrida and Foucault, and psychoanalytical theory (Austin 1962; Butler 1990, 1993).

22 Although Butler emphasizes the importance of language in producing gendered bodies, she does not argue that bodies are merely linguistic constructs (Butler 1993). Butler's argument must be considered as an epistemological rather than an ontological claim (Vasterling 1999: 19).

23 The U.K. seems to present an exception here. The historian Kate Fisher has described how, in the early decades of the twentieth century, working-class communities in the U.K. considered the use of contraceptives predominantly as a man's responsibility. In the 1920s and 1930s, the first birth control clinics in the U.K. failed to convince potential female clients of the attractiveness of cervical contraceptive caps and sponges. Kate Fisher has described this resistance as the result of "conflicting cultures of contraception." The idea that women should control their own fertility, first put forward in the U.K. by Mary Stopes and other feminist birth-control campaigners in Europe and the United States, and reiterated during the second wave of feminism in the 1960s and 1970s, clashed with the existing culture of contraception in working-class communities, where both women and men held men responsible for birth control. Kate Fisher described these contraceptive practices in the early decades of this century as "a clearly male culture." In those days, men "played a very significant role in all aspects of contraceptive use: in initiating discussions about birth control, in determining which methods to use, in making sexual advances and in deciding how frequently contraception would be employed, in finding out about methods, and in obtaining any appliances used" (Fisher 1998: 8). Today, traces of similar "male cultures" still exist in several African countries (Stokes 1980).

24 With the term technosociality, I am paraphrasing the concept of "biosociality" introduced by Paul Rabinow to describe social movements that focus on health conditions of specific groups. Rabinow defines biosociality as: "persons having specific conditions (illnesses) who are organized, coordinated, and who feel a kinship based on their shared experience" (Rabinow 1992). I prefer the term technosociality for explaining the emergence of the women's health movement because it was the emergence of contraceptive technologies rather than the condition of pregnancy that pushed women to organize themselves in women's health groups.

25 This does not imply that there are no men who actually practice contraception: many men use condoms and a minority have chosen vasectomy. As Connell has suggested, the cultural ideal of masculinity does not necessarily correspond to the actual activities of the majority of men. Hegemonic masculinity does not mean the total cultural dominance of one specific form of masculinity. Alternatives may exist, but they are subordinated in the dominant cultural narrative (Connel 1987, 1995). Actually, the past decade has seen a substantial increase in the use of condoms, not as contraceptives but to prevent HIV and sexually transmitted diseases (STDs). In the United States, condom use among heterosexual men and women at risk of HIV/STDs increased from 10 percent in 1990 to 23 percent in 1992, and then leveled off again at 20 percent in 1996 (Catania et al. 2001: 179). Another U.S. survey

shows how condom use among women increased significantly between 1988 and 1995 (Bankole, Darroc, and Singh 1999: 264). This survey also indicates that condoms cannot be considered as strictly male contraceptives because women also buy them and insist that their partners use them. Although the increase in condom use reflects important changes in attitudes and behavior toward the use of condoms among men to prevent diseases, it is not yet clear whether and how this will affect men's attitudes and behavior toward condoms as contraceptives, which would challenge the hegemonic view of masculinity by allowing men to take responsibility for contraception. See Tone 2001 for an analysis of male responsibility in birth control decisions.

26 Connell introduced his theory as a critique on previous gender theories, particularly sex role theory, which largely neglected questions of power. See Demetriou 2001 for a more detailed description of Connell's theoretical approach.

27 Although Connell's structuralist approach to gender and Butler's poststructuralist theory of the performativity of gender represent two different intellectual traditions, I have chosen to combine their conceptual vocabulary because both theories go beyond essentialism and avoid a voluntaristic position. Although Butler's early work (Butler 1990) has been identified with voluntarism, in her later work she addressed the limits of the performativity of gender and underscored that her view of gender implied substantial stability (Butler 1993: 94, 95). According to Butler, performativity "cannot be understood outside of a process of iterability, a regularized and constrained repetition of norms" (95). Like Butler, Connell's work also explicitly addresses the constraints on the performances of particular forms of gender (Connell 1987, 1995). In the last decade, a large body of research has emerged that seeks a common ground between structuralist and poststructuralist accounts of gender. See Saetnan, Oudshoorn, and Kirecjzyk 2000: 5–7 for a more detailed discussion of this literature. Recently, Butler's and Connell's work show even more convergence. In "Restaging the Universal: Hegemony and the Limits of Formalism," Butler discusses the merits of the Gramscian notion of hegemony, a notion which, as we have seen, is central to Connell's approach to understanding social transformations. Reflecting on the different ways to understand social transformations, Butler concluded that "the theory of performativity is not far from the theory of hegemony in this respect: both emphasize the way in which the social world is made—and new possibilities emerge—at various levels of social action through a collaborative relation with power" (2000: 14).

28 Connell (1987: 186), e.g., discusses Cynthia Cockburn's 1983 study of the printing industry.

29 Connell developed his "three-fold model of the structure of gender relations" in his first three books (Connell 1987: 90–118; 1995: 73–76; 1996: 161–62). In his most recent book, Connell identifies linguistic practices, which he calls "the structure of symbolism," as a fourth structuring principle of gender (Connell 2000: 26, 42–43, 150–55). See Demetriou 2001 for a detailed discussion of Connell's work.

30 For a nice exception, see the recent studies of Moore and Schmidt (1999) and Mamo and Fishman (2002). Moore and Schmidt have analyzed how discursive practices used by semen banks in the United States construct differences among men and simultaneously maintain hegemonic forms of masculinities. Mamo and Fishman have analyzed discourses on Viagra. Both studies are, however, largely restricted to the use of these technologies.

31 I borrow the term *articulation* from economic and social studies of technology, which have introduced the concept to describe the increasing importance of sounding out the cultural

and political acceptability of new technologies as part of socio-technical transformations (see Rip 1995). I employ the term *articulation* to refer to one aspect of creating the cultural feasibility of technology, namely the articulation of the gender identities of the end-users by the other actors in the sociotechnical network. In symbolic interactionist theory and computer-supported cooperative work, the term *articulation* is used as well to refer to the invisible work required to manage contingencies (Bowker and Star 2000: 310), and to plan and coordinate the different levels of work organization, including experiments, the laboratory, and the social world (Fujimara 1987: 258, 259). Although the cultural work I want to describe can be understood as the creation of alignments between the laboratory and the social world, I use the term *articulation* in a more specific manner, namely, to refer to the ways in which collective and individual actors construct and project the gender identities of the end-users of the technology.

32 The concept of "a niche" was first introduced in evolutionary theory of technological change to capture the dynamics of radical technological innovation (Dosi et al. 1988). *Niche* refers to a protected space in which technological innovation can take place. The protection is needed because the knowledge, expertise, techniques, market, and societal infrastructures still have to be developed (Schot, Hoogma, and Elzen 1994). I argue that protection is also required to articulate the cultural feasibility of the new technology.

33 Although the social and the cultural are always interwoven, I make an analytical distinction between the social and the cultural work involved in the development of technology because it enables me to address the specificities of these activities in more detail. I employ the term *social* to refer to all the work involved in establishing and transforming sociotechnical networks. With *cultural work*, I refer to the work involved in producing, sustaining, or transforming conventionalized performances of gender as inscripted in technological artifacts, social institutions, and the formation of gender identities. By making an analytical distinction between the social and the cultural work involved in changing contraceptive discourse, I can draw attention to the different kinds of actors and locations where this work takes place.

34 My research focuses exclusively on the so-called physiological means of contraception, particularly hormonal methods, because most work has been done on these methods. Innovation in male contraceptives also includes vas-based methods, which rely on "cutting, blocking, or otherwise limiting fertility in the vas deferens, the passage through which sperm travel from the epididymis (where they mature) to the penis" (Lissner 1992: 55). These methods include non-scalpel vasectomy, chemical injection, and injectable plugs. Heat methods are yet another type of contraceptive that have been included in the research agenda, although only by a very limited number of clinicians. Heat methods are effected by heating the testes. They are based on the observation that "the testes must be several degrees cooler than normal body temperature in order to maintain proper spermatogenesis" (Lissner 1992: 62). See Lissner 1992 for a detailed description of these last two types of male contraceptive methods.

35 The empirical data for this book were derived from a variety of sources. Chapters 2, 3, 4, 5, 8, 10, and 11 are based on an analysis of the scientific literature on laboratory and clinical research on male hormonal contraceptives included in Medline in the period January 1966– March 1993; an additional selection of relevant publications that appeared in key journals on reproductive and contraceptive research in the period 1993–2000; protocols, information

materials for volunteers of clinical trials, and press bulletins of clinical trials in the U.S. and the U.K; the archives of the World Health Organization (WHO), particularly the minutes of the Task Force on Methods for the Regulation of Male Fertility in the period 1972–1994, and the annual reports and other relevant publications of the WHO Special Programme for Research and Development and Research Training in Human Reproduction in the period 1972–1999. Chapters 6 and 7 are based on an analysis of publications in major social science journals in the field of family planning research included in Popline, the computerized program of abstracts of population-related publications in the period 1960–1998; publications of the U.S.-based, international non-governmental family planning organization, Access to Voluntary and Safe Contraception (AVSC); and newsletters of the Population Council. Chapter 9 is based on an analysis of articles in newspapers in the U.K. and The Netherlands in the period 1994–2000. Finally, all chapters include information derived from interviews with the most prominent university-based researchers and clinicians in the male contraceptive research community in Europe and the United States; with social scientists; with representatives of the World Health Organization; with representatives of the Population Council; with representatives of the AVSC and the Young Men's Clinic in New York; with public health students; and with representatives of the Dutch pharmaceutical firm, N. V. Organon (see Bibliography for complete details of the interviews).

2. How Man Came to be Included in the Contraceptive Research Agenda

1   The sterilization method for men (vasectomy) consists of an operation to block the muscular tube (the vas deferens) which carries spermatozoa from the testes to the outside. This technology differs from other contraceptive methods because it is meant to be permanent. In this book I restrict my discussion to reversible contraceptive methods.

2   The concept of path dependence, first developed by economic historians in the 1970s, has acquired increasing attention among many social scientists since the mid-1990s (see Hirsch and Gillespie 2001).

3   Until the late 1990s the literature on path dependence devoted relatively little attention to how specific technological paths have originated (Hirsch and Gillespie 2001). See Karnoe and Garud 2001 for a notable exception.

4   India, as a former British colony, even had the first government-sponsored birth-control clinic in the world, which was opened in 1930 (Clarke 1998: 184).

5   See Poel 1998 for an exception to the neglect of the role of social movements in studies of technological innovation.

6   In addition to these research groups, a small number of individual reproductive scientists were involved in male contraceptive research, among them Alan Jones at the University of Manchester and Roy L. Whistler at Purdue University in Indiana. The first articles on male contraceptive agents were published in the 1950s by the American researchers C. G. Heller, W. O. Nelson, and C. A. Paulsen (1950), B. J. Sieve (1952), and Gregory Pincus (1957). In England, reports on male contraceptive pharmaceuticals were published by Alan Parkes (1953) and H. Jackson (1959). The first paper to report on the contraceptive activity of a hormonal substance in men (testosterone proprionate) was published as early as 1940

(Heckel, Rosso, and Kestel 1951: 235). Nevertheless, the major concern of reproductive scientists and clinicians who studied male reproduction prior to the 1970s was the development of technologies to treat infertility rather than to control fertility (Pfeffer 1985; Warren and Bunge 1957; Heckel, Rosso, and Kestel 1951). For a more detailed analysis of the early history of contraceptive research in England, see Borell 1984: 8; for the history of the reproductive sciences in the United States, see Clarke 1998.

7 In the 1950s there existed a growing concern with the possible adverse effects of drugs on male fertility. Several classes of drugs were reported to cause unwanted infertility in man. Much attention was given to Furadantin, a drug widely used at that time for the treatment of urinary tract infections, which also appeared to interfere with spermatogenesis (Warren and Bunge 1957). One paper, published in the *Journal of Urology,* was the first to address the contraceptive effects of chemical drugs in man (Warren and Bunge 1957). The first clinical trial with a chemical contraceptive drug (bis dichloroacetyl diamines) took place in the early 1960s, but it was abandoned when it was noted "that ingestion of alcohol while taking the contraceptive drug caused severe flushing and irregular heart beats" (Bremner and De Kretser 1975: 391).

8 Pincus and his colleagues, who eventually developed the hormonal contraceptive Pill for women, initially included both sexes in the animal tests and even in one of the first clinical trials that preceded the licensing of the Pill by the FDA. Notwithstanding the fact that the hormone preparations had a definite contraceptive effect in these men (male patients from a mental institute), men were not included in later trials due to the occurrence of side-effects (Seaman and Seaman 1978: 84). Two other American research groups that reoriented their research to hormonal contraceptive agents for men were Maddock, Leach, and Paulsen at Wayne State University, and Heller, Laidlaw, Harvey, and Nelson at the University of Oregon Medical School and the Rockefeller Institute for Medical Research in New York (Paulsen 1977; Heller et al. 1958). Warren Nelson later tried to advocate male contraceptive research at the Population Council when he was named the first medical director of that organization (Heller et al. 1958).

9 See Clarke 1998 for an extensive analysis of the illegitimacy of the early attempts to develop female contraceptive methods and the field of reproductive sciences as a whole.

10 American firms included Syntex, Searle, Ortho, Parke-Davis, Merck Sharpe, Dohme, Upjohn, Mead Johnson, Wyeth-Ayerst, and Eli Lilli. In Europe, the pharmaceutical companies Organon, Schering A.G., and Roussel-Uclaf developed sizable contraceptive R&D programs (Gelijns and Pannenborg 1993: 216).

11 Djerassi described the litigation system in the United States in this manner: "Even though few pill suits that have gone to trial have been won by the plaintiffs, the legal defense cost for the drug and insurance companies has escalated to such an extent, especially because of liberalized discovery rules permitting plaintiff's attorneys to demand tens of thousands of documents, that out-of-court settlement of such litigation is often cheaper than defending it in court" (Djerassi 1989: 357).

12 Initially, the FDA requested that contraceptive research should include seven years of testing on beagles and ten years on monkeys (Djerassi 1989: 357). In reaction to criticism of these guidelines, the FDA simplified the regulatory requirements for contraceptives in 1990 by dropping the requirement of toxicology tests in dogs (Mastroianni, Donaldson, and Kane 1990: 483; Djerassi 1989: 357).

13 According to estimates made by Mercke & Sharpe (WHO/HRP 1990a: 14).

14 In 1988, "60 percent of all funding for contraceptive research in the United States came from the federal government, compared with 25 percent in 1970" (Fraser 1988).

15 In 1981 Diraddo and Wardell described how between 1963 and 1976 U.S. pharmaceutical firms studied twenty new contraceptive agents; of these, only two were eventually approved by the FDA (Harper 1983: 12–13).

16 For those pharmaceutical companies that have continued contraceptive R&D, the withdrawal of the other companies definitely had a positive effect: it reduced the number of competing companies (Bergink interview 1993).

17 In this respect, Organon seems to be an exception. The Dutch pharmaceutical firm continued to invest in basic research for contraceptives, including the development of vaginal rings and implants (Waites interview 1994). Recently, Organon reacted to the "crisis" in contraceptive development by publishing an article in *Human Reproduction* in which the authors emphasized the importance of industry in contraceptive research and development (Vemer and Bergink 1994: 376–79).

18 I borrow the term *reluctant actor* from Adele Clarke, who has described the reluctant attitude of reproductive scientists to becoming involved in contraceptive research in the early decades of the twentieth century (Clarke 1998: 205).

19 Clarke coined the term *recalcitrant market* to describe the constraints on markets for contraceptives in the first half of the twentieth century (Clarke 1998: 166).

20 See Ericsson for a description of the negative market assessment by the German pharmaceutical firm Schering A.G. in the early 1970s (Ericsson 1973: 300).

21 As I have described elsewhere, the late 1970s witnessed the emergence of new types of R&D organizations. In Europe, science policy stimulated the creation of intermediary organizations to promote or organize cooperative research between industry and the public sector. In a broader context, public sector agencies, such as UNESCO and WHO, launched research programs in the agricultural and health sectors (Oudshoorn 1997a: 41). Despite the growing importance of these intermediary organizations in scientific and technological developments, such research networks have generally been overlooked by scholars in science and technology studies. A notable exception is Laredo et al. 1992.

22 WHO was created as an intergovernmental organization in 1948 as a branch of the United Nations, and consists of three major organizations: an assembly of delegates from each member nation, which acts as the supreme policymaking body; an executive board, which is charged with carrying out the decisions of the Assembly; and the Secretariat, supervised by the Secretary General of the U.N., which is the chief technical and administrative office of WHO (Lee 1997: 25).

23 Besides contraceptive R&D, the HRP was given a number of tasks, including "the development of scientific institutions and manpower in Third World countries; the setting of scientific and technical standards; the provision of supplies and equipment needed for research; and establishment of information about the performance of existing methods of birth planning" (Atkinson and Schearer 1980).

24 In 1978 only 6 percent of funding for contraceptive development went into research on male contraceptive methods (Atkinson and Schearer 1980: 52).

25 Analysis of the Medline abstracts over the period January 1966 to March 1993.

26 In these early years the coordination of the work of the Male Task Force was largely concen-

trated in Paulsen's institute in Seattle, which accommodated a secretary for the coordination of task force activities. In 1977 the secretary was moved to WHO headquarters in Geneva and the Task Force was assisted by a WHO staff member, Dr. M. R. N. Prasad, an Indian pioneer in male contraceptive research, who was appointed as manager (WHO/HRP 1977; WHO/HRP 1973b).

27 See Kammen for a detailed analysis of how antifertility vaccine research became increasingly focused on the development of female rather than male contraceptive methods. The availability of specific hormones and animal models, as well as the differential access to male and female patients, facilitated the development of antifertility vaccines for women (Kammen 2000).

28 In the period between 1979 and 1982 other task forces initiated several activities with relevance for the development of male contraceptives. The Plants Task Force searched its computerized database for plants which could be used as male contraceptives. The result of this search illustrates the potential richness of this new source. The computer search yielded 170 plants; of these, 15 species were chosen for further screening for their efficacy. All plants were described as active, but some were noted to be toxic (WHO/HRP 1988: 6). A second major activity in this period was the production of a manual for the standardization of semen analysis, the WHO Laboratory Manual for the Examination of Human Semen and Semen-Cervical Mucus Interaction. The manual, which represented the first attempt to standardize semen analysis worldwide, described "simplified methods for the analysis of semen including sperm motility, density, morphology and the in vivo penetration of cervical mucus" (WHO 1992: 6). This project could only be realized because it was considered highly relevant by another, and in this period, much stronger, participant in the HRP—the Task Force on Diagnosis and Treatment of Infertility. A third major activity of the HRP during the period of the Male Task Force's suspension consisted of the organization of workshops to stimulate basic research to increase the understanding of the male reproductive system. The in-depth report described this initiative: "In recognition of the need to improve knowledge and technical awareness in the field of Andrology, the Special Program took the decision to initiate a series of Andrology Workshops of which the first took place in 1980 in Singapore. . . . The second workshop was held in 1981, also in Singapore. . . . This established the pattern for subsequent workshops and served as a partial response to the concerns about the number of investigators, especially in developing countries, able to do research in Andrology" (WHO/HRP 1988: 8).

29 Wei Wen, a Chinese scientist from Beijing, described how the Chinese first noticed the antifertility properties of Gossypol: "Its anti-fertility properties were discovered like so many other notable scientific breakthroughs—by accident. In the late 1950s, a doctor working in Jiangsu province, east China, was struck by the high incidence of childless marriages among people consuming large quantities of crudely-processed cottonseed oil. Later, doctors in central China's Hubei province found that girls brought up on a cottonseed oil diet who wed men from the same area remained childless. Medical research experts put two and two together and decided to test cottonseed oil for contraceptive possibilities" (Wen 1980: 195).

30 The results of the clinical trials with Gossypol were first published in a Chinese medical journal in 1978 (see National Coordinating Group 1978: 417).

31 The fact that the Population Council opted for a different research strategy than the WHO

illustrates the highly contested nature of the evaluation of adverse effect in contraceptive research. In 2000 the Population Council reported the results of an international study which concluded that Gossypol pills were effective in suppressing sperm production for 60 percent of the men in the trial, that there were no "undesirable" side effects, but that reversibility could not be guaranteed. A Brazilian company is trying to get approval from the Brazilian Ministry of Health to produce the pills as a substitute for surgical vasectomy (Segal 2000: 3).

32 During the late 1980s research on hormonal methods, including large-scale phase I and phase II multicenter clinical trials, came to the fore once again within the Male Task Force, especially after the Gossypol program was terminated in 1990 (WHO/HRP 1993: Appendix 5.2). The WHO/HRP 1992 Annual Report also discussed six lines of research: hormonal methods, drugs and plant products, vasectomy procedures, inhibin and FSH, sperm surface antigens, and a basic science program. Cost estimates for the period 1986–1991 reveal the renewed interest in hormonal methods: more than 55 percent of the total budget was allocated to hormonal research, whereas chemical drugs, *Trypterigium wilfordii*, and vasectomy were receiving respectively 14 percent, 11 percent, and 6 percent of the budget (WHO/HRP 1993: 24, Appendix 5.2).

33 The women's health movement was very active and strong in the late 1960s and 1970s. It was reponsible for preventing the FDA from licensing a newly developed long-acting injectable contraceptive (medroxy-progesterone, MDPA) for women. Feminist health advocates took the view that this new contraceptive threatened women's rights, since its use might easily be abused in certain societies. The "ban the jab" political lobby was an important factor in discouraging industry from further research of this kind (Matlin 1994a: 125).

34 In 1977 Barbara and Gideon Seaman devoted an entire chapter of *Women and the Crisis in Sex Hormones* to the male Pill (Seaman and Seaman 1977).

3. Creating a Worldwide Laboratory for Synthesizing Hormonal Contraceptive Compounds

1 Except for certain biologicals, e.g., special vaccines (Djerassi 1970: 943).

2 This does not imply that the availability of steroids was unproblematic for the pioneers in female contraception. The early history of R&D in the field of steroids shows how, before the Second World War, scientists "were severely handicapped by an insufficient supply of cheap and effective hormones. This was partially resolved during the 1940s by Marker's breakthrough in steroid chemistry with the Mexican yam and the rush for easier and cheaper ways of manufacturing progesterone for the development of the anti-arthritic drug cortisone after the Second World War" (Marks 2001: 87). By the early 1950s, when Gregory Pincus began to look for suitable hormones to develop a contraceptive for women, he could rely on a wide variety of cheaper synthetic hormones (Marks 2001: 60).

3 In medicine, the "proper" use of prescribed drugs is called patient compliance. The implanted contraceptive Norplant is, for example, advertised by Wyeth-Ayert as "compliance-free contraception" (Adele Clarke personal communication).

4 Stephen Matlin has been one of my major sources for information about the role of WHO in developing new contraceptives, and in particular about the HRP's synthesis program, cre-

ated to synthesize new contraceptive compounds. Matlin was one of the principal investigators of this program and worked at the Department of Chemistry of the City University in
London, a laboratory that played a central role in the synthesis program.

5　By taking the decision to develop long-acting contraceptives, WHO, like the pharmaceutical
firm Upjohn, had to face feminist criticism. Since the 1980s WHO has adopted the strategy to
invite representatives of women's health organizations to special meetings to discuss issues
such as safety and the acceptability of new contraceptives (Hardon 1997). Moreover, WHO
has appointed a special employee to maintain contact with women's health organizations,
"to help integrate women's perspectives into the research and the institution strengthening
work of the program" (Cottingham interview 1994).

6　Those present at the July meeting included Sidney Archer (Professor of Steroid Chemistry at
the Rensselaer Polytechnic Institute, who had worked with Sterling Winthrop); Giuseppe
Benagiano (Manager, Task Force for Long-acting Contraceptives, WHO, Geneva); Pierre
Crabbé (Professor of Chemistry at the University of Grenoble and, in the 1960s, General
Manager of the Research Division of Syntex in Mexico City), who was appointed coordinator
of the synthesis program; Egon Diczalusy (Professor of Reproductive Endocrinology at the
Karolinska Institute in Stockholm, also affiliated with industry); Carl Djerassi (a leading
chemist and Research President of Syntex at that time); and Josef Fried (Professor of Steroid
Chemistry at the University of Chicago, who had previously worked with Squibb).

7　Hoch introduced the concept of "boundary elites" to describe the role of scientists who have
regular and direct involvement with both business and academic scientists (Hoch 1989;
Crabbé, Diczalusy, and Djerassi 1980: 992).

8　The chemists were selected largely because they were known to the initiators of the synthesis
program. Djerassi, Fried, and Archer were all steroid chemists whose former Ph.D. students
worked in all parts of the world. Pierre Crabbé, who began his career in chemistry as a
student of Carl Djerassi, had a lot of experience in developing countries. The selected
chemists, most of them working in laboratories in developing countries, had thus been
trained mainly in the United States and Europe (Matlin interview 1994; Djerassi 1970).

9　The extension and strengthening of networks with investigators in developing countries has
been (and still is) a major goal of the HRP (Crabbé, Diczalusy, and Djerassi 1980: 992–93;
Atkinson and Schearer 1980).

10　The antimalarial program during World War II was organized by the military (Crabbé,
Diczalusy, and Djerassi 1980: 993).

11　Most participating scientists readily adopted the regime set by the program for synthesizing
the predesigned compounds, not least because alternative compounds would very likely have
cost extra money (Matlin interview 1994).

12　The criteria for testing the purity of the compounds were set by the Steering Committee. This
committee had set very strict purity limits of at least 99.5 percent, which is a much stricter
condition than is normally found in the pharmaceutical industry. "Part of the concern was
that as they were looking for very long-acting injectable agents, it was appreciated that the
physical form of the solid might have a critical bearing on the rate of release. So in order to
avoid artifacts and confusion they decided that they wanted such a high purity" (Matlin
interview 1994). Due to these strict limits, more than 50 percent of the synthesized steroids
failed to pass the test.

13　Although most participating laboratories developed esters of both progestins and testosterone in parallel, the androgens were given "a somewhat lower priority partly because it was mainly a female-oriented focus in the task force" (Matlin interview 1994). The fact that the Task Force for Long-acting Contraceptives was more interested in female contraceptives also resulted in a delay in the actual work on androgens: although 20 AET-1, which was eventually selected as an effective male compound, was first synthesized in 1979, it was only "during a reevaluation of the data at the end of the program that people realized that there was actually an androgen there that was looking very good" (Matlin interview 1994).

14 The injectable for men, testosterone buciclate (code name 20 AET-1), is a long-acting androgen replacement preparation. Many strategies envisaged for controlling male fertility necessitate androgen replacement therapy. The development of long-acting androgens is therefore a crucial part of the development of hormonal contraceptives for men (WHO/HRP 1993: 71).

15 Examples of such drugs mentioned by WHO include remedies for tropical diseases, rodenticides, and pesticides designed specifically for tropical pests (Crabbé et al. 1983: 252).

16 Since 1974, WHO has filed fourteen patent applications: seven were granted, six were abandoned, and one was rejected. I could not trace what happened with the other two applications (Waites interview 1994).

17 In the early 1980s, WHO's decision to patent its products was rather controversial, mainly because it involved ethical questions with respect to the organization's position as a public agency. According to Matlin, "There were huge debates at that time of what was the right approach because one of the things that was held to be true was that WHO as a public agency could not be sued by anybody. What would be the ethical and moral position of an agency developing a drug which might go wrong or which might be abused by somebody if they could not be sued. It has never happened." (Matlin interview 1994).

18 Two other firms were mentioned as becoming more interested in the field of contraceptives, and WHO compiled a list of pharmaceutical companies in developing countries to increase the number of potential candidates for this project (WHO/HRP 1992a: 26–27).

19 WHO expressed reservations about the financial basis of this firm and its capability in modern drug development (WHO/HRP 1992a: 28).

20 This happened, for example, in the case of the development of novel progestagen compounds. WHO could only choose a specific compound (norethisterone) as the parent progestagen to develop new compounds because this compound was no longer protected by patents (Crabbé et al. 1983: 243).

4. The Inaccessible Man: The Quest for Male Trial
Participants and Test Locations

1 The quest for "healthy patients" for the first oral contraceptive for women would have been much simpler if contraceptive research had not been constrained by political and moral taboos against birth control. If contraceptive research had not been prohibited, Pincus would not have been forced to find a test location outside the medical institutions. He might well have persuaded other gynecological clinics to participate in the clinical trials. Moreover, a solution for the problem of finding a suitable location for the clinical testing of the Pill did not necessarily imply a preference for Puerto Rico. It is very likely that the required test location might as well have been found among family planning clinics in the continental

United States that had no laws prohibiting birth control activities. Actually, one such trial was organized, in Los Angeles, at about the same time that the third trial in Puerto Rico took place. The choice of Puerto Rico must therefore be understood as resulting from a mixture of cultural imperialism and practical testing considerations. Since the contraceptive pill was called into existence mainly because it was considered a technological fix for the population problem in "underdeveloped countries," its testing required a population that reflected this ideology: poor, illiterate women. Puerto Rico, with its poorly educated and impoverished population, provided such a testing ground (Oudshoorn 1994a). Throughout the 1960s, Puerto Rico continued to serve as a laboratory for the testing of new contraceptives, including new brands and generations of hormonal oral contraceptives, hormonal skin patches, vaginal foams, and intrauterine devices (Ramirez de Arellano and Seipp 1983: 131).

2   For a more detailed analysis of the clinical testing of the Pill, see Oudshoorn 1994a.

3   For a more detailed analysis of the role of Chinese scientists in contraceptive R&D agenda, see chapter 2.

4   This analysis is based on the publications on male contraceptives included in the Medline database for the period from January 1966 to March 1993.

5   See chapter 2 for a more detailed description of China's policy with respect to population control and its involvement in male contraceptive research.

6   Dr. Kessler also established other organizational structures for the HRP, such as the task force concept and the steering committee concept (Waites interview 1994).

7   Results of both the WHO multicenter clinical trials indeed showed there was a difference in physiological reactions among different population groups. Asian men, particularly Chinese and Indonesian men, were suppressed to azoospermia by hormonal compounds more readily than non-Asian men (WHO/HRP 1990b; WHO/HRP 1996).

8   For a detailed analysis of how family planning discourse is gradually changing toward including men, see chapters 6 and 7.

9   The testing of the first hormonal contraceptive for women lasted for a period of just less than five years. The first clinical trials of hormonal compounds for women took place in 1953. The approval for marketing by the U.S. Food and Drug Administration (FDA), not as a birth control pill but as a treatment for menstrual disorders, dates from 1957. In May 1960 the FDA eventually granted its approval for the marketing of this hormonal compound (Enovid) explicitly for contraceptive purposes (Maisel 1965: 142; Oudshoorn 1994a: 120, 132, 133). In the case of the female contraceptive Pill, the major testing (aimed to establish the proper dosage and to monitor and reduce health risks) took place only after the drug had been introduced on the market (Maisel 1965; Vaughan 1972: 48, 49; Oudshoorn 1994 [1994a: 134–35). The use of hormones as contraceptives for women in the 1960s and the 1970s has therefore been portrayed as having been under continuous testing (Maisel 1965: 146; Oudshoorn 1994 [1994a: 135). Due to changes in the drug regulatory systems, history cannot repeat itself. The testing of new male (and female) contraceptives now takes place under conditions in which the testing of drugs, in general, and contraceptives, in particular, is subject to strict regulations for testing and approval for marketing by drug regulatory agencies such as the FDA, including long-term animal testing and the monitoring of side-effects in human subjects (Oudshoorn 2001). Although this has resulted in a more extensive period of clinical testing, the development of contraceptives for women usually covers a period of fifteen years. Clinical trials for Norplant, a hormonal contraceptive consisting of

rods that needs to be inserted under the skin of the upper arm, were conducted by the Population Council between 1970 and the early 1980s, and the new contraceptive was produced by the Finnish company Leiras Pharmaceuticals in 1983 (Mintzes, Hardon, and Hanhart 1993: 7).

5. The Co-construction of Technologies and Risks

1 In the late 1950s androgen therapy was mainly applied to the treatment of hypogonadism. Other clinical uses included therapy for undescended testes and infertility due to low sperm production (Brooks 1998).

2 See Bain et al. 1980 for an overview of these clinical trials.

3 For other review articles that emphasize sexual functions, see Davis 1977 and Gombe 1983.

4 For a reflection on these changes, see Greep 1976: 209.

5 See chapter 10 for a more detailed analysis of the acceptability studies.

6 In this respect, lipid chemistry evaluation was the least problematic. This test method could easily be added to the other clinical chemistry methods because it did not require other specialized skills.

7 The trial consisted of a collaborative effort among a department of gynecology and obstetrics, a laboratory for sperm analysis, a coagulation laboratory, a clinical chemistry laboratory, a department of anatomy, and a department of theoretical statistics. In these types of collaborations, researchers were increasingly confronted with problems of standardization of data due to the variety of sources. In this case, this task was delegated to theoretical statisticians (Foegh 1983: 18). For a detailed analysis of the problems of standardization in collaborative male contraceptive R&D, see chapter 3.

8 For a detailed analysis of the local variations that exist in routine laboratory methods, see Jordan and Lynch 1992.

9 The first phase II clinical trial for Norplant, for example, was organized five years after the first small-scale trials had been initiated (Mintzes, Hardon, and Hanhart 1993: 7).

10 A few notable exceptions are Jessika van Kammen, Anita Hardon, John Abrahams, and Steven Epstein. Jessika van Kammen has described the tactics reproductive scientists involved in the development of anti-fertility vaccines have used to safeguard the assessment of safety as their exclusive domain, thus disregarding risk assessments of women's health organizations (Kammen 2000). Adopting a similar focus, Hardon has described how contraceptive researchers prioritized efficacy of anti-fertility vaccines above the safety of these contraceptives (Hardon 1997). Steven Epstein has described the role of yet another social movement, the AIDS movement, and has showed how AIDS activists renegotiated the standards and procedures for testing the efficacy of drugs for the treatment of HIV (Epstein 1996). John Abrahams has analyzed the role of pharmaceutical companies in assessments of drug safety, concluding that the commercial interests of these firms profoundly shape the assessment of health risks (Abrahams 1994; Abrahams and Sheppart 1999). For a detailed analysis of the rise of clinical experimentation in the United States, see Marks 1997.

11 The problem is that the hormonal contraceptive agents are developed as injections, or more recently, as pills, whereas the current supplementary testosterone preparations require administration by injection, implant, or plaster. According to David Kinniburgh, an endocrinologist involved in clinical trials at the Edinburgh University that is testing combined

contraceptive agents consisting of pills and implants, many volunteers who followed the intake procedure to become accepted as trial participants decided to quit when they were informed about the implants (Kinniburgh interview 1998): "The main thing that puts people off in approaching to be interested is explaining what they need to do. And things that put them off are implants, which is one every twelve weeks. It's a very simple procedure but that can be enough for some people" (Kinniburgh interview 1998).

12 As has been described in the previous chapter, the efficacy of hormonal contraceptives in Asian men was higher than in non-Asian men. For Asian men, the percentage of men in which sperm production was completely suppressed was approximately 90 percent (WHO/ HRP 1990b).

13 This did not imply that the Population Council completely left the field of male contraceptive R&D; they continued their activities in developing immunological contraceptives, both for women and men (Thau interview 1993).

14 The negative media coverage of a pregnancy of the partner of a man in Manchester who participated in the second large-scale WHO clinical trial indicates the still-contested nature of the male contraceptive trials (Ringheim 1996b: 83; King 1999: 14).

15 Views that emphasize the independence and neutrality of scientific experts still largely dominate drug regulation policy, as has been described by Abrahams (Abrahams 1994: 495)

16 If we take this view literally, Organon's R&D director is right. The hormonal contraceptive discussed in this interview consisted of a combination of a pill and an injection. The latter was added to restore the negative interference with sexuality caused by the contraceptive compounds of the Pill. As a whole, however, the method did not have any negative influence on male sexuality.

17 This does not imply that the Pill had only a negative impact on female sexuality. Marks, for example, has described how women taking the Pill experienced an increase in sexual desire (Marks 2001). Other authors have described how the Pill enabled women to realize a better sex life because of the absence of fear of pregnancy (Seaman and Seaman 1978).

18 When in the early 1990s the effects of the Pill on sexuality were studied for the first time in a double-blind, placebo-controlled trial, 12 of 25 women in Scotland reported the side-effect of reduced sexual interest (Graham et al. 1995). According to a Finnish survey of Norplant users, 34 of the 207 participants reported a loss of libido, and 16 of these women rated their loss of libido as disruptive (Sihvo, Ollila, and Hemminki 1995). As for other contraceptive methods for women, at the time Norplant was first licensed for manufacture in 1983, no studies on the effects on libido had been carried out.

19 Actually, the discourse on risk assessment of female contraceptives show three different risk models: the assessment of side-effects as against the risk of unwanted pregnancy; an evaluation of the risks and benefits of a contraceptive as against those of other methods available in family planning programs; and the appraisal of contraceptive side-effects on the basis of women's experiences in daily-life situations. Elsewhere we have described how side-effects are rated differently according to the risk model that has been adopted. In the face of these different assessments, one aspect remains remarkably stable: the health risks of male contraceptives are considered to be more disruptive than those effects for women. The evaluation of side-effects of female methods such as Norplant and anti-fertility vaccines was settled by qualifying them as non-life-threatening, minor, and transient, whereas the opposite

tendency has been noted in the development of male hormonal methods (Kammen and Oudshoorn 2002).

20 Men themselves also seem to have a low tolerance for risk associated with hormonal contraceptives. A survey of 115 men in the U.K. in 1998 reported that a large number of men participating in the study (71 percent) responded that they were not prepared to tolerate any side-effects (Brooks 1998: 15).

21 Elsewhere we have described another important difference in the assessment of risks of male and female contraceptives. Based on a comparison of the clinical testing of physiological contraceptives for women and men in the last three decades, we have shown how the lay perspectives of men are taken more seriously by experts and policymakers than the lay perspectives of women. In the case of male contraceptives, men's well-being when using contraceptives was a central issue from the very beginning. Men's emotional well-being and sexuality have been put on the international research agenda by the reproductive scientists themselves, and the need for long-term data about male contraceptives has been emphasized by the pharmaceutical industry. In the case of female contraceptives, the concern for the long-term effects of contraceptives was put forward by the women's health movement, and research into women's mental health and libido when using hormonal contraceptives was initiated only at the instigation of women's health advocates. We therefore concluded that the incorporation of lay interests in the experts' methods of risk assessment shows a clear gender pattern. Whereas the perspectives of male contraceptive users have been emphasized and negotiated by authoritative spokespersons within the medical establishment, the incorporation of the interests and needs of female contraceptive users depended on women's health advocates (Kammen and Oudshoorn 2002).

6. The Politics of Language: Changing Family Planning Discourse to Include Men

1 A similar shift has taken place in the attention for men's health. In the early 1990s men's health became included as a specific topic on policy agendas, particularly in the United States (London Dept. of Health 1992).

2 According to Stycos, the family planning community suffered from a "medical bias." The dominance of medical discourse in the ideology of family planning had framed the "advantages" of family planning largely in terms of health, rather than economic benefits. The latter, as Stycos suggested, would have been more attractive to men. The medical "bias" also implied a reliance on medically approved contraceptives and on the distribution of contraceptives through clinics that were rarely attended by men. In addition, Stycos indicated a "feminist bias" in family planning due to the women's movement's efforts to increase women's control over contraception. These biases explained, Stycos concluded, the almost exclusive focus on women in family planning services and a "depreciation" of male contraceptives (Stycos 1996: 2).

3 The authors were referring to the U.N. Conference on Population and Development that took place in Cairo in 1994.

4 These figures are based on an analysis of Popline, a computerized program of abstracts of population-related publications developed by Stycos, who made a search for the number of

published articles whose keywords mentioned "family planning" and "male," or "family planning" and "female" (Stycos 1996: 22).

5 Quite remarkably, many surveys have only focused on married women, thus reinforcing the image that unmarried women are not sexually active, as has been noted by Cynthia Lloyd, Director of the Research Division of the Population Council (Lloyd 1993: 17). It was only in 1991 that the United Nations first collected data on contraceptive use among unmarried women, concluding that these women were a "potentially important group of users in many countries" (Lloyd 1993: 17).

6 A 1997 evaluation of the quality of care and adherence to reproductive rights in family planning settings in eight countries from Africa, Asia, Europe, and Latin America concluded that there still existed a huge gap between Cairo's emphasis on reproductive rights and the practice of family planning services: five of the eight countries still had demographic targets as their major incentives for family planning policies (Hardon and Hayes 1997: 20).

7 For an extensive overview of the organizations involved in promoting men's reproductive health activities, see the HIM CD-ROM provided by POPLINE Digital Services, Center for Communication Programs, Johns Hopkins School of Public Health, Baltimore, Md. (e-mail: popline@jhuccp.org).

8 Kenya and Mexico are still exceptions. Most countries don't have specific policies for men, or "have policies that allow men to veto the use of contraceptives by their wives" (Hardon and Hayes 1997: 19).

9 Actually, the assumption that high-fertility attitudes and values are more dominant among non-white men does persist in the research community, as exemplified by Anderson's research in the early 1990s (Anderson 1989; 1990).

10 See Grady et al. 1996 for a review of the following studies: Beckman 1978a; Bertrand et al. 1987; Bulatao 1984; Edwards 1994; Gerrard, Breda, and Gibbons 1990; Kane and Sivasubramaniam 1989; Meekers and Oladosu 1996; Nyblade 1991; Shah 1994; and Williams 1992.

11 This analysis is based on the bibliography, "Readings on Men," compiled by Ann Biddlecom of the Population Council in 1996. Although this bibliography does not include all articles published on men and family planning, it is a suitable resource to indicate changes in objectives and vocabulary in the family planning literature in this area.

12 Susan Leigh Star has described the powerful role of metaphor by suggesting that "power is about whose metaphor brings worlds together" (Star 1991: 52).

13 The change in objective toward including men to prevent sexually transmitted diseases cannot be credited to feminist activism, but was initiated by national and international health agencies, family planning organizations, and governmental policies.

7. Making Room for Men: Configuring Men as Clients of Family Planning Clinics

1 I would like to thank Bruce Armstrong, Diana Diazgranados, and Kelly McKracken of the Young Men's Clinic in New York City for granting me interviews.

2 Although andrology as a discipline emerged in the late 1960s, andrological clinics are still very rare and marginal in the medical community (Oudshoorn 1994a).

3   The United States is the world's largest donor to international reproductive health services (Danforth and Green 1997: 1). Since the late 1980s organizations such as the MacArthur Foundation, USAID, and UNFPA have provided funding for programs that serve men (AVSC 1997b: 9–10). USAID-funded Cooperating Agencies estimated in 1997 that they spent an average of 12 percent of their USAID project funds on services for men (Danforth and Green 1997: vii).

4   The Young Men's Clinic is not a free-standing clinic; it is part of a very large family planning clinic that has allocated some money to male-specific services (Armstrong interview 1997).

5   Profamilia was motivated to open men's clinics because male visitors to their clinics felt "intimidated and uncomfortable entering waiting rooms that were filled with women." Again, the major incentive for creating men's clinics was to provide better services for men rather than to protect the privacy of women.

6   For its clinics, Profamilia has adopted a strategic planning of services to generate income for male services. Clinics offer a broad array of medical services for men to attract enough male clients. In this manner, they can generate revenues to subsidize vasectomies and other reproductive health services for men. Services for men that generate income include physical examinations needed for employment, urology services, ambulatory surgery, circumcision, hernia repair, male infertility diagnosis, and treatment for sexual dysfunction (UNFPA 1995: 31). The clinics in Bogotá and Medellín are not only self-sufficient but produce profits that are used to cover the costs of clinics which are not self-sufficient and to help clients, including women, who cannot afford to pay full fees for services. The clinics are not only successful in generating income but also in increasing the number of men reached for reproductive services and the incidence of vasectomies in Colombia. Due to the opening of its first two clinics, Profamilia was able to perform 77 percent more vasectomies in 1986 than in 1985 (AVSC 1997f: 22; Vernon, Ojeda, and Vega 1991: 55).

7   This argument has also been articulated in debates on improving health care in prostate cancer programs (Cameron and Bernardes 1998: 684).

8   For a more detailed analysis of machismo in Colombia, see Gillmore 1990 and AVSC 1997b: 6.

9   My analysis of the practices of men's clinics in Colombia is based on a case-study carried out by the AVSC, which provided rich material on current developments in these clinics (AVSC 1997b).

10   Profamilia's staff has suggested that this may be related to the stronger macho attitudes younger men tend to have. Other barriers mentioned by young men themselves include problems with getting time off from work and their lack of experience in seeking urological and reproductive health services (AVSC 1997b: 25).

11   Again, a case study by the AVSC of this clinic in 1996 has been extremely useful for my analysis. In addition, I have used material taken from interviews with the founder and director of the clinic, Dr. Bruce Armstrong, and two public health students, Diana Diazgranados and Kelly McKracken, who worked at the clinic in October 1997.

12   This is at least the program I witnessed when I visited the clinic on 27 October 1997.

13   Male nurses more readily receive positive reactions from patients, they are more readily nominated for promotions, and they are more likely to receive higher salaries (Otten 1985).

8. "The First Man on the Pill": Disciplining Men as Reliable Test Subjects

1 Adele Clarke and Theresa Montini have made the important point that users can be configured in their absence, thus creating what they have called "implicated actors" who experience the consequences of being configured as users (Clarke and Montini 1993). This has been very common in the history of female contraceptives.

2 Since the late 1970s, noncompliance has become an important concern in the medical community (Epstein 1996: 205).

3 See Cockburn and Ormrod 1993, who defined the distinction between subjective identity (the gendered sense of self as created and experienced by the individual) and projected identity (the potential, actual, or desired gender identity as others perceive or portray it).

4 The age limit has been legitimated by the assumption that young men will be able to adapt to the hormonal changes induced by the contraceptive (Wu interview 1994).

5 Due to the lobby of women's health advocates and AIDS activists who criticized the fact that drugs are only tested among a very selective group of people, the FDA has introduced criteria for the selection of trial participants in which it is required that the test populations should be representative of the general population in terms of gender, sexual preference, and ethnic background (Epstein 2002).

6 A similar practice exists in the treatment of infertility in men where clinicians have constructed the couple as a new category of patient (Kirejczyk 1993; Ploeg 1998).

7 This representation of trial participants as unreliable is not restricted to male participants of contraceptive trials. Clinical trials of Thalidomide among women show a similar representation of trial participants and the introduction of elaborate measures to assure patient compliance (Timmermans and Leiter 2000: 54–55).

8 These investigations are specified as mandatory tests for male hormonal contraceptive trials in the WHO *Guidelines for the Use of Androgens in Men* (WHO/HRP 1992b). The manual also includes a number of optional tests, such as psychological tests and bone density measurements. For a more detailed analysis of the tests used in clinical trials in the 1970s, 1980s and 1990s, see chapter 5.

9 A similar role of clinical trials as a means to have access to medical care has been described by Jessika van Kammen for Southern women who participated in the testing of contraceptive vaccines (Kammen 2000).

10 See Griffith 1998, who has described a similar role of humor in creating specific relationships in health care, in this case, among healthcare professionals.

11 See Timmermans and Leiter 2000 for a similar account on how trial participants are constructed as unreliable and the extensive measures required to discipline test subjects, in this case women who participated in clinical trials of Thalidomide in the United States. Extensive measures to control the participants' sexual behavior were introduced to avoid the risk of fetal exposure to Thalidomide.

12 For a further analysis of the scepticism of journalists, see chapter 9.

13 Western women participating in clinical trials of contraceptive vaccines have articulated similar altruistic incentives, that is, they are participating in the trial so as to help women in developing countries (Kammen 2000).

14 This part of my research is based on an analysis of the results of so-called acceptability studies, which are based on questionnaires and focus group discussions among male con-

traceptive trial participants that were carried out by Karin Ringheim, a social scientist at USAID, as part of two large-scale, multicenter clinical trials organized by WHO in the late 1980s and early 1990s. My original plan to interview male trial participants failed because researchers were reluctant to cooperate in facilitating contacts with these men because they expected a negative interference with their own research. Although there are some disadvantages in relying on secondary data (particularly the fact that I have not been able to ask my own questions), Ringheim's published and unpublished reports of the interviews with men who participated in the WHO clinical trials included very detailed and extensive quotes from these interviews, which enabled me to make my own analysis of the experiences and opinions of these men. Moreover, the WHO trials were the first large-scale clinical trials of new male contraceptives and included men from different geographical contexts, which made these trials an interesting case study for my analysis.

15 To be sure, not all participants in the group discussions in which these self-images were expressed considered themselves to be different from other men. Men in Singapore and Bangkok considered themselves to be like "any other man on the street" or "more or less the same" as other men (Ringheim 1993a: 22).

16 A poll carried out among women in Europe for the European Society of Human Reproduction and Embryology in 1997 reported that almost half of married women were dissatisfied with their current contraceptive method (Arlidge 1997).

17 I would like to thank David Kinniburgh at the Centre for Reproductive Biology in Edinburgh for being so kind to give me a copy of this poster.

18 This heroic imagery is also visible in flyers used to recruit homosexual men for clinical trials for the testing of anti-HIV vaccines in The Netherlands in the late 1990s (Keuken 2000).

9. On Masculinities, Technologies, and Pain: The Testing of Male Contraceptives in the Clinic and the Media

1 In this context, the work of Donald MacKenzie on the testing of the ballistic missile is an exception because he included non-experts (the manned-bomber lobby in the United States) in his analysis (MacKenzie 1989).

2 The issues addressed in the science and media literature include the public understanding of science and the ways in which newspapers influence communications and debates within science itself (see Lewenstein 1995 for an extensive review of the science and media literature).

3 See Hagendijk and Meeus 1993 for this criticism of the asymmetry in studies of science–media relations.

4 Whereas Collins and Gieryn have focused on the media as the site of the construction of knowledge claims, and Hagendijk and Meeus have analyzed the role of scientists and journalists in the closure of a controversy, I perform a symmetrical analysis of scientific and journalistic texts in order to understand the dynamics of testing a technology. For a similar approach to the study of controversies, see Engels, Pansegrau, and Weingart 1996.

5 For other studies on the construction of users by scientists and engineers, see Woolgar 1991, Akrich 1992, and Akrich 1995.

6 My analysis is based on a quantitative and qualitative assessment of the texts, in which I have focused on the following topics: the thematic structure of the text (more specifically the

organization of topics dealt with in the text); the information presented in the various sections of the text; the space devoted to a particular issue (how many accounts deal with a given issue); and the strategies used to present the information. I have used the analysis of these topics to reconstruct how these elements contribute to the overall story, or "storyline," of the text. I have borrowed the term *storyline* from Hagendijk and Meeus, who have made a similar symmetrical analysis of journalistic and scientific texts of a public controversy over a claim about a possible cure for AIDS (Hagendijk and Meeus 1993: 394).

7   I would like to thank William Bremner, Alvin Paulsen, Geoffrey Waites, and Fred Wu for sharing their experience in doing research in the field of male contraceptives; also the participants in the "Gender, Science, and Technology" workshop held at the Norwegian University of Science and Technology in Trondheim in May 1997; the participants of the Science and Technology Dynamics Conference at the University of Amsterdam in September 1997; and colleagues and students of the Department of Science and Technology Studies at Cornell University for their useful comments on an earlier version of this paper. Last but not least, I thank Daniel Kleinman and the three anonymous reviewers of *Science, Technology & Human Values* for their suggestions for revisions to this chapter.

8   As we saw in chapter 6, the representation of users as "contraceptive couples" can be understood in the context of the changes in family planning policies that were made during the U.N. International Conferences on Population and Development of the last two decades.

9   The fact that the article published in *Fertility and Sterility* did not include a detailed discussion of the assessment of the acceptability of the method may also reflect publication practices in the field of reproductive sciences, where trial results on acceptability and efficacy (or other technical aspects) are usually published in separate journals. However, WHO's decision to claim authorship of the efficacy paper and not the acceptability paper indicates that the organization is less interested in the latter. Moreover, the WHO press bulletin of the trial only refers to the article in *Fertility and Sterility*.

10   As we saw in chapter 5, the fact that the occurrence of pregnancies is used as criteria to determine the efficacy of contraceptive methods for men has been a highly controversial issue in the early years of clinical testing. In the 1970s, WHO was very reluctant to cooperate in clinical testing of contraceptives for men because there was too much risk involved for women.

11   WHO collected more than 150 newspaper articles and TV and radio programs in the United States, Europe, and China that reported the results of the clinical trial (WHO 1996a).

12   Due to practical considerations, I have restricted my analysis to Dutch and British newspapers. The analysis of the British newspapers was conducted by Catherine King as part of her dissertation at the University of Durham, Faculty of Human Sciences (King 1999). As Catherine King has described, a major difference between the Netherlands and the U.K. is that, unlike in Holland, there were ongoing trials in Britain, that is, in Edinburgh and Manchester. This must have made the issue more immediate for the British journalists and readers because they were dealing with British researchers and trial participants (King 1999: 14). The researchers at Manchester University conducted one of the nine single-country studies of the multicenter clinical trial sponsored by WHO, which is the subject of my analysis in this chapter. The Dutch newspapers included four of the five leading national

daily newspapers that are distributed in the Netherlands: *Algemeen Dagblad, De Volkskrant, Trouw,* and *De Telegraaf;* and one weekly journal, *Haagse Post/De Tijd.* These newspapers reach large audiences in all socioeconomic classes of the Dutch population and cover the major political currents in the Netherlands. *Trouw* and *De Volkskrant* traditionally aim at the more progressive, left-wing-oriented public, whereas *Algemeen Dagblad* and *De Telegraaf* are mainly targeted to audiences with more conservative, right-wing political preferences. *Haagse Post/ De Tijd* attracts both progressive and conservative readers. All of them can be characterized as "serious" newspapers; I have not included the tabloid press in my analysis. Catherine King's analysis of the British press included the national quality journals: the *Guardian,* the *Independent,* the *Times,* and the *Daily Telegraph,* and their Sunday counterparts: the *Observer,* the *Independent on Sunday,* the *Sunday Times,* and the *Sunday Telegraph.* In addition, one daily tabloid paper was included: the *Daily Mail* (and the *Daily Mail on Sunday*), along with several newspapers from the areas where the trials of male contraceptives had taken place: the *Manchester Evening News,* the *Scotsman* (and *Scotland on Sunday*), and the Scottish tabloid, the *Daily Record* (King 1999: 10–11). The media coverage of the WHO trial consisted of two types of texts. Most newspapers devoted a short article in their news sections to report the news of the completion of the testing of the new male contraceptive technology. These texts basically summarized the main results of the test, as described in the WHO press bulletin. The newspapers also included longer articles in their "background to the news" sections. I have focused specifically on these background articles because they provide a much richer source for studying the role of non-experts in the construction of scientific claims. Such articles do not just repeat the news as it is formulated in scientific press releases or by national or international news agencies, but relate the news to much broader contexts than indicated in these sources. Remarkably, the Dutch journalists were all women, except for those working for *Haagse Post/De Tijd.* The same was true of the British news media coverage, particularly the longer, reflective articles. As Catherine King has suggested, the news media thus represented male contraceptives as a women's issue (King 1999: 23).

13 The journalist might as well have used another, more recent survey reporting that 67 percent of Dutch women stress the need for new male contraceptives (Vennix 1990).

14 Most strikingly, the discussion in the media focused particularly on the fact that the contraceptive is an injection. This is rather peculiar because injections are widely accepted as a mode of administration for the treatment of all kinds of diseases. The negative attitude in the media may be related to the fact that it concerns an injection meant to be used as a contraceptive by healthy people, rather than a medication for an illness. Moreover, journalists paid much attention to the site of the injection, which was not mentioned in the WHO press release. The contraceptive was frequently described as the "buttock injection," and the very act of injecting the contraceptive in the buttock was represented as a somewhat embarrassing activity. One may wonder whether an injection in the arm would have evoked similar reactions in the media.

15 The fact that side-effects were highlighted in the British press and not in the Dutch press may be related to the fact that British journalists have interviewed the British researchers involved in the WHO trials, most notably Fred Wu from the University of Manchester, who provided more extensive information in answer to the questions of the journalists. As King described, in these interviews Wu played down worries about side-effects by emphasizing

that these were dose-related and that clinicians were already working toward reducing the dosage and testing combined compounds of progesterone and testosterone.

16 This concern is also frequently articulated in the British press coverage of other clinical trials of male contraceptives that have taken place in Britain between 1990 and 1998 (King 1999: 32, 41). As King has described, the British press coverage in this period showed the same patterns as the press coverage of the 1996 WHO press release, described in this chapter. For an extensive analysis of these journalistic texts, see King 1999.

17 See Gilmore 1993 and Stycos 1996 for a further analysis of cultural views of the relationships between masculinity, contraception, and fertility.

18 A browse through the media coverage of the press bulletin, as collected by WHO (WHO 1996a), indicates that the U.S. press also voiced criticism of the acceptability of the hormonal contraceptive injection, although they seem to have adopted a less critical attitude than the Dutch and British press. The New York Times (7 April 1996, Sunday Late Edition) covered the WHO press bulletin and concluded that "men might not relish the discomfort" (WHO 1996a: 4). Criticism of the painful nature of the contraceptive injection was also voiced in Associated Press (International News section) stories that quoted two experts who described the technology as "a painful injection in the buttock" and "an effective contraceptive, the only drawback being the painful method" (WHO 1996a: 38). Several radio reports in the United States raised the issue of the unreliability of men. The Good Day Wake Up program, broadcast on WNYW in New York, quoted a spokesperson of Marie Stopes International, a major international family planning organization, who concluded: "This research still has a long way to go. . . . Getting men to take responsibility will be the real test" (WHO 1996a: 2). Finally, CNN devoted a program to the results of the clinical trial. The highlight of this program ran as follows: "Officials at the World Health Organization say a pill form of a male contraceptive is unlikely in the near future. Experts believe cultures will have to change before men will take the hormones" (WHO 1996a: 40).

19 This is in sharp contrast to the media coverage of reproductive technologies for women, particularly IVF technologies, where the media have played a crucial role in the articulation of the need and acceptability of this technology (Kirejczyk 1996: 217).

20 The fact that the Dutch pharmaceutical company AKZO Organon recently initiated the testing of a hormonal contraceptive pill (not an injection) indicates that the discussions in the media had a definite impact on the R&D agenda (Suppression of spermatogenesis 1997). See chapter 10 for a more extensive analysis of how Organon has become involved in male contraceptive R&D.

21 In the Netherlands, most national journals have a special section on science, with stories that summarize the scientific claims reported in journals such as Science and Nature.

22 Collins and Pinch have suggested that journalists only deconstruct scientific claims of fringe sciences, that is, of sciences at the margins of the spectrum of respectability. In this view, mainstream science is less likely to be subjected to a contest for authority in deciding the credibility of scientific results. Or, to quote Harry Collins: "Only when the subject matter is fringe science will the production team [journalists] offer their own substantive contribution to the debate, or their own expert comments" (Collins 1987: 709).

23 See Clarke 1998 for a detailed analysis of how the reproductive sciences have gained credibility and status by focusing on fundamental research and, in the case of contraceptive R&D, high-tech approaches.

1   See Ringheim 1993b and Davidson et al. 1985 for an overview of this literature.

2   The field of social science research shows an interesting debate on the different methods used to study acceptability. Acceptability studies of men participating in clinical trials have been criticized because the participants in these studies may not be representative of men in larger populations. Social scientists have suggested that subjects in clinical trials are often atypical "because they are self selected and because they are given more staff attention than is normal in family planning programs" (Keller 1979: 232). Their views may therefore not be representative of acceptability under "ordinary conditions" (Marshall 1977). In response to this criticism, WHO articulated the legitimacy of acceptability studies with clinical trial participants by suggesting that clinical trials provided the only possibility to study actual users (WHO/HRP 1976: 7). The organization emphasized the advantage of such studies, since the views of acceptability are obtained from men with "first-hand experiences with the method," whereas field surveys assess the acceptability of "hypothetical rather than directly experienced methods" (WHO 1980: 121, 123). This view became generally accepted within the WHO Task Force for the Acceptability of Fertility Regulating Methods in the late 1970s. Acceptability studies as a part of clinical trials thus came to be represented as more valuable because they assessed the original experience of people with specific methods rather than attitudes toward methods that don't exist (Mundigo interview 1994).

3   See WHO/HRP 1976, WHO 1980, WHO/HRP 1994, and Ringheim 1995 for protocols and reports of these acceptability studies. Although acceptability studies became a priority within the WHO's HRP rather early, this did not imply that social science research became firmly embedded in the organization. Social scientists remained marginal compared to biomedical experts. Although the HRP had established a special task force for social science research as early as 1972, collaborative projects between this task force and the Task Force for the Regulation of Male Fertility initially remained restricted to the 1970s. In the 1980s, no acceptability studies were conducted at all. Social science research on the acceptability of male hormonal contraceptives on trial was only reinitiated in the 1990s as part of the two large-scale multicenter clinical trials. In the last two decades, social science research within the HRP has been largely redirected to reproductive health services research (Mundigo interview 1994).

4   The protocol mentioned yet another objective, namely, the improvement of measurement instruments and experimental design, as well as "strategies for collaboration with biomedical scientists" (WHO/HRP 1976: 3). The latter illustrates the still fragile relationship between social and biomedical scientists.

5   See Oudshoorn 1995b for a further analysis of this R&D effort.

6   The most extreme forms of technical delegates, suggested by reproductive scientists who adopt the population discourse, are the distribution of contraceptives through the tap or as a food additive, a strategy described by Carl Djerassi as the use of "Orwellian agents" (Djerassi 1989: 948; Hermite, Hubinont, and Schwers 1976: 310).

7   Moreover, the first oral contraceptive for women consisted of very high doses compared to current contraceptive pills. Such high amounts of hormones could never be approved for marketing in the current drug regulatory climate (Oudshoorn 1994a).

8   In an interview in the Dutch journal De Volkskrant in December 2000, Organon announced the

start of a clinical trial with 120 men in Germany, England, Scotland, Finland, and Belgium (Ekkelboom 2000).

11. Technologies of Trust

1   Actually, Margaret Sanger sponsored the development of a number of female contraceptives. In the 1910s and 1920s she championed the diaphragm and spermicides (see Clarke 1998 for a detailed analysis of the history of contraceptives).

2   Other social movements that have played an important role in contraceptive development, particularly in the early decades of the twentieth century, include the eugenic movement and the population control movement. See Clarke 1998 for a detailed analysis of the role of these social movements in this period.

3   This point has also been made by historians of birth control technologies; see, for example, Marks 2001.

4   Of course, there were some individual men, particularly in the United States and most notably Joseph Pleck, Roy Greep, and Carl Djerassi, who played an important role in advocating the development of new contraceptives for men. Although they, and their graduate students, hardly figure as a movement, Pleck and Djerassi were considered "heroes" of the American anti-sexist men's movement (Raphael Allen personal communication). Moreover, the British men I described in chapter 8 who shared feminists' views about sharing responsibility for contraception can also be considered important change agents. Their voices, however, only emerged in the 1990s as part of the clinical testing of male hormonal contraceptives and thus cannot be considered instrumental in initiating technological innovation.

5   My discussion of the configuration strategies is largely restricted to the United States and Western Europe because I have not analyzed data from other parts of the world. Given its different cultural and political context, the Chinese case, in particular, may very well diverge here, even though China continues to participate in numerous university- and industry-organized clinical trials.

6   Similar images of men seem to be present in discourses in the public health domain and in the gay community regarding sexually transmitted diseases and safe sex.

7   For other studies which portray masculinity as multiple, see Morgan 1992 and Hearn and Collinson 1994.

8   This discussion took place on the cyber-fem discussion list from 11 to 17 January 2000.

9   See Garfinkel 1967 and Kessler and McKenna 1978, who have described how people tend to extrapolate from the inspectable to the uninspectable in making sense of the world.

10 See Berg and Lie 1993 for a detailed discussion of the gender politics of technology.

11 Sometimes technologies are designed in such a way that users cannot escape the intended use and the script of the artifact. Norplant, a hormonal implant requiring women to go to a healthcare provider to have it inserted under the skin or have it removed, creates dependencies between providers and users that women cannot resist except by not using it (Oudshoorn 1995b).

Bibliography

• • • •

Interviews

Armstrong, Bruce. Founder and Director, Young Men's Clinic of New York. 27 October 1997.

Baird, David T. Centre for Reproductive Biology, University of Edinburgh. 15 June 1998.

Bennink, Herjan Coelingh. Director, Reproductive Medicine Programme, N. V. Organon. 10 December 1999.

Bergink, Willem. Program Manager, Reproductive Medicine, N. V. Organon. 1 July 1993.

Biddlecom, Ann. Editor *(Toward a New Partnership)*, Programs Division, Population Council. 28 October 1997.

Bremner, William. Division of Endocrinology, Department of Medicine, University of Washington, Seattle. 18 October 1994.

Bruce, Judith. Program Director (Gender, Family, and Development), Programs Division, Population Council. 28 October 1997.

Cottingham, Jane. Social Scientist, WHO. 14 February 1994.

Diazgranados, Diana, and Kelly McKracken. Public Health Students, Young Men's Clinic of New York. 27 October 1997.

Farley, T. M. M. Statistician, WHO Special Programme for Research and Development and Research Training in Human Reproduction. 17 February 1994.

Griffin, David. Manager (since 1995), WHO Special Programme for Research and Development and Research Training in Human Reproduction, Task Force on Methods for the Regulation of Male Fertility. 17 February 1994.

Grootegoed, Anton. Faculty of Medicine, Erasmus University, Rotterdam. 6 May 1993.

Johansson, Elof. Director, Center for Biomedical Research, Population Council. 27 October 1997.

Kersemaekers, Wendy. Project Manager, Medical Research, N. V. Organon. 10 December 1999.

Kinniburgh, David. Centre for Reproductive Biology, University of Edinburgh. 15 June 1998.

Kloosterboer, Herman. Head of the Department of Endocrinology, N. V. Organon. 7 July 1993.

Matlin, Stephen. Warwick University, Coventry. 28 November 1994.

Matsumoto, Alvin. Division of Endocrinology, Department of Medicine, University of Washington, Seattle. 18 October 1994.

Mundigo, Alex. Social Scientist, WHO Special Programme for Research and Development and Research Training in Human Reproduction. 17 February 1994.

Nieschlag, Eberhard. Clinical Research Institute of Reproductive Medicine, Max Planck University, Münster. 24 May 1995.

Paulsen, Alvin. Division of Endocrinology, Pacific Medical Center, School of Medicine, University of Washington, Seattle. 18 October 1994.

Rubino, Diana. Publications, Programs Division, Population Council. 28 October 1997.

Stycos, J. Mayone. Department of Population and Development Studies, Cornell University. 21 October 1997.

Swerdloff, Ronald. Medical Center, University of California, Los Angeles. 4 April 1993.

Thau, Rosemary. Director (early 1990s), Contraceptive Development Program, Population Council. 16 April 1993.

Waites, Geoffrey. Manager (1983–1994), WHO Special Programme for Research and Development and Research Training in Human Reproduction, Task Force on Methods for the Regulation of Male Fertility. 14 and 15 February 1994.

Wang, Christina. Division of Endocrinology and Metabolism and Reproductive Biology, Cedars-Sinai Medical Center, Los Angeles. 9 April 1993.

Weber, J. Faculty of Medicine, Erasmus University, Rotterdam. 19 May 1993.

Wegner, Mary Nell. Director (Men as Partner's Initiative), Access to Voluntary and Safe Contraception. 28 October 1997.

Wu, Fred. Department of Medicine, University of Manchester. 22 April 1994.

Published Sources

Abrahams, J. 1994. Distributing the benefit of the doubt: Scientists, regulators, and drug safety. Science, Technology, and Human Values 19 (4): 493–522.

Abrahams, J., and J. Sheppard. 1999. Complacement and conflicting scientific expertise in British and American drug regulation: Clinical risk assessment of triazolam. Social Studies of Science 29 (6): 803–45.

Access for Voluntary and Safe Contraceptives International (AVSC). 1996. AVSC International Publications. New York: AVSC International.

——. 1997a. Programming for male involvement in reproductive health. New York: AVSC International.

——. 1997b. Profamilia's clinics for men: A case study. New York: AVSC International.

——. 1997c. Men as partners in reproductive health. Workshop report, Mombasa, Kenya. New York: AVSC International.

——. 1997d. Selected U.S. reproductive health clinics serving men: Three case studies. New York: AVSC International.

——. 1997e. Reaching out to men as partners in reproductive health. Video. New York: AVSC International.

——. 1997f. Men as partners initiative: Summary report of literature review and case studies. New York: AVSC International.

——. 1997g. The Family Planning Association of Pakistan's Faisalabad Program for Men: A case study. New York: AVSC International.

——. 1997h. Improving men's reproductive health benefits both women and men. AVSC International News Release, 13 June.

Aitken, R. J., ed. 1986. *The zona-free hamster oocyte penetration test and the diagnosis of male fertility.* Proceedings of a workshop sponsored by the World Health Organization, Special Programme of Research Development and Research Training in Human Reproduction, 3 May 1985, at Boston. Copenhagen: Scriptor.

Aitken, R. J., E. M. Wallace, and F. C. W. Wu. 1992. Residual sperm function in oligospermia induced by testosterone enanthate administered as a potential steroid male contraceptive. *International Journal of Andrology* 15: 416–24.

Aitken, R. J., and F. C. W. Wu. 1989. Suppression of sperm function by depot medroxyprogesterone acetate and testosterone enanthate in steroid male contraception. *Fertility and Sterility* 51 (4): 691–98.

Akhtar, F. B., E. Michel, H. Bents, W. H'nigl, U. A. Knuth, J. Sandow, and E. Nieschlag. 1985. Failure of high-dose sustained release luteinizing hormone releasing hormone agonist (Buserelin) plus oral testosterone to suppress male fertility. *Clinical Endocrinology* 23: 663–65.

Akrich, M. 1992. The de-scription of technical objects. In *Shaping technology—building society: Studies in sociotechnical change,* ed. W. Bijker and J. Law, 205–44. Cambridge, Mass.: MIT Press.

——. 1995. User representations: Practices, methods, and sociology. In *Managing technology in society: The approach of constructive technology assessment,* ed. A. Rip, T. J. Misa, and J. Schot, 167–84. London: Pinter Publishers.

Akrich, M. and B. Latour. 1992. A summary of human and nonhuman assemblies. In *Shaping Technology/Building Society: Studies in Sociotechnical Change,* ed. W. E. Bÿker and J. Law. Cambridge, Mass.: MIT Press.

Aldhous, P. 1990. Contraception: Equality for the sexes? *Nature* 347: 701.

Anderson, E. 1989. Sex codes and family life among poor inner-city youth. *Annals of the American Academy of Political and Social Science* (January), edited by William Julius Wilson.

——. 1990. *Streetwise: Race, class, and change in an urban community.* Pennsylvania: University of Pennsylvania Press.

Anderson, R. A., J. Bancroft, and F. C. W. Wu. 1992. The effects of exogenous testosterone on sexuality and mood of normal men. Medical Research Council Biology Unit, Centre for Reproductive Biology. Typescript.

Androgens, lipids, and cardiovasular risk. 1992. *Annals of Internal Medicine* 117 (10): 871–72.

Archer, S., G. Benagiano, P. Crabbé, E. Diczfalusy, C. Djerassi, J. Fried, and T. Higuchi. 1983. Long-acting contraceptive agents: Design of the WHO chemical synthesis programme. *Steroids* 41 (3): 243–53.

Arlidge, J. 1997. First man on the pill "can't wait to start." *Manchester Evening News,* 6 October.

Arnold, K., D. Jones, S. O'Neill, and R. Porter. 1998. *Needles in medical history: An exhibition at the Wellcome Trust History of Medicine Gallery, April 1998.* London: The Wellcome Trust.

Arthur, W. B. 1989. Competing technologies, increasing returns, and lock-in by historical events. *Economic Journal* 899: 116–31.

Ashmore, M., M. Mulkay, and T. Pinch. 1989. *Health and efficiency: A sociology of health economics.* Miltone Keynes: Open University Press.

Atkinson, L., and S. B. Shearer. 1980. Prospects for improved contraception. *International Family Planning Perspectives* 6: 2.

Austin, J. L. 1962. *How to do things with words.* Cambridge, Mass.: Harvard University Press.

Babiak, J., and L. L. Rudel. 1987. Lipoproteins and atherosclerosis. *Bailliere's Clinical Endocrinological Metabolism* 1: 515–50.

Bain, J., Z. Khait, V. Rachlis, and E. Robert. 1980. The combined use of oral medroxyprogesterone acetate and methyltestosterone in a male contraceptive trial programme. *Contraception* 21 (4): 365–79.

Balswick, J. O. 1972. Attitudes of lower class males toward taking a male birth control pill. *National Council on Family Relations: The Family Coordinator* 21: 195–99.

Bankole, A., J. E. Darroc, and S. Singh. 1999. Determinants of trends in condom use in the United States, 1988–1995. *Family Planning Perspectives* 31 (6): 264–71.

Barfield, A., J. Melo, E. Coutinho, F. Alvarez-Sanchez, A. Faundes, V. Brache, P. Leon, J. Frick, G. Bartsch, W.-H. Weiske, P. Bremner, D. Mishell Jr., G. Bernstein, and A. Ortiz. 1979. Pregnancies associated with sperm concentrations below 10 million/ml in clinical studies of a potential male contraceptive method: Monthly depot medroxyprogesterone acetate and testosterone esthers. *Contraception* 20 (2): 121–27.

Baughmann, N. C, J. T. Bertrand, B. Djunghu, M. P. Edwards, B. Makani, and K. L. Niwembo. 1996. The male versus female perspective on family planning: Kinshasa, Zaire. *Journal of Biosocial Science* 28: 37–55.

Beach, L. R., and J. R. Udry. 1972. Powerlessness and regularity of contraception in an urban negro male sample: A research note. *Journal of Marriage and the Family* 34: 112–14.

Beckman, L. J. 1978a. Communication, power, and the influence of social networks in couple decisions on fertility. In *Determinants of fertility in developing countries: Fertility regulation and institutional influences,* ed. R. A. Bulatao and R. D. Lee, 2:415–43. New York: Academic Press.

——. 1978b. Couples' decision-making process regarding fertility. In *Social Demography,* ed. L. B. I. K. Taeuber and J. Sweet, 57–81. New York: Academic Press.

Behre, M., W. Hubert, D. Nashan, and E. Nieschlag. 1992. Depot gonadotropin-releasing hormone agonist blunts the androgen-induced suppression of spermatogenesis in a clinical trial of male contraception. *Journal of Clinical Endocrinology and Metabolism* 74 (1): 84–90.

Belkien, L., U. A. Knuth, E. Nieschlag, and T. Schrmeyer. 1984. Reversible azoospermia induced by the anaboloic steroid 19-nortestosterone. *The Lancet* (25 February): 417–20.

Benditt, J. M. 1980. Current contraceptive research. *Family Planning Perception* 12 (3): 149–55.

Berelson, B. 1969. Beyond family planning. *Science* 163 (16): 533–43.

Berends, L. 1998. De erectie van de alchemist. *Het Parool* (9 June): 2–3.

Berer, Marge. 1996. Men. *Reproductive Health Matters* 7: 7–10.

Berg, A. 1996. Digital feminism. Report no. 28. Ph.D. diss., Norwegian University of Science and Technology, Centre for Technology and Society, Trondheim.

Berg, A. J., and M. Lie. 1993. Feminism and constructivism: Do artifacts have gender? *Science, Technology, and Human Values* 20 (3): 332–51.

Berg, M. 1992. The construction of medical disposals: Medical sociology and Medical problem solving in clinical practices. *Sociology of Health and Illness* 14 (3): 151–80.

Bernardes, J., and E. Cameron. 1998. Gender and disadvantage in health: Men's health for a change. *Sociology of Health and Illness* 20 (5): 73–93.

Bertrand, Jane T., M. P. Edwards, and K. L. Niwembo. 1987. Evaluation of a communications program to increase adoption of vasectomy in Guatemala. *Studies in Family Planning* 18 (6): 361–70.

Bertrand, J. T., B. Makani, M. P. Edwards, N. C. Baughmann, K. L. Niwembo, and B. Djunghu. 1996. The male versus female perspective on family planning: Kinshasa, Zaire. *Journal of Biosocial Science* 28: 37–55.

Bhasin, S., D. J. Handelsman, and R. S. Swerdloff. 1985. Hormonal effects of GnRH agonist in the human male: An approach to male contraception using combined androgen and GnRH agonist treatment. *Journal of Steroid Biochemistry* 23 (5b): 855–61.

Bialy, G., and D. J. Patanelli. 1981. Potential use of male antifertility agents in developed countries. *Chemotherapy* 27 (2): 102–6.

Bijker, W. E. 1987. The social construction of fluorescent lighting, or how an artifact was invented in its diffusion stage. In *The social construction of technological systems: New directions in the sociology and history of technology*, ed. W. E. Bijker, T. P. Hughes, and T. J. Pinch, 75–102. Cambridge, Mass.: MIT Press.

——. 1994. Toward a theory of sociotechnical change. Lecture in the Colloquium Series of the Department of Science Dynamics, University of Amsterdam. 8 May.

——. 1995. *Bicycles, bulks, and Bakelite: Towards a theory of sociotechnical change.* Cambridge, Mass.: MIT Press.

Bijker, W. E., T. P. Hughes, and T. J. Pinch, eds. 1987. *The social construction of technological systems: New directions in the sociology and history of technology.* Cambridge, Mass.: MIT Press.

Bijker, W. E, and J. Law. 1992. Shaping technology—Building society. Cambridge, Mass: MIT Press.

Bogue, D. J. 1967. *Sociological contributions to family planning research.* Chicago: University of Chicago Press.

Borell, M. 1987. Biologists and Birth Control 1918–1930. *Journal of the History of Biology* 19: 51–87.

Bouchard, P., and E. Garcia. 1987. Influence of testosterone substitution on sperm suppression by LHRH agonists. *Hormone Research* 28: 175–80.

Bowker, G. 1994. *Science on the run: Information management and industrial geophysics at Schlumberger, 1920–1940.* Cambridge, Mass.: MIT Press.

Bowker, G. C., and S. L. Star. 2000. *Sorting things out: Classification and its consequences.* Cambridge, Mass.: MIT Press.

Brand, A. van, and K. Schwartz. 1999. De pillen voor plezier. *Trouw* (21 April): 17.

Briggs, M., and M. Briggs. 1974. Oral contraceptive for men. *Nature* 252 (December 13): 585–86.

Bremner, W. J., and D. M. de Kretser. 1975. Contraceptives for males. *Signs: Journal of Women in Culture and Society* 1 (21): 387–96.

Brooks, M. 1998. Men's views on male hormonal contraception: A survey of attenders at a fitness centre in Bristol, U.K. *The British Journal of Family Planning* 24: 7–17.

Bruce, J., A. Leonard, and J. B. Lloyd. 1995. *Families in focus: New perspectives on mothers, fathers, and children.* New York: Population Council.

Bulatao, R. A. 1984. Content and process in fertility decisions: A psychosocial perspective. *Fertility and Family* 16: 159–99.

Butler, J. 1990. *Gender trouble: Feminism and the subversion of identity.* New York: Routledge.

——. 1993. *Bodies that matter: On the discursive limits of "sex."* New York: Routledge.

——. 1995. Melancholy gender/Refused identification. In *Constructing Masculinity*, ed. M. Berger, B. Wallis, and S. Watson, 21–37. New York: Routledge.

Callon, M. 1987. The sociology of an actor-network: The case of the electric vehicle. In *Mapping the dynamics of science and technology*, ed. M. Callon, J. Law, and A. Rip, 19–34. Basingstoke, U.K.: MacMillan.

Catania, J. A., J. Canchola, D. Binson, M. M. Dolcini, P. P. Paul, L. Fisher, K.-H. Choi, L. Pollcak, J. Chang, W. L. Yarber, J. R. Heima, and T. Coates. 2001. National trends in condom use among at-risk heterosexuals in the United States. *Journal of Acquired Immune Deficiency Syndromes* 27: 176–82.

Check, W. 1999. Stripping away cultural taboos: The Kinsey Institute for Research into Sex, Gender, and Reproduction, Orgyn. *Organon's Magazine on Women and Health* 1: 18–24.

Chikamata, D. 1997. Male needs and responsibilties in family planning and reproductive health. *Toward a New Partnership* 2:7–8.

Ching, C. L. 1983. The male role in contraception: Implications for health education. *Journal of School Health* (March): 197–201.

Christian Johnson, R. 1977. Feminism, philanthropy, and science in the development of the oral contraceptive pill. *Pharmacy in History* 19 (2): 63–79.

Clark, K. B. 1985. The interaction of design hierarchies and market concepts in technological evolution. *Research Policy* 14: 235–51.

Clarke, A. 1990. Controversy and the development of reproductive sciences. *Social Problems* 37 (1): 18–37.

——. 1998. *Disciplining reproduction: Modernity, American life, and "the problem of sex."* Chicago: University of Chicago Press.

Clarke, A. E., and T. Montini. 1993. The many faces of RU 486: Tales of situated knowledges and technological contestations. *Science, Technology, and Human Values* 18 (1): 42–78.

Clarke, A., and L. J. Moore. 1995. Clitoral conventions and transgressions: Graphic representations in anatomy texts, c. 1900–1991. *Feminist Studies* 21 (2): 255–301.

Cleland, J., and C. Scott, eds. 1987. *The world fertility survey.* Oxford: Oxford University Press.

Cockburn, C. 1983. *Brothers: Male dominance and technological change.* London: Pluto.

——. 1992. The circuit of technology: Gender, identity, and power. In *Consuming technology: Media and information in domestic spaces*, ed. S. Silverstone and E. Hirsch, 32–47. London, Routledge.

Cockburn, C., and S. Ormrod. 1993. *Gender and technology in the making.* London: SAGE Publications.

Colborn, T., D. Dumanski, and J. P. Meyers. 1996. *Our stolen future: Are we threatening our fertility, intelligence, and survival? A scientific detective story.* London: Dutton Signet.

Collins, H. M. 1987. Certainty and the public understanding of science: Science on television. *Social Studies of Science* 17: 689–713.

Collins, H. M., and T. J. Pinch. 1979. The construction of the paranormal: Nothing unscientific is happening. In *On the margins of science: The social construction of rejected knowledge*, ed. R. Wallis, 237–70. Sociological Review, monograph 27. Keele, U.K.: University of Keele.

Connell, R. W. 1987. *Gender and power.* Cambridge: Polity Press.

——. 1995. *Masculinities.* Cambridge: Polity Press.

——. 1996. New directions in gender theory, masculinity research, and gender politics. *Ethnos* 61: 161–62.

——. 2000. *The men and the boys.* Cambridge: Polity Press.

Constant, E. W. 1983. Scientific theory and technological testability: Science dynameters and water turbines in the nineteenth century. *Technology and Culture* 24: 183–98.

Contraceptive Development Branch, Center for Population Research, National Institute of Child

Health and Human Development, Special Programme of Research, Development and Research Training in Human Reproduction World Health Organization. 1985. *Consultation on the chemical synthesis of fertility regulating agents.* Bethesda, Typescript.

Corner, G. W. 1965. The early history of oestrogenic hormones. *Proceedings of the Society of Endocrinology* 33: 3–18.

Coutinho, E. M. 1974. Male contraception and the unisex pill. *International Planned Parenthood Federation Medical Bulletin* 8 (3): 3–4.

Coutinho, E. M., and J. F. Melo. 1973. Succesful inhibition of spermatogenesis in man without loss of libido: A potential new approach to male contraception. *Contraception,* 8 (3): 207–17.

Cowan, R. S. 1987. The consumption junction: A proposal for research strategies in the sociology of technology. In *The social construction of technological systems: New directions in the sociology and history of technology,* ed. W. E. Bijker, T. P. Hughes, and T. J. Pinch. Cambridge: MIT Press.

Crabbé, P., S. Archer, G. Benagiano, E. Diczfalusy, C. Djerassi, J. Fried, and T. Higuchi. 1983. Long-acting contraceptive agents: Design of the WHO chemical synthesis programme. *Steroids* 41 (3): 243–53.

Crabbé, P., E. Diczalusy, and C. Djerassi. 1980. Injectable contraceptive synthesis: An example of international cooperation. *Science* 209: 992–95.

Cussins, C. 1998. Ontological choreography: Agency for women patients in an infertility clinic. In *Differences in medicine: Unravelling practices, techniques, and bodies,* ed. M. Berg and A. Mol. Durham, NC, Duke University Press.

Danforth, N. 1994. AVSC men's program strategy. *AVSC News* 32 (2): 6.

Danforth, N., and C. P. Green. 1997. Involving men in reproductive health: A review of Usaid-funded activities. POPTECH, report no. 96-079-050. Arlington: Population Technical Assistance Project.

Das, P. ad J. Oerdemans. 1984. *De wereld sinds 1870.* Groningen: Wolter-Noordhoff.

Davidson, A. R., K. C. Ahn, S. Chandra, R. Diaz-Guerrero, D. C. Dubey, and Amir Mehryar. 1985. *Contraceptive choices for men: Existing and potential male methods.* Report prepared for presentation at the Seminar on Determinants of Contraceptive Method Choice, 26–29 August, East-West Population Institute, Honolulu, Hawaii.

Davis, J. E. 1977. Status of male contraception. *Obstetrics and Gynaecology Annual* 6: 355–69.

Demetriou, D. Z. 2001. Connel's concept of hegemonic masculinity: A critique. *Theory and Society* 30: 337–61.

D'Emilio, J., and E. B. Freedman. 1997. *Intimate matters: A history of sexuality in America.* 2d ed. Chicago: University of Chicago Press.

Deys, C., and M. Potts. 1977. Factors affecting patient motivation. International Reference Centre for Abortion Research, London, England. Typescript.

Diczfalusy, E. 1985. Contraceptive futurology or 1984 in 1984. *Contraception* 31 (1): 1–10.

———. 1986. World Health Organization, Special Programme of Research, Development, and Research Training in Human Reproduction—The First Fifteen Years: A Review. *Contraception* 34 (1): 18–119.

Diller, L., and W. Hembree. 1977. Male contraception and family planning: A social and historical review. *Fertility and Sterility* 28 (12): 1271–79.

Djerassi, C. 1970. Birth control after 1984. *Science* 169: 941–51.

———. 1989. The bitter pill. *Science* 245: 356–61.

———. 1992. *The pill, Pygmy chimps, and Degas' horse.* Oxford: Oxford University Press.

———. 2001. *This man's pill: Reflections on the fiftieth birthday of the pill.* Oxford: Oxford University Press.

Dosi, G. 1982. Technological paradigms and technological trajectories: A suggested interpretation of the determinants and directions of technical change. *Research Policy* 11: 147–62.

Dosi, G., C. Freeman, R. Nelson, G. Silverberg, and L. Soete. 1988. *Technical change and economic theory.* London: Pinter Publishers.

Duden, B. 1991. *The woman beneath the skin: A doctor's patients in eighteenth-century Germany.* Cambridge, Mass.: Harvard University Press.

Dyck, J. van. 1995. *Manufacturing babies and public consent: Debating the new reproductive technologies.* New York: New York University Press.

Ebin, V. 1996. African men want more children than their wives. *Population Today* 24 (10): 15–32.

Edwards, S. R. 1994. The role of men in contraceptive decision-making: Current knowledge and future implications. *Family Planning Perspectives* 26 (2): 77–82.

Ekkelboom, J. 2000. Mannenpil legt ballen in de luren. *De Volkskrant,* 12 December.

Elzen, B., B. Enserink, and W. A. Smit. 1996. Socio-technical networks: How a technology studies approach may help to solve problems related to technical change. *Social Studies of Science* 26: 95–141.

Epstein, S. 1996. *Impure science: Aids, activism, and the politics of knowledge.* Berkeley: University of California Press.

———. 1997. Activism, drug regulation, and the politics of therapeutic evalution in the AIDS era: A case study of ddC and the "surrogate makers" debate. *Social Studies of Science* 27 (5): 691–727.

———. 2002. Inclusion, diversity, and biomedical knowledge-making: The multiple politics of representation. In *How users matter: The co-construction of users and technologies,* ed. N. E. J. Oudshoorn and T. J. Pinch. Cambridge, Mass.: MIT Press.

Engels, A., P. Pansegrau, and P. Weingart. 1996. *Kommunikationen uber Klimawandel zwischen Wissenschaft, Politik und Massamedien.* DFG-Projekt, IWT paper, no. 13. Institut für Wissenschafts und Technikforschung, Universität Bielefeld.

Ericsson, J. 1973. Conceptual contraception. In *Advances in the Biosciences,* vol. 10: *Schering workshop on contraception: The masculine gender, Berlin, November 29 to December 2, 1972,* 299–309. Oxford: Pergamon Press.

Faulkner, W. 2000. The power and the pleasure? A research agenda for making gender stick to engineers. *Science, Technology, and Human Values* 25 (1): 87–119.

———. 2001. The technology question in feminism: A view from feminist technology studies. *Women's Studies International Forum* 24 (1): 79–95.

Fawcett, D. W. 1978. Prospects for fertility control in the male. In *Hormonal contraceptives, estrogens, and human welfare,* ed. M. C. Diamond and C. C. Korenbrot. New York: Academic Press.

Ferdinand, L. S. 1996. Another side of quality. *Reproductive Health Matters* 7 (special issue: Men): 144–45.

Fisher, K. 1998. Conflicting cultures of contraception: Birth control clinics and the working-classes in Britain between the wars. Paper presented at the workshop on Cultures of Medicine, June 1998, at the Wellcome Institute for the History of Medicine, London.

Foegh, M. 1983. Evaluation of steroids as contraceptives in men. *Acta endocrinologica,* supp. 260.

Foegh, M., K. Nicol, J. Bruunhuus Petersen, and G. Schou. 1980. Clinical evaluation of long-term treatment with levo-norgestel and testosterone enanthate in normal men. *Contraception* 21 (6): 631–40.

Fox, R. C., and J. Swazey. 1992. *Spare parts*. Oxford: Oxford University Press.

Franklin, S., C. Lury, and J. Stacey. 1991. Feminism and cultural studies: Pasts, presents, futures. *Media, Culture, and Society* 13: 171–92.

Franklin, S., and H. Ragne. 1998. *Reproducing reproduction: Kinship, power, and technological innovation*. Philadelphia: University of Pennsylvania Press.

Fraser, L. 1988. Pill politics. *Mother Jones* 12 (5): 30.

Frye Helzner, J. 1996. Men's involvement in family planning. *Reproductive Health Matters* 7: 146–54.

Frykman, J. 1996. Space for a man: The transformation of masculinity in twentieth century culture. *Reproductive Health Matters* 7: 11–18.

Fujimura, J. H. 1987. Constructing doable problems in cancer research: Articulating alignment. *Social Studies of Science* 17: 257–93.

——. 1988. The molecular biological bandwagon in cancer research: Where social worlds meet. *Social Problems* 35: 261–83.

——. 1992. Crafting science: Standardized packages, boundary objects, and translation. In *Science as practice and culture*, ed. A. Pickering, 168–215. Chicago: University of Chicago Press.

Galison, P. 1987. *How experiments end*. Chicago: University of Chicago Press.

Gallen, M. E., L. Liskin, and N. Kok. 1986. Men: New focus for family planning programs. *Population Reports* 1 (33): 889–919.

Garfinkel, H. 1967. *Studies in ethnomethodology*. Englewood Cliffs, N.J.: Prentice Hall.

Garschagen, O. 1998. Amerikanen in de rij voor "penispil." *Volkskrant*, 1 May.

Geest, S. van der, and A. Hardon. 1994. De kracht van injecties: sociale en culturele aspecten. In *De macht der dingen: medische technologie in cultureel perspectiel*, ed. S. van der Geest, P. ten Have, G. Nÿhof, and P. Verbeek-Heicla. Amsterdam: Spinhuis.

Gelijns, A, and C. Pannenborg. 1993. The development of contraceptive technology: Case studies of incentives and disincentives of innovation. *International Journal of Technology Assessment in Health Care* 9 (2): 210–32.

Geurts, P. 1998. The first world congress on the aging male, Geneva, 1998, Orgyn. *Organon's Magazine on Women and Health* 4: 30–31.

Gerrard, M., C. Breda, and F. X. Gibbons. 1990. Gender effects in couples' sexual decision making and contraceptive use. *Journal of Applied Social Psychology* 20: 449–64.

Gieryn, T. F. 1992. The ballad of Pons and Fleischmann: Experiment and narrative in the (un)making of cold fusion. In *The social dimensions of science*, ed. E. McMullin, 217–43. Notre Dame, Ind.: University of Notre Dame Press.

Gilbert, G. N., and M. Mulkay 1984. *Opening Pandora's box: a sociological analysis of scientists' discourse*. Cambridge: Cambridge University Press.

Gilmore, D. 1990. *Manhood in the making: Cultural concepts of masculinity*. New Haven, Ct.: Yale University Press.

——. 1993. *De man als mythe: Mannelijkheid in verschillende culturen*. Amsterdam: Maarten Muntinga.

Glander, H.-J. 1987. Bemerkungen zur nichtnormalen reversiblen Kontrazeption beim Man. *Der Hautarzt* 38 (6): 321–26.

Goffman, E. 1976. *Gender advertisements*. Cambridge, Mass.: Harvard University Press.

Goldstein, L., ed. 1991. *The female body: Figures, styles, speculations*. Ann Arbor: University of Michigan Press.

Gombe, S. 1983. A review of the current status in male contraceptive studies. *East African Medical Journal* 6 (4): 203–11.

Gomes, W., and N. L. Van Demark. 1974. The male reproductive system. *Annual Review of Physiology* 36: 307–30.

Gordon, P., and L. J. DeMarco. 1984. Reproductive health services for men: Is there a need? *Family Planning Perceptives* 1: 44–49.

Gossypol: A new antifertility agent for males. 1979. *Gynaecological and Obstetric Investigations* 10 (4): 163–76.

Gossypol prospects. 1984. *The Lancet* 8386: 1108–09.

Gough, H. H. 1992. Some factors related to men's stated willingness to use a male contraceptive pill. *Journal of Sex Research* 15 (1): 27–37.

Grady, W. R., K. Tanfer, J. O. G. Billy, and J. Lincoln-Hanson. 1996. Men's perceptions of their roles and responsibilities regarding sex, contraception, and childrearing. *Family Planning Perspectives* 28 (5): 221–26.

Graham, C. A., R. Ramos, J. Bancroft, C. Maglaya, and T. M. M. Farley. 1995. The effects of steroidal contraceptives on the well-being and sexuality of women: A double blind, placebo-controlled, two-center study of combined and progesterone-only methods. *Contraception* 52: 363–69.

Greep, R. O. 1976. Some reflections on male reproductive biology and contraception. In *Regulatory Mechanisms of Male Reproductive Physiology: Sixth Brook Lodge Workshop on Problems of Reproductive Biology*, ed. C. Spilman, T. J. Lobl, and K. T. Kirton. New York: American Elsevier Publishing Co.

Greep, R. O., M. A. Koblinsky, and F. S. Jaffe. 1976. *Reproduction and human welfare, a challenge to research: A review of the reproductive sciences and contraceptive development.* Cambridge, Mass.: MIT Press.

Griffith, L. 1998. Humour as resistance to professional dominance in community mental health teams. *Sociology of Health and Illness* 20 (6): 874–95.

Guerin, J. R. 1988. Inhibition of spermatogenesis in men using various combinations of oral progestagens and percutaneous or oral androgens. *International Journal of Andrology* 11: 187–99.

Guille, J. L., D. le Lannou, B. Lobel, and F. Olivo. 1989. Contraception in men: Efficacy and immediate toxicity, a study of 18 cases. *Acta Urologica Belgica* 57 (1): 117–24.

Hagendijk, R. 1996. Wetenschap, constructivisme en cultuur. Ph.D. diss., University of Amsterdam.

Hagendijk, R., and J. Meeus. 1993. Blind faith: Fact, fiction, and fraud in public controversy over science. *Public Understanding of Science* 2: 391–415.

Halffman, W. 2002. Boundaries of regulatory science: Eco/toxicology and aquatic hazards of chemicals in the U.S., England, and the Netherlands, 1970–1995. Ph.D. diss., University of Amsterdam.

Handelsman, D. J. 1991. Bridging the gender gap in contraception: Another hurdle cleared. *The Medical Journal of Australia* 154 (4): 230–33.

Handy, B. 1998. The Viagra craze. *Time*, 4 May: 38–45.

Hardon, A. 1993. *Reproduktieve rechten, reproduktieve gezondheid en family planning.* Lecture at the workshop Family Planning, Human Rights, and Reproductive Healthcare. Amsterdam: University of Amsterdam.

———. 1995. *User studies on hormonal contraceptives: Towards gender aware and experience-near approaches.* Paper presented at the WHO/HRP meeting, n.d., Geneva.

——. 1997. Contesting claims on the safety and acceptability of anti-fertility vaccines. *Reproductive Health Matters* 10: 68–82.

Hardon, A., and E. Hayes, eds. 1997. *Reproductive rights in practice: A feminist report on the quality of care.* London: Zed Books.

Harper, M. J. K. 1983. *Birth control technologies: Prospects by the year 2000.* Austin: University of Texas Press.

Harper, J., and T. W. Jezowski. 1991. Men and family planning: A special initiative. *AVSC News,* October.

Harper, P. B. 1994. Cairo conference sets new directions. *AVSC News* 32 (4): 6–7.

Haspels, A. A. 1985. Hormonen en de pil. *Cahiers Bio-wetenschappen en Maatschappij* 10 (1): 19–27.

Haws, J. M., M. N. Wegner, and C. S. Carigan. 1997. *Men as partners, men as clients: A meeting to develop a model for men's reproductive health services.* New York: AVSC International.

Hearn, J., and D. J. Collinson. 1994. Theorizing unities and differences between men and between masculinities. In *Theorizing masculinities,* ed. H. Brod and M. Kaufman. London: Sage.

Heath, D. 1997. Bodies, antibodies, and modest interventions. In *Cyborgs and citadels: Anthropological interventions in emerging sciences and technologies,* ed. G. L. Downey and J. Dumit. Santa Fe, N.M.: School of American Research Press.

Heckel, N. J. 1939. *Proceedings of the Society for Experimental Biology and Medicine* 40: 658.

Heckel, N. J., W. A. Rosso, and L. Kestel. 1951. Spermatogenic rebound phenomenon after administration of testosterone propiate. *Journal of Clinical Endocrinology* 11 (3): 235–45.

Heller, C. G., et al. 1950. Improvement in spermatogenesis following depression of the human testis with testosterone. *Fertility and Sterility* 1 (5): 415–23.

Heller, C. G., W. M. Laidlaw, H. T. Harvey, and W. O. Nelson. 1958. Effects of progestational compounds on the reproductive processes of the human male. *Annals of the New York Academy of Sciences* 71: 649–65.

Hermite, L., P. O. Hubinont, and J. Schwers. 1976. Sperm action. *Progress in Reproductive Biology* Basel: S. Karger.

Hippel, E. von. 1976. The dominant role of users in the scientific instrument innovation process. *Research Policy* 5: 212–39.

——. 1988. *The sources of innovation.* Oxford: Oxford University Press.

Hirsch, P., and J. Gillespie. 2001. Unpacking path dependence: Differential valuations accorded history across disciplines. In *Path dependence and creation,* ed. R. Garud and P. Karnoe. London: LEA Press.

Hoch, P. K. 1989. The crystallization of a strategic alliance: The American physics elite and the military in the 1940s. In *Science, technology, and the military,* ed. E. Mendelsohn, M. R. Smith, and P. Weingart, 87–116. Dordrecht: Kluwer.

Hubbard, R. 1981. The emperor doesn't wear any clothes: The impact of feminism on biology. In *Men's studies modified: The impact of feminism on the academic disciplines,* ed. D. Spender, 213–37. Oxford: Oxford University Press.

Hulton, L., and J. Falkingham. 1996. Male contraceptive knowledge and practice: What do we do? *Reproductive Health Matters* 7: 90–100.

International Women's Health Coalition. 1994. Women's voices '94: Women's declaration on population policies. Report prepared for the 1994 United Nations International Conference on Population and Development in Cairo.

Jackson, H. 1959. Antifertility substances. *Pharmacological Reviews* 11: 135–72.

——. 1972. Chemical methods of male contraception. In *Reproduction in mammals*, vol. 5: *Artificial control of reproduction*, ed. C. R. Austin and R. V. Short. Cambridge: Cambridge University Press.

——. 1975. Progress towards a male oral contraceptive. *Clinics in Endocrinology and Metabolism* 4 (3): 643–63.

Jezowski, T. 1994. Men's program: Cairo-Male involvement in family planning. *AVSC News* 32 (4): 8–9.

Johnson, A. 1996. It'll be a pain in the bum. *The Guardian*, 3 April.

Jordan, K., and M. Lynch. 1992. The sociology of a genetic engineering technique: Ritual and rationality in the performance of the "plasmid prep." In *The right tools for the job*, ed. A. Clarke and J. Fujimura, 77–114. Princeton, N.J.: Princeton University Press.

Jourdan, T. 1997. Race for male pill. *Scottsman*, 2 July.

Kammen, J. van. 1998. Integrating users into the design of anti-fertility vaccines. University of Amsterdam, Department of Science Dynamics. Typescript.

——. 2000. Conceiving contraceptives: The involvement of users in anti-fertility vaccine development. Ph.D. diss., University of Amsterdam.

Kammen, J. van, and N. Oudshoorn. 2002. Gender and risk assessment of contraceptive technologies. *Sociology of Health and Illness* 24 (4): 436–61.

Kane, T. T., and S. Sivasubramaniam. 1989. Family planning communication between spouses in Sri Lanka. *Asian and Pacific Population Forum* 3 (1/2): 1–10.

Karnoe, P., and R. Garud. 2001. Path creation and dependence in the Danish wind turbine field. In *Constructing industries and markets: Essays in cognition, institutions, and economy*, ed. M. Ventresca and J. Porac, New York: Elsevier Science.

Kaufman, M. 2000. Testosterone gel: Elixer of youth or risk of health? *The Herald Tribune*, May 29.

Keller, A. 1979. Contraceptive acceptability research: Utility and limitations. *Studies in Family Planning* 10 (8/9): 230–37.

Kessler, A. 1991. Establishment and early development of the Programme. In *Biennial Report, 1990–1991: Special Programme of Research, Development, and Research Training in Human Reproduction*, 43–59. Geneva: World Health Organization.

Kessler, S., and W. McKenna. 1978. *Gender: An ethnomethodological approach*. New York: Wiley.

Ketting, E. 1993. *De wereldwijde behoefte aan Family Planning*. Lecture at the workshop Family Planning, Human Rights, and Reproductive Healthcare, 5 November, Stichting Wereld en Bevolking.

Ketting, M., and B. Wieringa. 1996. Geen PRIK in mijn bil: Mannen voelen niets voor eigen "pil." *De Telegraaf*, 10 April: T17.

Keuken, D. 2000. De zoektocht naar een HIV vaccin. Masters thesis, University of Amsterdam.

Khanna, J. 1996. Fax from J. Khanna, Technical Officer, Special Programme of Research, Development, and Research Training in Human Reproduction, WHO, Geneva, 21 August.

King, C. C. 1999. *Men and the male pill: Representations of a new male contraceptive and contemporary masculinities in the British press*. Ph.D. diss., University of Durham, U.K.

Kirejczyk, M. 1993. Shifting the burden onto women: The gender character of in vitro fertilization. *Science as Culture* 3 (17): 507–22.

——. 1996. *Met technologie gezegend? Gender en de omstreden invoering van in vitro fertilisatie in de Nederlandse gezondheidszorg*. Utrecht: Jan van Arkel.

Kleinman, D. L. 1994. Layers of interests, layers of influence: Business and the genesis of the National Science Foundation. *Science, Technology, and Human Values* 19 (3): 5–22.

Kline, R., and T. Pinch. 1996. Users as agents of technological change: The social construction of the automobile in the rural United States. *Technology and Culture* 37: 763–95.

Klinge, I. 1998. *Gender and bones: The production of osteoporosis, 1941–1996.* Ph.D. diss., University of Utrecht, Netherlands.

Knight, J., and J. C. Callahan. 1989. Male contraception and future prospects. In *Preventing birth: Contemporary methods and related moral issues,* ed. J. Knight and J. C. Callahan, 285–345. Salt Lake City: University of Utah Press.

Knorr-Cetina, K. 1993. Strong constructivism—From a sociologist's point of view: A personal addendum to Sismondo's paper. *Social Studies of Science* 23: 555–59.

Knuth, U. A., and E. Nieschlag. 1987. Endocrine approaches to male fertility control. *Baillieres Clinical Endocrinology and Metabolism* 1 (1): 113–31.

Knuth, U. A., C. H. Yeung, and E. Nieschlag. 1989. Combination of 19-nortestosterone-hexyloxyphenylpropionate (Anadur) and depot-medroxyprogresterone-acetate (Clinovir) for male contraception. *Fertility and Sterility* 51 (6): 1011–18.

Kole, E. 1999. *Organizing the transfer of electronic network technology to meet the objectives of NGPs in the South.* Research proposal, University of Amsterdam, September. Typescript.

Kretser, D. M. de. 1974. The regulation of male fertility: The state of the art and future possibilities. *Contraception* 9 (6): 561–600.

——. 1976. Towards a pill for men. *Proceedings of the Royal Society in London* 195 (6): 161–74.

——. 1978. A fertility regulation in the male. *Bulletin of the World Health Organization* 56 (3): 353–60.

Laird, J. 1994. A male pill? Gender discrepancies in contraceptive commitment. *Feminism and Psychology* 4: 458–69.

Laqueur, T. 1990. *Making sex: Body and gender from the Greeks to Freud.* Cambridge, Mass.: Harvard University Press.

Laredo, P. 1994. EC and EUREKA-promoted networks: Toward a redefinition of european public-interventions? Paper presented at the Science Dynamic's Progress Conference, June 1994, University of Amsterdam.

Laredo, P., B. Kahane, J. B. Meyer, and D. Vinck. 1992. *The networks built by the fourth Medical and Health Services Research Programme.* Bruxelles: CCE Bruxelles.

Latour, B. 1987. *Science in Action: How to follow scientists and engineers through society.* Milton Keynes, U.K.: Open University Press.

Latour, B., and S. Woolgar. 1979. *Laboratory life: The social construction of scientific facts.* Beverly Hills: Sage.

Law, J. 1988. On the art of representation: Notes on the politics of visualization. In *Picturing power: Visual depiction and social relations,* ed. G. Fyfe and J. Law. London: Routledge.

Lawson, T. 1997. Men will be on the pill in five years. *Daily Mail,* 3 February.

Leclair, A. 1996. Waar blijft het gejuich om de bilprik? *HP/De Tijd,* 12 April: 8–10.

Lee 1997. WHO and the developing world: The contest for ideology. In *Western medicine as contested knowledge,* ed. A. Cunningham and B. Andrews. Manchester: Manchester University Press.

Lente, H. van. 1993. *Promising technology: The dynamics of expectations in technological development.* Delft: Eburon.

Leonard, A., and K. Moore. 1996. *Men: What are we going to do about them?* New York: Population Council.

Lewenstein, B. V. 1995. Science and the media. In *Handbook of science and technology studies,* ed. S. Jasanoff, G. E. Markle, J. C. Peterson, and T. J. Pinch, 343–61, Thousand Oaks: Sage.

Lie, M. 1995. Technology and masculinity: The case of the computer. *European Journal of Women's Studies* 2: 379–94.

Lie, M., and K. H. Sørenson. 1996. *Making technology our own? Domesticating technology into everyday life.* Oslo: Scandinavian University Press.

Liebenau, J. 1987. *Medical science and medical industry: The formation of the American pharmaceutical industry.* London: Macmillan Press, in association with Business History Unit, University of London.

Lissner, E. A. 1992. Frontiers in nonhormone male contraceptive research. In *Issues in reproductive technology I: An anthology,* ed. H. B. Holmesed. New York: Garland Publishers.

Lloyd, C. B. 1993. *Family and gender issues for population policy.* New York: The Population Council.

Lohan, M., and W. Faulkner. Forthcoming. Masculinities and technologies: Some introductory remarks. In *Men and Masculinity.*

London Department of Health. 1992. *The annual report of the chief medical officer.* London: Department of Health.

Lowy, I. 1994. Introduction to *The invisible industrialist: Manufacturers and the production of scientific knowledge.* Paris: INSERM/CNRS Workshop.

Lynch, M. 1985. *Art and artifact in laboratory science: A study of shop work and shop talk in a research laboratory.* London: Routledge & Kegan Paul.

Lynn, F. M. 1986. The interplay of science and values in assessing and regulating environmental risks. *Science, Technology, and Human Values* 11: 40–50.

Lyotard, J.-F. 1984. *The post-modern condition: A report on knowledge.* Minneapolis: University of Minnesota Press.

MacKenzie, D. 1989. From Kwajalein to Armageddon? Testing and the social construction of missile accuracy. In *The uses of experiment,* ed. D. Gooding, T. J. Pinch, and S. Schaffer, 409–36. Cambridge: Cambridge University Press.

MacKenzie, D., and J. Wajcman, eds. 1999. *The social shaping of technology.* 2d ed. Buckingham/Philadelphia: Open University Press.

Maisel, A. Q. 1965. *The hormone quest.* New York: Random House.

Male participation and responsibility in fertility regulation. 1995. WHO, *Progress in Human Reproduction,* 35.

Mamo, L., and J. R. Fishman. 2001. Potency in all the right places: Viagra as a technology of the gendered body. *Body and Society* 7 (4): 13–37.

Marks, H. M. 1997. *The progress of experiment: Science and therapeutic reform in the United States, 1900–1990.* Cambridge: Cambridge University Press.

Marks, L. 2001. *Sexual chemistry: A history of the contraceptive pill.* New Haven, Conn.: Yale University Press.

Marlin, E. 1998. But will I grow tits? *New Woman* (August), 5.

Marshall, J. 1977. Acceptability of fertility regulating methods: Designing technology to fit people. *Preventive Medicine* 6: 65–75.

Martin, C. W., R. A. Anderson, R. Anakwe, A. Glasier, and D. T. Baird. 1997. *Human Reproduction* 12. Abstract Book I. Mastroianni, L., P. J. Donaldson, and T. T. Kane. 1990. Development of contraceptives: Obstacles and opportunities. *New England Journal of Medicine* 322: 482–85.

Matlin, S. 1994a. The pill—40 Years On. *Education in Chemistry* (September): 123–27.

———. 1994b. Prospects of pharmacological male contraception. *Drugs* 48 (6): 851–63.

———. 1991. P. Crabbé. Memorial oration. Paper presented at the First International Conference of Andrology, n.d. Nenjiing, China.

Matsumoto, A. M. 1988. Is high dosage testosterone an effective male contraceptive agent? *Fertility and Sterility* 60 (2): 324–28.

Maugh, T. H. 1981. Male "pill" blocks sperm enzyme. *Science* 212 (17): 314.

McLaughlin, L. 1982. *The pill, John Rock, and the Church: The biography of a revolution*. Boston: Little, Brown.

Meekers, D., and M. Oladosu. 1996. Spousel communication and family planning decision-making in Nigeria. Ph.D. diss. Pennsylvania State University.

Men as partners: Happenings around the globe. 1997. *AVSC News* 35 (2): 2.

Men's programs series. 1994. *AVSC News* 32 (2): 6.

Men's roles and responsibilities in reproduction. 1996. *Arrows for change: Women's and gender perspectives in health policies and programmes* 2 (1): 1–2.

Michel, E., H. Bents, F. B. Akhtar. 1985. Failure of high-dose sustained release luteinizing hormone releasing hormone agonist (Buserelin) plus oral testosterone to suppress male fertility. *Clinical Endocrinology* 23: 663–65.

Millman, N., and C. G. Hartman. 1956. Oral control of conception: A contemporary survey. *Fertility and Sterility* 7: 110–22.

Mintzes, B., ed. 1991. *A question of control: Women's perspectives on the development and use of contraceptive technologies*. Amsterdam: Wemos, Women and Pharmaceuticals Project, and Health Action International.

Mintzes, B., A. Hardon, and J. Hanhart, eds. 1993. *Norplant: Under her skin*. Amsterdam: Women and Pharmaceuticals Project, Women's Health Action Foundation, and Wemos.

Mishra, B. D. 1967. Correlates of males' attitudes toward family planning. In *Sociological contributions to family planning research*, ed. D. J. Bogue. Chicago: Community and Family Study Center, University of Chicago.

Mokyr, J. 1990. *The lever of riches*. New York: Oxford University Press.

Mondigo, A. I. 1995. Men's roles, sexuality, and reproductive health. Paper presented at the International Lecture Series on Population Issues, n.d. São Paulo, Brazil.

Moore, J. J., and M. A. Schmidt. 1999. On the construction of male differences: Marketing variations in technosemen. *Men and Masculinities* 1 (4): 331–51.

Morgan, D. 1992. *Discovering men*. London: Routledge.

Moscucci, O. 1990. *The science of woman: Gynaecology and gender in England, 1800–1929*, Cambridge: Cambridge University Press.

Mouritzen, J., and N. Deehow. 2001. Technologies of managing and the mobilization of paths. In *Path dependence and creation*, ed. R. Garud and P. Karnoe. London: LEA Press.

Naald, W. van der. 1996. Silent sperm: Wetenschappelijke "detective" schetst ingrijpende effecten van milieuvervuiling. *Greenpeace* 2: 34–36.

Nahon, D., and N. Lander. 1993. The masculine mystique. *Canadian Pharmacological Journal* 126: 458–59.

National Coordinating Group on Male Antifertility Agents. Gossypol: A New Antifertility Agent for Males. 1979. Gynecology and Obstetrics Investigation 10: 163–176.

Nicoll, V. 1998. Record woman. *Daily Record* (Edinburgh), 3 April.

Niemi, S. 1987. Andrology as a specialty: Its origins. *Journal of Andrology* 8: 201–3.

Nieschlag E., A. Lerch, and S. Nieschlag. 1994. *Institut for Reproduktionsmedizin der Westfälischen Wilhelms-Universitat Munster*. Munster: Westfalischen Wilhelms-Universitat.

Nieuw optimisme over mannenpil. 1997. *De Volkskrant*, Amsterdam, 28 June.

Noble, D. 1984. *Forces of production: A social history of industrial automation*. New York: Knopf.

———. 1985. Science for sale. *Etcetera, A Review of General Semantics* 41: 375.

Nowak, R. 2000. Life in the old dog. *New Scientist* (22 July): 36–41.

Nyblade, L. 1991. Husband-wife communication: Mediating the relationship of household structure and polygyny to contraceptive knowledge, attitudes, and use. Manuscript.

O'Connell, J. 1993. Metrology: The creation of universality by the circulation of particulars. *Social Studies of Science* 23: 129–73.

Oldenziel, R. 1999. Making technology masculine: Men, women and modern machines in America. Amsterdam: Amsterdam University Press.

Oost, E. van. 2000. Making the computer masculine. In *Women, work, and computerization: Charting a course to the future*, ed. E. Balka and R. Smith, 9–16. Amsterdam: Kluwer Academic Publishers.

Otten, M. 1985. *Assepoesters en kroonprinsen: Een onderzoek naar de minderheidspositie van agentes en verplegers*. Amsterdam: Socialistische Uitgeverij Amsterdam.

Oudshoorn, N. E. J. 1993. United we stand: The pharmaceutical industry, laboratory, and clinic in the development of sex hormones into scientific drugs, 1920–1940. *Science, Technology, and Human Values* 18 (1): 5–24.

———. 1994a. *Beyond the natural body: An archeology of sex hormones*. London: Routledge.

———. 1994b. From family planning politics to chemicals: The role of WHO in creating translocal laboratory practices. Paper presented at the 4S/EASST Conference, October 1994, New Orleans.

———. 1995a. Discourse coalitions in contraceptive technologies: The case of male contraceptives. Paper presented at the Science Dynamics Internal Conference, July 1995, University of Amsterdam.

———. 1995b. Technologie en zorg: Vriendinnen of vijanden? Het voorbeeld van nieuwe anticonceptiemiddelen voor vrouwen en mannen. *Gezondheid: Theorie en Praktijk* 3: 278–89.

———. 1996. *Gender scripts in Technologie: Noodlot of Uitdaging*. Enschede: Inaugurele rede Universiteit Twente.

———. 1997a. From population control politics to chemicals: The WHO as an intermediary organization in contraceptive development. *Social Studies of Science* 27: 41–72.

———. 1997b. From private to public bodies: The transformation of male bodies into test subjects for contraceptive R&D. Manuscript.

———. 1997c. The making of the new man: Symbolic interventions to change family planning discourses towards including men. Paper presented at the Annual Meeting of the Society for Social Studies of Science, November, Tucson, Arizona.

———. 1997d. Menopause, only for women? The social construction of menopause as an exclusively female condition. *Journal of Psychosomatic Obstetrics and Gynaecology* 18: 137–44.

———. 1999. On masculinities, technologies and pain: The testing of male contraceptive technologies in the clinic and the media. *Science, Technology, and Human Values* 24 (2): 265–89.

———. 2000. Imagined men: Representations of masculinities in discourses on male contraceptive technology. In *Bodies of technology: Women's involvement with reproductive medicine*, ed. A. Saetnon, N. E. J. Oudshoorn, and M. Kirejczyk, 123–46. Columbus: Ohio University Press.

———. 2002. Drugs for healthy people: The culture of testing hormonal contraceptives for women and men. In *Biographies of remedies: Drugs, medicines, and contraceptives in Dutch and Anglo-American healing cultures*, ed. G. M. van Heteren, M. Gijswit-Horstra, and E. M. Tansey, 79–92. Amsterdam: Rodopi.

Oudshoorn, N. E. J., M. Brouns, and E. van Oost. Forthcoming. Diversity and agency of users in the design of medical video-communication technologies. In *The Politics within Technology*, ed. H. Harbers. Cambridge, Mass.: MIT Press.

Oudshoorn, N. E. J., and T. J. Pinch, eds. 2003. *How users matter: The co-construction of users and technologies*. Cambridge, Mass.: MIT Press.

Oudshoorn, N. E. J., A. R. Saetnan, and M. Lie. 2002. On gender and things: Reflections on an exhibition on gendered artifacts. *Womens' Studies International Forum* 859 (1): 1–13.

Parkes, A. S. 1953. The quest for the ideal contraceptive. *Proceedings of the Society for the Study of Fertility* 5: 20–26.

Paulsen, C. A. 1977. Regulation of male fertility. In *Frontiers in reproduction and fertility control: A review of the reproductive sciences amd contraceptive development*, ed. R. O. Greep and M. A. Koblinsky, 458–65. Cambridge, Mass.: MIT Press.

Paulsen, C. A., W. J. Bremner, and J. M. Leonard. 1982. *Male contraception: Clinical trials*. New York: Raven Press.

Paulsen, C. A., W. J. Bremner, and A. M. Matsumoto. 1994. *Male contraceptive development*. Seattle: Population Center for Research in Reproduction, Department of Medicine, University of Washington and Veterans Administration Medical Center.

Paulsen, C. A., J. M. Leonard, E. C. Burgess, and L. F. Ospina. 1978. Male contraceptive development: Re-examination of testosterone enanthate as an effective single agent. In *Hormonal control of male fertility*, ed. D. J. Patanelli, 17–36. Bethesda: Department of Health, Education and Welfare, National Institute of Health.

Pavlou, S. N., K. Brewer, M. G. Farley, J. Lindner, M. C. Bastias, B. J. Rogers, L. Swift, J. E. Rivier, W. W. Vale, P. M. Conn, and C. M. Herbert. 1991. Combined administration of a gonadotropin-releasing hormone antagonist and testosterone in men indures azoospermia without loss of libido. *Journal of Clinical Endocrinology and Metabolism* 73 (6): 1360–69.

Pfeffer, N. 1985. The hidden pathology of the male reproductive system. In *The sexual politics of reproduction*, ed. H. Homans, 31–45. London: Gower.

Pinch, T. 1993. Testing—one, two, three . . . testing!: Toward a sociology of testing. *Science, Technology, and Human Values* 18 (1): 25–42.

———. 2001. Why you go to a piano store to buy a synthesizer: Path dependence and the social construction of technology. In *Path dependence and creation*, ed. R. Garud and P. Karnoe, 381–400. London: LEA Press.

Pinch, T., M. Ashmore, and M. Mulkay. 1992. Technology, testing, text: Clinical budgeting in the U.K. National Health Service. In *Shaping technology/Building society: Studies in sociotechnical change*, ed. W. E. Bijker and J. Law. Cambridge, Mass.: MIT Press.

Pinch, T. J., and W. E. Bijker. 1987. The social construction of facts and artefacts. In *The social construction of technological systems: New directions in the sociology and history of technology*, ed. W. E. Bijker, T. P. Hughes, and T. J. Pinch, 3–25. Cambridge, Mass.: MIT Press.

Plata, M. I. 1996. Bringing men and women together in family planning clinics. In *Learning about sexuality: A practical beginning*, ed. S. Zeidenstein and K. Moore. New York: Population Council and International Women's Health Coalition.

Ploeg, I. van de. 1998. Prosthetic bodies: Female embodiment in reproductive technologies. Ph.D. diss., University of Maastricht, Netherlands.

Poel, I. van de. 1998. Changing technologies. Ph.D. diss., University of Twente.

Population Council, 1996. Male involvement: A challenge for the Bangladesh National Family Planning Program, Policy Dialogue Series, June, nr. 3. New York: The Population Council.

Population Council. 1995a. *Annual Report*. New York: Population Council.

———. 1995b. *Newsletter: Men and families*, vol. 1, February.

———. 1995c. *Newsletter: Men and families*, vol. 2, September.

———. 1996. *Towards a new partnership: Encouraging the positive involvement of men as supportive partners in reproductive health*. New York: Population Council.

———. 1997. *Newsletter*, vol. 2.

Population Reference Bureau, Inc. 1995. *Conveying concerns: Women write on male participation in the family*. Washington, D.C.: Population Reference Bureau.

Potts, D. M. 1976. The implementation of family planning programmes. *Proceedings of the Royal Society London*: 213–24.

Prentice, T. 1990. Are we ready for the male pill? *Times* (of London), 22 October.

Prikpil voor mannen is geen pretje, maar wel betrouwbaar. *Trouw* (Amsterdam). 6 April 1996.

Rabinow, P. 1992. Artificiality and enlightment: From sociobiology to biosociality. In *Incorporations*, ed. J. Crary and S. Kwinter, 234–52. New York: Zone.

Ramirez de Arellano, A. B., and C. Seipp. 1983. *Colonialism, Catholicism, and contraception: A history of birth control in Puerto Rico*. Chapel Hill: University of North Carolina Press.

Raspé, G., and S. Bernhard. 1973. *Advances in the Biosciences. Schering Workshop on Contraception: The Masculine Gender, Berlin 29 November to 2 December 1972*, New York: Pergamon Press.

Reddy, P. R. K., and J. M. Roo. 1972. Reversible antifertility action of testosterone propionate in human males. *Contraception* 5 (1): 295–301.

Richards, E. 1988. The politics of therapeutic evaluation: The vitamin C and cancer controversy. *Social Studies of Science* 18 (4): 653–701.

Righart, H. 1996. Het mannelijk schuldgevoel: Het moderne leven wordt er ook met de prikpil niet gemakkelijker op. *HP/De Tijd* (12 April): 12.

Ringheim, Karin. 1993a. Factors that determine prevalence of use of contraceptive methods for men. *Studies in Family Planning* 24 (2): 87–99.

———. 1993b. Guidance for future social science research on hormonal methods for men: Findings from followup questionnaires and focus group discussions with former clinical trial participants. Report to the Steering Committee of the Task Force on Methods for the Regulation of Male Fertility. Geneva: WHO.

———. 1995. Evidence for the acceptability of an injectable hormonal method for men. *International Family Planning Perspectives* 21 (2): 75–80.

———. 1996a. Male involvement and contraceptive methods for men: Present and future. Paper presented at the American Public Health Association session, "Toward Gender Partnership in Reproductive Health," 19 November, New York City.

———. 1996b. Whither methods for men? Emerging gender issues in contraception. *Reproductive Health Matters* 7: 79–89.

Rip, A. 1995. Introduction of new technology: Making use of recent insights from sociology and economics of technology. *Technology Analysis and Strategic Management* 7 (4): 417–31.

Robey, B., S. O. Rutstein, L. Morris, and R. Blackburn. 1992. The reproductive revolution: New Survey Findings. *Population Reports*, series M, no. 11: 1–2.

Rommes, E., E. van Oost, and N. Oudshoorn. 1999. Gender in the design of a digital city. *Information, Communication, and Society* 2 (4): 476–95.

Sachs, A. 1994. Men, sex, and parenthood in an overpopulating world. *World Watch* 7 (2): 12–19.

Saetnan, A., N. E. J. Oudshoorn, and M. Kirecjzyk. 2000. *Bodies of technology: Women's involvement with reproductive medicine*. Athens: Ohio University Press.

Scale, D. 2002. The male pill and the science museum: Creating consumers for male hormonal contraceptives. Thesis, Department of History and Philosophy of Science, Cambridge University.

Scarria, J. J., C. Markland, and J. J. Speidel, eds. 1987. *Control of male fertility: Proceedings of a workshop*. Hagerstown, Md.: Medical Department, Harper & Row.

Schally, A. V., and A. M. Comaru-Schally. 1987. Male contraception involving testosterone supplementation: Possible increased risks of prostate cancer? *The Lancet* (21 February): 448.

Schearer, S. B. 1977. Pharmacological approach to contraception in men. *Drug Therapy* 5 (2): 72–77.

Schmidt, M., and L. S. Moore. 1998. Constructing a good catch, picking a winner: The development of technosemen and the deconstruction of the monolithic male. In *Cyborg babies: From techno-sex to techno-nots*, ed. R. Davis-Floyd and J. Dumit. New York: Routledge.

Schot, J., and A. Rip. 1997. The past and future of constructive technology assessment. *Technological Forecasting and Social Change* 65: 251–68.

Schot, J., R. Hoogma, and B. Elzen. 1994. Strategies for shifting technological systems. The case of the automobile system. *Futures* 26 (10): 1059–76.

Schoysman, R. 1976. Etat actuel de la contraception masculine. *Schweizerische Medizinische Wochenschrift* 106 (10): 329–33.

Schulte, M. M., and F. L. Sonensteinn. 1995. Men at family planning clinics: The new patients? *Family Planning Perspectives* 27 (5): 212–25.

Schwartz, N. B. 1976. Comment on Bremner and de Kretser's Contraceptives for Males. *Signs* 2 (1): 247–48.

Seaman, B. 1972. *The doctor's case against the pill*. New York: P. H. Wyden.

Seaman, B., and G. Seaman. 1978. *Women and the crisis in sex hormones: An investigation of the dangerous uses of hormones—from birth control to menopause and the safe alternatives*. Toronto: Bantam Books.

Secord, J. A. 1989. Extraordinary experiments: Electricity and the creation of life in Victorian England. In *The Uses Of Experiment*, ed. D. Gooding, T. Pinch, and S. Schaffer, 337–83. Cambridge: Cambridge University Press.

Seex, J. 1996. Making space for young men in family planning clinics. *Reproductive Health Matters* 7 (special issue Men, May): 22–40.

Segal, S. J. 1971. Beyond the laboratory: Recent research advances in fertility regulation. *Family Planning Perspectives* 3 (3): 17–21.

———. 1972. Contraceptive research: A male chauvinist plot? *Family Planning Perspectives* 4 (3): 21–25.

———. 2000. A male contraceptive pill by 2000? A follow-up. *Toward a New partnership. Encouraging the Positive Involvement of Men as Supportive Partners in Reproductive Health* 6: 3–5.

Service, R. F. 1994. Barriers hold back new contraception strategies. *Science*, 266 (2 December): 1489.

Setchell, B. P., ed. 1984. *Male reproduction: Benchmark papers in human physiology* 17. New York: Van Nostrand Reinhold.

Shah, N. M. 1974. The role of interspousal communication in adoption of family planning methods: A couple approach. *Pakistan Development Review* 13: 454.

Shankland, L. 1993. Putting the male "pill" to the test. *Western Mail* (Edinburgh), 15 July.

Shapin, S. 1994. *A social history of truth: Civility and science in seventeenth century England*. Chicago: University of Chicago Press.

Shapin, S., and S. Schaffer. 1985. *Leviathan and the air pump: Hobbes, Boyle, and the experimental life*. Princeton, N.J.: Princeton University Press.

Sheldon, J. S. 1972. Contraceptive research: a male chauvinist plot? *Family Planning Perspectives* 4 (3):21–25.

Sieve, B. F. 1952. A new antifertility factor: A preliminary report. *Science* 116: 373–85.

Silverstone, R., and L. Haddon. 1996. Design and the domestication of information and communication technologies: Technical change and everyday life. In *Communication by design: the politics of information technologies*, ed. R. Silverstone and R. Mansell, New York: Oxford University Press.

Sihvo, S., E. Ollila, and E. Hemminki. 1995. Perceptions and satisfaction among Norplant users in Finland. *Acta Obstetricia Gynecologica Scandinavica* 74: 441–45.

Singh, S. 1987. Additions to the questionnaire. In *The world fertility survey*, ed. J. Cleland and C. Scott. Oxford: Oxford University Press.

Singleton, V. 1996. Feminism, sociology of scientific knowledge, and postmodernism: Politics, theory, and me. *Social Studies of Science* 26: 445–68.

Skibiak, J. P. 1993. Male barriers to the use of reproductive health services: Myth or reality? Paper presented at the 121st Annual Meeting of the American Public Health Association, May 21, San Francisco.

Skoglund, R. D., and A. A. Paulsen. 1973. Danazol-testosterone combination: A potentially effective means for reversible male contraception: A preliminary report. *Contraception* 7 (5): 357–65.

Smart, B. 1992. *Modern conditions, postmodern controversies*. London: Routledge.

Smith, G. 1997. Male pill is off the menu. *Daily Record* (Edinburgh), 26 December.

Soufir, J. C., P. Jouannet, J. Marson, and A. Soumach. 1983. Reversible inhibition of sperm production and gonadotrophin secretion in men following combined oral medroxyprogesterone acetate and percutaneous testosterone treatment. *Acta Endocrinologica* 102 (4): 625–32.

Spilman, C., T. J. Kirton, and K. T. Kirton, eds. 1976. *Regulatory Mechanisms of Male Reproductive Physiology: Sixth Brook Lodge Workshop on Problems of Reproductive Biology*. New York: American Elsevier Co.

Star, S. L. 1989. *Regions of the mind: Brain research and the quest for scientific certainty*. Stanford, Calif.: Stanford University Press.

———. 1991. Power, technology, and the phenomenology of conventions: On being allergic to onions. In *A sociology of monsters: Power, technology, and the modern world*, ed. J. Law, 25–56. Oxford: Basil Blackwell.

Steele Verme, C., M. N. Wegner, and T. Jerzowski. 1996. The language of male involvement: What do you mean by that? *Populi* 23 (2): 10–11.

Steinhauer, J. 1995. At a clinic young men talk of sex. *New York Times*, 6 September.

Stokes, B. 1980. Men and family planning. *Worldwatch Paper* 41 (December).

Stycos, J. M. 1996. Men, couples, and family planning: A retrospective look. Working papers series of the Population and Development Program of Cornell University, New York.

Stycos, J. M., K. Back, and R. Hill. 1956. Problems of communications between husbands and wives on matters relating to family limitation. *Human Relations* 1: 207–15.

Suppression of spermatogenesis by desogestrel with testosterone pellets: An international study. 1997. Case record form. Contraceptive Development Network.

Swann, J. P. 1988. *Academic scientists and the pharmaceutical industry.* Baltimore, Md.: Johns Hopkins University Press.

Sweetenham, E. 1994. Good health: Male pill made me more virile—How a simple injection may revolutionise birth control. *Daily Mail* (London), 26 April.

Swerdloff, R. S., D. J. Handelsman, and S. Bhasin. 1985. Hormonal effects of GNRH agonist in the human male: an approach to male contraception using combined androgen and GNRH against treatment. *Journal of Steroid Biochemistry* 23: 855–61.

Swerdloff, R. S., L. A. Campfield, A. Palacios, and R. D. McClure. 1979. Suppression of human spermatogenesis by depot androgen: Potential for male contraception. *Journal of Steroid Biochemistry* 11: 663–70.

Swerdloff, R. S., and D. Heber. 1983. Superactive gonadotropin-releasing hormone agonists. *Annual Revieuw of Medicine* 34: 491–500.

Swerdloff, C., S. Wang, and S. Bhasin. 1992. Developments in the control of testicular function. *Bailliaere's Clinical Endocrinology and Metabolism* 6 (2): 451–83.

Timmermans, S., and V. Leiter. 2000. The redemption of Thalidomide: Standardizing the risk of birth defects. *Social Studies of Science* 30 (1): 41–73.

Tom, L., S. Bhasin, W. Salameh, B. Steiner, M. Peterson, R. Z. Sokol, J. Rivier, W. Vale, and R. Swerdloff. 1992. Induction of azoospermia in normal men with combined nalgluonadotropin-releasing antagonist and testosterone enanthate. *Journal of Clinical Endocrinology and Metabolism* 75 (2): 476–83.

Tone, A. 2001. *Devices and desires: A history of contraception in America.* New York: Hill and Wang.

United Nations. 1984. International Conference on Population, Mexico City. *Recommendations for the further implementation of the World Population Plan of Action.* New York: United Nations.

———. 1994a. International Conference on Population and Development. Report on the International Conference on Population and Development, document no. Cairo A/Conf. 171/13. New York: United Nations.

———. 1994b. International Conference on Population and Development. Program of Action. New York: United Nations.

———. 1995. Family Planning Association. Male involvement in reproductive health, including family planning and sexual health. New York: United Nations.

University of Manchester. Communications Office. 1993. Press Bulletin. 14 July.

Vasterling, V. 1999. Butler's sophisticated constructivism: A critical assessment. *Hypatia* 14 (3): 17–38.

Vaughan, P. 1972. *The pill on trial.* Harmondsworth, U.K.: Penguin Books, Ltd.

Vemer, H., and W. Berginik. 1994. The role of industry in contraceptive research and development. *Human Reproduction* 9 (2): 32–40.

Vennix, P. 1990. De pil en haar alternatieven. *Nisso studies nieuwe reeks* 6, Utrecht: Eburon.

Vernon, R., G. Ojeda, and A. Vega. 1991. Making vasectomy services more acceptable to men. *International Family Planning Perspectives* 17 (2): 45–70.

Vries, C. de. 1996. Mannenpil? *Volkskrant* (4 April): 17.

Waites, G. M. H. 1986. Male fertility regulation: Recent advances. *Bulletin of the World Health Organization* 64 (2): 151–58.

Waites, G. M. H., C. Wang, and P. D. Griffin. 1998. Gossypol: Reasons for its failure to be accepted as a safe, reversible male antifertility drug. *International Journal of Andrology* 21: 8–12.

Wajcman, J. 1991. Feminism confronts technology. Cambridge, Mass.: Polity Press.

Wallace, E. M., and F. C. W. Wu. 1990. Effect of depot medroxyprogesterone acetate and testosterone enanthate on serum lipoproteins in man. *Contraception* 41 (1): 63–71.

Ward, M. C. 1986. *Poor women and powerful men: America's great experiment in family planning.* Boulder, Colo.: Westview Press.

Warren, O., and R. G. Bunge. 1957. The effect of therapeutic dosages of nitrofurantoin (furadantin) upon spermatogenesis in man. *Journal of Urology* 77 (2): 275–81.

Watson, J. 2000. *Male bodies: Health, culture, and identity.* London: Routledge.

Wegner, M. N. 1997. Improving men's reproductive health benefits both women and men. AVSC International News Release, 13 June.

Wen, Wei. 1980. China invents male birth control pill. *American Journal of Chinese Medicine* 8 (2): 195–97.

West, C., and D. H. Zimmerman. 1987. Doing gender. *Gender and Society* 1: 125–251.

Wilkinson, H. 1996. Men: The most powerful "minority" ever. *Reproductive Health Matters* (special issue: Men) 7: 155–57.

Williams, L. B. 1992. *Who decides? Determinants of couple cooperation and agreement in U.S. fertility decisions.* Ann Arbor: University of Michigan Press.

Woolgar, S. 1991. Configuring the user: The case of usability trials. In *A sociology of monsters: Essays on power, technology, and domination,* ed. J. Law. London: Routledge.

World Health Organization. 1996a. Office of Information. Lexis/Nexis: A collection of the media coverage of the WHO press bulletin. 2 April. Archive WHO/HRP, Geneva.

——. 1996b. WHO completes international trial of a hormonal contraceptive for men. Press Release no. WHO/26, 2 April.

——. 1973a. Special Program for Research and Development and Research Training in Human Reproduction (HRP). Task Force on Methods for the Regulation of Male Fertility. Abstract of 1973 Annual Report. Archive WHO/HRP, Geneva.

——. 1973b. Minutes of the Fourth Meeting of the Steering Committee of the Male Task Force, 26–28 August, Geneva. Archive WHO/HRP, Geneva.

——. 1976. Task Force on Acceptability of Fertility Regulation Methods. Protocol: Acceptability of male antifertility methods in clinical trial. Archive WHO/HRP, Geneva.

——. 1977. Minutes of the Fifteenth Meeting of the Task Force on Methods for the Regulation of Male Fertility, 6–8 September, Geneva. Archive WHO/HRP, Geneva.

——. 1979a. Minutes of the Twenty-first Meeting of the Steering Committee, 2–5 October. Archive WHO/HRP, Geneva.

——. 1979b. Task Force on Psychosocial Research in Family Planning. Acceptability of drugs for male fertility regulation: A prospectus and some preliminary data. *Contraception* 21 (2): 121–34.

———. 1980. Special Programme of Research, Development, and Research Training in Human Reproduction. Ninth Annual Report. Geneva, November.

———. 1981a. Task Force on Long-Acting Agents for Fertility Regulation. Minutes of Meeting of Investigators Participating in the Chemical Synthesis Programme, Singapore. Archive WHO/HRP, Geneva.

———. 1981b. Minutes of the Tenth Annual Report, Archive WHO/HRP, Geneva.

———. 1982. Task Force on Psychosocial Research in Family Planning. Hormonal contraception for men: Acceptibility and effects on sexuality. *Studies in Family Planning* 13 (11): 328–42.

———. 1983. *Twelfth Annual Report.* November, Geneva: WHO.

———. 1986a. Minutes of Steering Committee Meeting of the Task Force on Methods for the Regulation of Male Fertility, 14–17 April, Geneva. Archive WHO/HRP, Geneva.

———. 1986b. Task Force on Methods for the Regulation of Male Fertility. *Evaluation of the requirement for azoospermia in an antifertility method based on suppression of sperm production with testosterone enanthate in normal men.* Geneva, November. Geneva: WHO.

———. 1987a. Task Force on Methods for the Regulation of Male Fertility. Minutes of Steering Committee Meeting, 21–24 September, Geneva. Archive WHO/HRP, Geneva.

———. 1987b. Task Force on Methods for the Regulation of Male Fertility. Scientific and Technical Review Committee. *In-depth review report prepared for the Scientific and Technical Advisory Group,* September, Geneva. Archive WHO/HRP, Geneva.

———. 1988. Task Force on Methods for the Regulation of Male Fertility (1987). Scientific and Technical Review Committee. In-Depth Review Report Prepared for the Scientific and Technical Advisory Group, 29 February–4 March, Archive WHO/HRP, Geneva.

———. 1989. Task Force on Methods for the Regulation of Male Fertility. Minutes of Steering Committee Meeting, 30 November–3 December, Geneva. Archive WHO/HRP, Geneva.

———. 1990a. Inter-Agency Consultation on Meeting the Challenges of the 1990s in Human Reproduction Research, Geneva. Archive WHO/HRP, Geneva.

———. 1990b. Task Force on Methods for the Regulation of Male Fertility. Contraceptive efficacy of testosertone-induced azoospermia in normal men. *Lancet* 336: 955–59.

———. 1991. Task Force on Methods for the Regulation of Male Fertility. Minutes of Steering Committee Meeting, 30 September–2 October, Geneva. Archive WHO/HRP, Geneva.

———. 1992a. Task Force on Methods for the Regulation of Male Fertility. Minutes of Steering Committee Meeting, 21–25 April, Geneva. Archive WHO/HRP, Geneva.

———. 1992b. *Guidelines for the use of androgens in men.* Geneva: WHO.

———. 1992c. *WHO laboratory manual for the examination of human semen and sperm-cervical mucus interaction.* 3d ed. Published on behalf of the World Health Organization by Cambridge University Press.

———. 1992–1993. Biennial Report. Geneva: WHO.

———. 1993. Annual Technical Report, 1992. Archive WHO/HRP, Geneva.

———. 1994. Task Force for Social Science Research on Reproductive Health, in collaboration with the Task Force on Methods for the Regulation on Male Fertility of the Human Reproduction Program. Protocol: Study of the acceptability of an injectable hormonal contraceptive method for men. Archive WHO/HRP, Geneva.

———. 1996. Task Force on Methods for the Regulation of Male Fertility. Contraceptive efficacy of testosterone-induced azoospermia and oligospermia in normal men. *Fertility and Sterility* 65 (4): 821–29.

——. 1990–1999. Biennial Report. Geneva: WHO.

Wu, F. C. W. 1988. Male contraception: Current status and future prospects. *Journal of Clinical Endocrinology* 29: 443–65.

Young Men's Clinic. n.d. Flyer.

Zotti, M. E., and E. Siegel. 1995. Preventing unplanned pregnancies among married couples: Are services for only the wife sufficient? *Nursing and Health* 18: 133–42.

Zuckerman, C. B. 1956. Physiological control of population growth. *Nature* 177: 58–60.

Index

• • • •

Abortion pill, research on, 29–30

Abortion politics, pregnancy risk in contraceptive testing and, 81–82

Abrahams, John, 79, 87, 105, 257 n.10

Acceptability of contraception: articulation of, 209–24; assessment of, 214–18; male contraceptive research, 91–92, 94–97; masculine identity and, 182–86, 202–4, 262 n.14, 266 n.18; pharmaceutical firm's studies, 219–24; studies as cultural tools, 210–14, 267 n.2

Access to Voluntary and Safe Contraception (AVSC), 118, 131–34, 136, 138–39, 141–42, 249 n.35; Young Men's Clinic case study, 155–64, 261 n.11

Actor-network theory: alternative sociotechnical networks and, 229–32; cultural change and, 232–38, 268 n.5; pharmaceutical industry's contraceptive research and, 30, 218–24, 251 n.18; sociotechnical networks and, 11–12, 244 n.14

Adolescent health care, men's health services as component of, 165–70

Adolescents, health services for: in Colombia, 154–55, 261 n.10; in family planning clinics, 117, 123–24, 144, 261 n.4; Young Men's Clinic as model for, 155–64

Afzal, Mobeen (Dr.), 146–47

Age criteria, male contraceptive clinical trials, 173–77, 262 n.4

Agency: establishment in contraceptive research of, 62–65; sociotechnical and cultural change and, 226–28

Agency for International Development, 34

Aggressive behavior, hormone use and increase in, 97

Aging, male reproductive function and, 4, 243 n.3

AIDS research: male contraceptives and, 180–81; risk reduction in AIDS therapy and, 257 n.10

Aitken, R. John, 25, 71, 99, 101

Akrich, Madeleine, 12, 98–99, 192, 219, 241

Algemeen Dagblad, 202, 265 n.12

Androgens: cooperative research on, 64–65; health risks of, 92–93, 96; male contraceptive research and role of, 27, 72, 88, 257 n.1; oral administration, 216; pharmaceutical firms' research on, 220–22; standardized testing of, 93–94, 254 n.13, 255 n.14

Andrology: clinics for, 260 n.2; evolution of, 6, 244 n.5; marginalization of, 26–27

Antifertility vaccines: gender bias in risk assessment for, 258 n.19; research on, 29, 36–37, 252 n.27; risk reduction strategies for use of, 257 n.10

Sexual function and behavior: acceptability assessment based on, 214–18; clinical trial subject reliability and, 180, 262 n.11; control and responsibility issues, 117–19, 124–25, 234–38; female contraceptives' impact on, 107, 110, 258 nn.17–18, 259 n.21; male contraceptives and impact on, 88–99, 103–4, 106–7, 110, 258 n.16, 259 n.21; Thalidomide testing and, 262 n.11; Young Men's Clinic programs on, 159–64

Sexually transmitted diseases (STDs): adolescent health care and, 156–64; condom protection and, 246 n.25; family planning policy and, 124–25; men's health services including, 142, 154–55; Young Men's Clinic services for, 160–64

Sexual stimulants, history of, 243 n.3

Shapin, Steve, 57, 87

Side-effects of contraceptives: clinical trials and monitoring of, 92–93; gender bias in assessment of, 108–9, 258 n.19; male lack of tolerance for, 109, 259 n.20; media coverage of, 194–97, 200–208, 265 n.15; pharmaceutical industry research policies concerning, 104–10; risk reduction strategies and minimization of, 98; technology/risk co-construction and, 86–110

Silicone plug (Vasoc), research on, 43

Silverstone, Roger, 245 n.18

Single-parent families, family planning policies and, 123–25. *See also* Couples-oriented family research

Social science research: acceptability studies and cultural feasibility, 210–14, 267 n.2; feminist advocacy of male contraceptives and, 48–51; hegemonic masculinity and contraceptive technology, 15–17; male attitudes toward family planning, 119–23; male contraceptive technology and, 249 n.35; risk reduction strategies in clinical trials, 97–104, 257 n.10; sociotechnical networks, 11–12, 244 n.14

Sociotechnical networks, 11–12, 17, 244 n.14; alternative networks, development of, 31–44, 52–68, 228–32; contraceptive technol-

ogy and, 14–15, 246 n.24; cultural change and, 226–28; male-oriented transformation in, 113; technology/risk co-construction and, 86–87

Space design and allocation: in Colombia family planning clinics, 152–55; in family planning clinics, 141–49; in Young Men's Clinic, 159–64

Speech act theory, gender as performance and, 13, 246 n.21

Spermicides, chemical effects of, 24

Sperm production and reduction: as efficacy criteria, 195–97; ethnic differences in, during clinical trials, 80, 256 n.7, 258 n.12; hormonal effects on, 70–74, 88, 98–99, 176, 257 n.1

Sports physicals, male client recruitment using, 156–64

Staffing policies and trends: in Colombia family planning clinics, 153–55; dominance of women as, in family planning clinics, 145–49; Young Men's Clinic case study, 159–64

Standardization, in contraceptive research, 56–62; clinical trial monitoring procedures, 90–97, 257 n.7; Male Task Force manuals for, 83–84, 93–94

Star, Susan Leigh, 136, 260 n.12

Steroids: aggression linked to use of, 97; as contraceptive agents, 24, 29, 37, 253 n.2; health risks of, 92–93, 106; long-acting contraceptives using, 54–56, 254 n.6

Steroid Synthesis Program, 37, 53–62, 253 n.2

Storyline analysis, in scientific journals, 192, 263 n.6

Structuralism, gender identity and, 247 n.27

Stycos, J. Mayone, 115–16, 119–22, 259 nn.2, 4

Sweden, male contraceptive research in, 34

Swedish International Development Authority, 129

Swerdloff, Ronald, 71, 73, 89, 96, 98, 174

Task analysis, in family planning clinics, 141–49

"Technical delegates": acceptability studies,

215–16, 267 n.6; long-acting contraceptives, 53–62, 253 n.4, 254 nn.5, 13, 255 n.14

Technology research: articulation of need for, 16, 247 n.31; culture niche for, 16–17, 248 nn.32–33; gender dynamics and innovation in, 13–17, 113–15, 245 nn.19–20, 246 nn.21–25, 247 nn.26–31, 248 nn.32–33; news media coverage of, 191–92, 204–8, 263 n.2; path dependence in evolution of, 20–21, 249 n.2; risk co-constructed with, 86–110; role of trials in, 191–92, 263 n.1; social and cultural construction of, 11–12

Terminology of family planning, disputes concerning, 125–31

Testicles: extracts from, 243 n.3; hormonal effects on, 71; undescended testes, therapy for, 257 n.1; Young Men's Clinic services for diseases of, 161–64

Test locations, for clinical trials, 69–85

Testosterone: as contraceptive, clinical trials of, 88–89, 98–99; delivery system design for, 99, 216, 257 n.11; health risks of, 103; pharmaceutical firms' research on, 221; replacement therapy, 4, 243 n.3; standardized testing of, 254 n.13, 255 n.14

Test subjects: cooperativity of men as, 18; male contraceptive research, recruiting issues, 69–85, 89, 95, 153–64, 174–75, 177, 179, 182, 186–90, 268 n.5

Thalidomide testing, 262 nn.7, 11

Thau, Rosemary (Dr.), 72, 100, 174

Three-phase testing model, in clinical trials of male contraceptives, 93–97

Thrombosis: androgen use and risk of, 92–93; oral contraceptives and risk of, 96–97, 109

Title X program, men's health services and, 142

Tripterygium wilfordii, research on, 43

Trouw, 202, 265 n.12

Trust, technology and, 225–41

United Kingdom: contraceptive use in, 246 n.23; media coverage of male contraception in, 200, 203–8, 237–38, 264 n.12, 265 n.15

United Nations, contraceptive research and role of, 32, 198. *See also* World Health Organization (WHO)

United Nations Family Planning Association (UNFPA), 35

United Nations Fourth World Conference on Women, 125, 131

United Nations International Conference on Population and Development, 117–18, 124–25, 131, 137, 167

United Nations Population Fund, 131, 142–43, 261 n.3

United States, media coverage of contraceptive research in, 266 n.18

United States Agency for International Development (USAID), family planning survey and funding, 141–42, 146, 261 n.3

Unmarried women, bias in survey data concerning, 117, 260 n.5

Upjohn, 40, 53, 254 n.5

Urology, contraceptive research in field of, 76–77

User representations: acceptability studies and, 212–18; clinical trial subjects' reliability, 171–90; in contraceptive clinical trials, 88–97; cultural change and technology and, 12, 233–38, 245 n.18; "implicated actors" concept, 191 n.1; male clients in family planning, 119–23, 140–70; in news media, 192; in scientific journals, 194–97, 205–8

Vaccines: antifertility vaccines, 29, 36–37, 252 n.27, 257 n.10, 258 n.19; contraceptive vaccines, 262 n.13

Vas deferens, male sterilization involving, 248 n.34, 249 n.1

Vasectomy: acceptability studies on, 210–14; Chinese research on, 41, 43; hegemonic masculinity and, 15, 246 n.25; international promotion of, 133–34; medical provision of, 114; non-scalpel techniques, 248 n.34. *See also* Male sterilization

Viagra: hegemonic masculinity and discourses on, 190, 234, 247 n.30; popularity of, 3, 243 n.1

Waites, Geoffrey M., 264 n.7; Chinese contraceptive research, 41, 103–4; clinical trial recruitment efforts and, 74, 76–78; efficacy research of male contraceptives, 97, 99, 101; on Gossypol research, 43; on long-acting contraceptives, 54–55; pregnancy risk in contraceptive testing, 81–83; press bulletins in contraceptive research discussed by, 197–98; risk assessment issues, 108–9

Wang, Christina, 41, 80, 83–84, 103

Wen, Wei, 78, 103, 252 n.29

Whistler, Roy L., 249 n.6

Women's health advocacy: acceptability studies and, 217–18; articulation of women's health issues by, 149; emergence of, 14–15, 246 n.24; family planning policies and, 114–15, 117–19; health risks of oral contraceptives and, 27–28; language changes in family planning discourse and, 126–31, 138–39, 261 n.13; male contraceptive research and, 44–51, 201–8, 253 n.33, 265 n.13; men's health services in family planning and, 131–39, 142–49; news media's role in, 206–8; resistance to long-acting contraceptives from, 53–54, 254 n.5; selection criteria for clinical trials and, 262 n.5; sociotechnical and cultural change and, 226–28. See also Feminist movement

World Bank, 32, 198

World Congress on Aging, 4

World Congress on Fertility and Sterility (1962), 32

World Fertility Survey (WFS), 116–17

World Health Organization (WHO): acceptability studies by, 210–18, 267 nn.2–3; clinical trial infrastructure development, 77–84, 229–32; contraceptive research and, 31–38, 49–50, 251 n.22, 252 n.28; cultural stereotypes of men in, 119–20; efficacy testing of hormonal compounds, 101–4, 195–97; evaluation of contraceptive research by, 47–48; large-scale clinical trials of, 93–97; long-acting contraceptives research and, 53–57; male contraceptive research by, 122–23, 192–95, 264 n.9; patent applications for contraceptives filed by, 62–63, 66–68, 255 nn.16–17; pharmaceutical industry partnerships, 63–65, 220–24, 255 nn.16–19; Plants Task Force, 252 n.28; press bulletins of, 197–200, 206–8, 264 n.11, 266 n.18; Scientific Review Group, 81; selection criteria for clinical trials, 173–77; Steroid Synthesis Program, 37, 53–62, 67–68, 253 n.2; Task Force on Acceptability of Fertility Regulating Methods, 91, 210–14, 267 n.2; Task Force on Methods for the Regulation of Male Fertility, 193, 249 n.35; translocal laboratory practices, standardization of, 56–62; World Congress on Aging, 4. See also Human Reproduction Program (HRP) (WHO); Male Task Force (WHO); United Nations

Worldwatch Institute, 121–22

Wu, Fred C. W., 7, 94, 104; efficacy testing of male contraceptives, 99–101; female contraceptive research, 108; male contraceptive research, 25–26, 73, 264 n.7; male recruitment for clinical trials, 75–77, 175, 177; on pharmaceutical industry, 104–5; on side-effects of contraceptives, 265 n.15

Young Adult Reproductive Health Survey (ARHS), 117

Young Men's Clinic, 144, 155–70, 261 n.4

Zero risk, as research goal, 109–10